THE DANCE OF NURTURE

Food, Nutrition, and Culture

Series Editors: Rachel Black, Connecticut College
Leslie Carlin, University of Toronto

Published by Berghahn Books in association with the *Society for the Anthropology of Food and Nutrition* (SAFN).

While eating is a biological necessity, the production, distribution, preparation, and consumption of food are all deeply culturally inscribed activities. Taking an anthropological perspective, this book series provides a forum for thought-provoking work on the bio-cultural, cultural, and social aspects of human nutrition and food habits. The books in this series bring timely food-related scholarship to the graduate and upper-division undergraduate classroom, to a research-focused academic audience, and to those involved in food policy.

Volume 1
GREEK WHISKY
The Localization of a
Global Commodity
Tryfon Bampilis

Volume 2
RECONSTRUCTING OBESITY
The Meaning of Measures and
the Measure of Meanings
Edited by Megan B. McCullough
and Jessica A. Hardin

Volume 3
RE-ORIENTING CUISINE
East Asian Foodways in the
Twenty-First Century
Edited by Kwang Ok Kim

Volume 4
FROM VIRTUE TO VICE
Negotiating Anorexia
Richard A. O'Connor
and Penny Van Esterik

Volume 5
THE HERITAGE ARENA
Reinventing Cheese in
the Italian Alps
Cristina Grasseni

Volume 6
THE DANCE OF NURTURE
Negotiating Infant Feeding
Penny Van Esterik and
Richard A. O'Connor

The Dance of Nurture

Negotiating Infant Feeding

Penny Van Esterik and Richard A. O'Connor

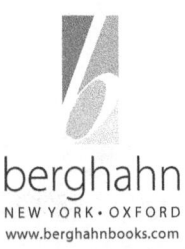

First published in 2017
Berghahn Books
www.berghahnbooks.com

© 2017, 2022 Penny Van Esterik and Richard A. O'Connor

First paperback edition published in 2022

Except for the quotation of short passages for the purposes
of criticism and review, no part of this book may be reproduced
in any form or by any means, electronic or mechanical,
including photocopying, recording, or any information
storage and retrieval system now known or to be invented,
without written permission of the publisher.

Library of Congress Cataloging-in-Publication Data

Names: Van Esterik, Penny, author. | O'Connor, Richard A., author.
Title: The dance of nurture : negotiating infant feeding / Penny Van Esterik and Richard A. O'Connor.
Description: New York : Berghahn Books, 2017. | Series: Food, nutrition, and culture ; volume 6 | Includes bibliographical references and index.
Identifiers: LCCN 2017010906 (print) | LCCN 2017016397 (ebook) | ISBN 9781785335631 (eBook) | ISBN 9781785335624 (hardback : alk. paper)
Subjects: LCSH: Infants—Nutrition—Social aspects. | Infants—Food—Social aspects. | Nurturing behavior in children.
Classification: LCC RJ216 (ebook) | LCC RJ216 .V37 2017 (print) | DDC 649/.3—dc23
LC record available at https://lccn.loc.gov/2017010906

British Library Cataloguing in Publication Data

A catalogue record for this book is available from the British Library.

ISBN 978-1-78533-562-4 hardback
ISBN 978-1-80073-456-2 paperback
ISBN 978-1-78533-563-1 ebook

https://doi.org/10.3167/9781785335624

Contents

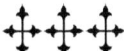

Acknowledgements vii

Introduction 1

Part I. Challenges
Chapter 1. Recovering Nurture 9
Chapter 2. Studying Nurture 23

Part II. Contexts
Chapter 3. Tracing the Human Story 45
Chapter 4. Entering the Commensal Circle 73

Part III. Diversities
Chapter 5. Customizing Nurture in Southeast Asia 109
Chapter 6. Modernizing Nurture: A Global Shift 137

Part IV. Interventions
Chapter 7. Mastering Nurture: Trying to Get Nurture Right 159
Chapter 8. Negotiating Nurture: Yesterday's Lessons, Tomorrow's Hope 193

References 223
Index 245

Acknowledgments

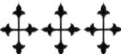

What began as a book about breastfeeding became a book about anthropology and the human condition. It was inspired by the work of all the networks and blogs hosted by people who have a scientific and empathetic commitment to breastfeeding and the nurture of the next generation. It would be impossible to list all the people and experiences that informed our work since so many of them live online. We are particularly grateful to the series editors of the Food, Nutrition and Culture series at Berghahn, Rachel Black and Leslie Carlin, who championed the project as a subject of interest to the broader community in food studies. Thanks to the anonymous reviewers who saw flaws and strengths in the manuscript in time to let us improve the book.

Penny: Nurturing practices can be scarce in academia; friends and colleagues nudged us to finish this work and provided generous assistance at those moments when it felt like the task was overwhelming, in particular I thank Cecilia Tomori, Alison Linnecar, Julie Smith, Dian Borek, and Naomi Duguid. The ideas expressed in this book were born from decades of experience watching and, whenever possible, helping the ongoing work of WABA (World Alliance for Breastfeeding Action) and IBFAN (International Baby Food Action Network). The hardworking individuals in these global networks who wear multiple hats play extraordinarily diverse roles in making it possible to nurture the next generation. I thank them for tolerating an anthropologist in their midst. My work has been inspired by the life and accomplishments of Dr. Michael Latham, International Nutrition, Cornell University, who taught me the importance of integrating research and advocacy.

Richard: Some books take on lives of their own. This one did. Exciting as a newborn and demanding as a child, its adolescence was—well we survived that, barely—and now it goes out into the world trailing debts deeper than words. For your heartfelt support and kindnesses, thank you first and always to Carolyn, and to my kids and their spouses—John and Kellie, Daniel and Kathy, Amorn and Harrison. And to the kids of my kids—Liam, Stella, Lewis, and Maeve—thank you for enlivening my life and keeping me alive to why this book matters. I am grateful to Sewanee for its institutional support, colleagues like Dan Backlund, and fine students who believe in their teacher and his projects. And thank you Penny and John for the many visits that birthed this book.

To John Van Esterik and Carolyn O'Connor who have nurtured us for so long in so many ways, our heartfelt thanks.

Introduction

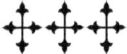

Broken Links

I began advocating for breastfeeding a couple of years after the birth of my daughter, Chandra, and later, began writing about breastfeeding for advocacy groups and academic audiences. Elsewhere (Van Esterik 1989: 20–27) I explained how my breastfeeding experiences influenced my interpretation of the infant-feeding controversy, and shaped my personal biases. Chandra's hospital birth was uncomplicated but unpleasant. My dominant memories are of being too cold to hold my newborn, and being ravenously hungry, but left unfed for many hours. I was not breastfed, but given lactic acid milk mixed with corn syrup. My mother was unable to help me with breastfeeding. In fact, she was more enthusiastic about the new convenient ready-to-feed infant formula samples we received, standard marketing practices in the 1970s. She thought I was breastfeeding to save money. As a foreign graduate student studying in the United States, I had minimal health insurance covering only one day in the hospital after my daughter's birth. The nurses were no help with breastfeeding, flicking Chandra's cheek to try and make her latch on, and I left the hospital before Chandra was breastfeeding properly. But I had an unusually supportive pediatrician who assumed I would have no problems with breastfeeding, and practical help from the wife of a fellow graduate student who was a La Leche League leader. When I complained that I had no milk on the third day, she took Chandra and breastfed her while her experienced six-month-old baby latched on to my engorged breasts forcefully and showed me how it was done. My friend helped me deal with engorgement, let down problems, and Chandra's tongue-tied latch. Looking back, I see that the support I needed to succeed with breastfeeding happened by chance, and the story could easily have gone the other way (which would have made my mother happy). Breastfeeding

> Chandra taught me to nurture; my mother nurtured me but never breastfed me; there was very clearly a broken link between the generations, and I had no embodied experience of being breastfed. As all mothers do, I adapted to the contingencies of my life as a graduate student by using personal and social resources to fill the gap left by the broken link. Only in retrospect can I see the commonalities between my experiences and those of other women. For example, reading Annette Beasley's (1996: 53) book reminded me of similar difficulties I had with Chandra favoring one side, and clicking her tongue with every swallow. (PVE)

The story of this broken link drew my attention to the importance of viewing breastfeeding, infant feeding, and nurture as links across generations. Forty years of advocacy work around breastfeeding provided endless numbers of stories about the complexity of breastfeeding and breastfeeding activism, some of which are included here. I wanted to use my past experiences in breastfeeding advocacy work to raise the arguments explored in this book. And I looked to anthropology for help.

Breastfeeding experience and advocacy work were not sufficient to develop the argument in this book, although it prepared me for addressing infant-feeding activism from the perspective of both NGOs and bilateral bureaucracies. It was clear to me that anthropology informed some of the best research in the field of infant feeding, but less clear why breastfeeding questions were also at the heart of anthropology. That is where Richard comes in to the story.

> I admire Penny's activism. That is not easy in anthropology. Although the discipline has a long tradition of intellectual activism, we eagerly want to change what people think. We shy away from changing how they live. That temerity rightly honors cultural relativism. Yet what is a civic-minded scholar to do when a culture's everyday doings crush its enduring values? That happens sometimes with breastfeeding and always with anorexia. That got us involved as anthropologists. We figured knowing how culture works would equip us to see and challenge how today's culture works against itself. We know other professionals battle these same problems. We wish them well. We do, however, worry when a profession's Cartesian logic creates the problems it sets out to solve. That, in a nutshell, is why eating disorders frustrate treatment and why breastfeeding is regularly misunderstood and wrongly politicized. Getting out of these traps is not easy. So we ask your indulgence as readers. Hang in there with all the theoretical and methodological moves. We have to go back to basics to do better. We hope the rethinking repays your efforts. (ROC).

Since Richard had already worked out arguments concerning why anorexia was an important case for anthropology, our collaboration was an opportunity to add another case study. We already knew that we attended to the same things in anthropology long before we began formal collaboration on *From Virtue to Vice* (2015) and *The Dance of Nurture*. Fieldwork in Thailand was foundational for us both. Although we carried out different ethnographic projects over the years, we both used Thailand to educate ourselves about other times and places. Consequently, we are both influenced by Thai concepts of nurture, an approach widespread in Southeast Asia. This is a shared narrative voice; when we speak separately, it is in notes followed by our initials.

Why use eating disorders and breastfeeding as instances of nurture or the failure of nurture? Both processes are activities that function as wholes and that interact with a person's unique constitution and with cultural scripts that organize modern life. Both subjects require holistic thinking, not reductionist binary oppositional thinking. Dividing mind from body, reason from emotion, public from private, and individual from society makes both eating disorders and breastfeeding incomprehensible. Both topics are difficult to study ethnographically. Both have uneasy relations with feminist explanations, and require what we call a relaxed feminist analysis. The path to breastfeeding and eating disorders are both long causal chains reflecting complex motivations entangling both reason and emotion.

Breastfeeding support is one of the most financially efficient interventions for reducing infant morbidity and mortality, but no interventions can force a mother to breastfeed against her will, as the Nazis and Italian fascists discovered. Such coercive interventions are rare and go against the logic and moral imperative to nurture others. In spite of decades of efforts to promote breastfeeding, few women follow the World Health Organization (WHO) recommendations for exclusive breastfeeding for six months, a key part of the Global Infant and Young Child Feeding Strategy.

The stories of anorexics detailed in *From Virtue to Vice* introduce us to North American women who are driven to succeed in many arenas of life; their self-regulatory rules to never give up, and to try harder even if it hurts, may sound familiar to breastfeeding mothers in Western societies. Mommy blogs introduce Euro-American mothers who write of struggling to breastfeed, and how they persevered in the face of pain and persistent problems. These progressive modern women who treat breastfeeding as an extreme sport have few counterparts in other parts of the world where nurture is still a dance, not a fight.

Why focus on nurture as an object of anthropological investigation? Because it is important both theoretically and practically; it is part of both the little and the large—global food security and grumbling stomachs. This book offers an explanation for why nurture is so basic to the human condition. Everyone takes it for granted that we must deal with the vulnerability of newborns, but we have underestimated the foundational importance of that nurturing work. Its impact stretches forward and backward, linking the generations.

An online publication in *Nature* (2011) identified the top ten questions that are both foundational and transformative (and difficult) for social scientists to tackle. Of course, nurture was nowhere to be seen. But the argument of our book resonated with the top ten questions about how to persuade people to adopt healthier behaviors, how to improve society's ability to get the important things approximately right, and how and why the social becomes biological. Nurture addresses these questions. The profound interdependence and need for social relatedness necessary to pass nurturing practices across the generations resides in this social universal: mother–infant interaction. An anthropological examination of nurture opens up possibilities for new research questions about our primate heritage, biocultural models in anthropology, and the limits of human adaptability.

Our reviewers pointed out that we were not clear about the potential audiences for this book; they were right. We want every reader to be as interested in infant feeding and nurture as we are. In fact, we should be more specific. We hope anthropologists, particularly medical anthropologists, will see breastfeeding and infant feeding as a lens for understanding the human condition, and that biological and cultural anthropologists will find that nurture as a biocultural hybrid could be a basis for working together on human commonalities. We hope that the New Ethnology will provide some guidance as to how to work across differences. But we are very conscious of the fact that this book, and particularly Chapter 3, is the result of two cultural anthropologists wading into the world of biological anthropology selectively, trying to understand the vast research emerging on lactation and breastfeeding. Ours is not the reading of insiders. But if we are to extend a hand across the subdivision divide, we must be able to understand how others make sense of less familiar fields and risk the misunderstandings that may result, or the integration we all seek will never happen.

Breastfeeding activists and those who work supporting new mothers in their infant-feeding practices will meet themselves on most pages. We hope they can tolerate the anthropological framing throughout. Health care professionals, particularly those working in public health and maternal and child health, may share some of our concerns about the complexities of applying global health policy in local contexts. We hope the subject of infant feeding will also be of interest to development workers who struggle with many of the same issues. Most of all, we hope readers will find a way to apply some of the ideas about nurture in their own lives.

We both love to dance—to celebrate, exercise, and relieve stress. We never noticed when or how it waltzed in to the book and became a guiding metaphor for nurture.

Plan of the Book

Anthropology is well placed to answer the broadest of questions about the human condition—in this case, nurture. In Part I, we document the challenges to breastfeeding and nurture (Chapter 1), and to studying both processes realistically (Chapter 2). Part II explores two important contexts for understanding nurture, first how breastfeeding is embedded in biocultural contexts (Chapter 3), and then how infant feeding is embedded in systems of food sharing and commensality (Chapter 4). Part III then examines the incredible diversity of nurture by showing how infant feeding is embedded in regional systems, specifically Southeast Asia (Chapter 5), and positioned in relation to modernity (Chapter 6). Finally, Part IV shows how infant feeding is handled by modern bureaucracies (Chapter 7) and negotiated by mothers and groups struggling to nurture the next generation (Chapter 8).

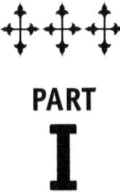

PART
I

Challenges

The first chapter opens with the crisis orientation that draws attention away from the importance of nurture and care in the development of our species and all humans. Anthropology has an important role to play in developing a biocultural model of nurture. We use the metaphor of dance to avoid the dualistic thinking that has polarized and impoverished the way breastfeeding is thought and talked about in popular, feminist, and biomedical discourses. Chapter 2 develops the model we use to shift the logic from distorting binaries to a unitary biocultural perspective, and explains how we define and use key concepts like culture, life cycle, and constitution used in the book. We end with a proposal for the development of the New Ethnology.

CHAPTER 1

Recovering Nurture

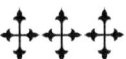

The world is not doing well—poverty, disease, violence, pollution, terrorism, hunger, and global warming producing floods, droughts, and typhoons, while experts quarrel and leaders dither about how to solve these problems. We seem to lurch from crisis to crisis, many of them interconnected, such as war and famine, ecological disasters and refugee flows, financial collapse and poverty. Many authors document the big picture that ties world politics and economics together, finding the large patterns that identify a tipping point for world-changing crises, and the collapse of civilizations (cf. Diamond 2005; Klein 2007; Graeber 2011). Potential political, ecological, and economic catastrophes in our globalized world are unpredictable, suggesting that extremes of turbulence threaten the limits of adaptability, as societies become more complex and more rigid (cf. Homer-Dixon 2006). From a global perspective, changes in complex systems can be rapid and dramatic, leading to environmental degradation and climate change or the collapse of financial systems. Human societies, disoriented following massive collective shocks of war, terrorism, and natural disasters, are vulnerable to abrupt system failures, as well as to the global conspiracies that are complicit in free-market economies that thrive on disaster.

Women are nowhere to be seen in these explorations of why past civilizations failed, but technology is front and center. Much as we try, these problems cannot be solved by technical ingenuity—a new vaccine, better fertilizers, or so-called humanized cow's milk, for example. Nor are they necessarily problems of modernity: "Disease, pollution and disasters multiply with a potency that cannot be consigned to the misguided epistemology of modernity" (Bessire and Bond 2014: 446). The Western world developed technologies that allowed them to dominate the modern world (Diamond 1997), but these technologies have done little to solve interconnected synergistic global problems, and have often made the situation worse, particularly in the context of corporate globalization.

Often the authors who write of the future of the world, look to corporations and technology to solve modern problems, rather than looking to them as the cause of modern problems. Diamond writes: "To me, the conclusion that the public has the ultimate responsibility for the behavior of even the biggest businesses is empowering and hopeful, rather than disappointing" (2005: 465). Somehow this does not ring true for food industries—particularly the baby food industry. When experts tell us we are on the brink of the third global food crisis in five years, a global catastrophe driven by droughts and the overconsumption of cheap industrial food, hunger and food insecurity just feels like the new normal.

These apocalyptic global scenarios, these expanding crises, are historically masculine in subject and scope, emphasizing aggression and competition. They ignore nurture as a critical part of human development. The grand narratives of epoch change do not resonate with the daily cycles of nurture more familiar to women. Nevertheless, cataclysmic disasters like the earthquake in Haiti (2010), floods in Bangladesh, tsunamis in Japan and Indonesia, and typhoons in the Philippines encourage acts of nurture, regardless of their political or ideological contexts. This suggests that while attention is focused on these big disaster stories, or oscillating epochs, in Graeber's (2011) words, they still bring out empathy and nurture in us—characteristics that are deeply embedded in what it means to be human. But the fundamental patterns of catastrophe that explain why past civilizations failed generally ignore women, children, care, and nurture.

The silences in these grand sweeps of history reveal a great deal about where nurture fits in the fate of human societies. In short, nowhere. These authors give us the warnings, raise the fears of existential threats to our existence. But they ignore a fundamental truth; our capacity to nurture the earth cannot be separated from our ability to nurture ourselves and nurture the next generation. Nurturing practices like breastfeeding and food sharing are like the canary in the mine; their absence warns us what needs to be fixed about systems out of control. It is not too late to set one system back on track and recognize the importance and the vulnerability of nurturing practices to human survival.

Humans always seek to solve problems, to intervene to try and improve conditions. But when faced with these crises, where do we start? In local communities? In global centers of power? At the UN? The search for solutions often comes down to problems of scale. Psychologist Judith Rodin argues in her book, *The Resilience Dividend* (2014) that we adapt to crises because of our tremendous capacity for resilience. This is a useful starting point for a psychologist. But anthropologists want to know where that resilience comes from, whether there are limits to our ability to adapt and how resilience develops in different communities. Starting points are often arbitrary—chosen for disciplinary, ideological, or political purposes. Economic models are popular approaches to these global crises. Proposed solutions are seldom generated out of historical or anthropological theory or life-embracing views of the world. So why not start at the beginning—with practices that embrace life—breastfeeding, nurture, and sharing food—and see where that takes us.

What if the world's problems relate to the breakdown of systems of nurture and care—foundational systems underlying other systems? Nurture refers to building social relations to support activities that help someone or something grow, flourish, and develop to its full potential by feeding it, caring for it responsively, and giving it support. With humans, well-being requires emotional, psychological and social support (cf. Gleason and Narvaez 2014: 336). Nurture is the subset of care most concerned with feeding and eating. Perhaps some answers to the big questions lie in the way we nurture each generation, and the way customs develop the resilience that help us adapt to familiar and unfamiliar circumstances—even crises.

Nurturing practices link the little and the large, and link one generation to the next, connecting global crises to the smaller moments in the life cycle, what is on hand for the next meal, for example. Erikson (1964: 96) expressed the relation between the little and the large in this way:

> The danger of any period of large-scale uprooting ... is that exterior crises will ... upset the hierarchy of developmental crises ... and that man will lose those roots that must be planted firmly in life cycles. For man's true roots are nourished in the sequence of generations.

The use of "man" in this equation is ironic, since the generations are nourished and linked through women.

When we attempt to capture the large, dramatic, macro-shifts of history, the "oscillating epochs," we lose the little, the daily details and micro-changes that are absorbed in the work of nurture. Below in the invisible substratum, the daily work of nurture and care proceeds almost unnoticed and certainly undervalued. Empathy, cooperation, care, and nurture have been considered less important than aggression and competition as factors driving human evolution until recently (cf. Hrdy 2009; Howell 2010; Fuentes 2013: 57). Our intellectual fascination with aggression, suffering, violence, and fear perpetuates an androcentric bias that has devalued the study of care and nurture. Sarah Hrdy (2009: 7) writes:

> New findings about how irrational, how emotional, how caring, and even how selfless human decisions can be are transforming disciplines long grounded in the premise that the world is a competitive place where to be a rational actor means being a selfish one.

It is tempting to consider this gap as willful ignorance, what Proctor (2008) calls agnotology. Perhaps care and nurture are too intimate, too local, too little, and too associated with women to rate as objects of global concern and scrutiny. The grand narratives of human history have left no place for nurture. But what if nurturing practices are at the root of complex global problems? What would happen if we put nurture back, right where it belongs—at the center of the human condition? Doing so would draw us to reconsider breastfeeding in the modern world. Taking nurture as the central process would shift the question from how to increase breastfeeding rates to how men, women, and non-breastfeeding mothers would benefit from conditions designed to support all nurturing practices including breastfeeding. Would more people be able to nurture themselves, the next generation, communities, and our planet?

Shifting perspective to the everyday small adjustments and negotiations attached to the work of feeding each other every day, day in and day out, feels much less dramatic than global warming or terrorism or even violence against women. Like the frog that gradually adjusts to rising temperatures until it boils to death, we barely notice the erosion of customs of nurture or empathy. These systems are so delicate, so vulnerable, yet so vital that—to quote an insightful pop song, you "don't know what you've got til' it's gone" (Joni Mitchell, 1970, *Big Yellow Taxi*).

Our capacity to nurture the next generation is in decline, even in crisis. The historical inheritance of customs that support nurture is rapidly disappearing from the human repertoire. Only if we acknowledge the critical role of nurture in human societies and individual development can we reverse the decline. The loss of customs of care and nurture are not dramatic—more breastfeeding problems here, some elder abuse there; hungry child soldiers here, prostitutes selling their bodies for food, everywhere; bullying, everywhere. War leaves more visible scars on landscapes and bodies than the erosion of nurture. But we are losing social tools that are not easily replaced, and erasing customs that could matter more than we think—customs that could be lynchpins of whole ecologies; think of postpartum rituals, feasting practices, fasting practices, shared meals, foster care, or even potluck suppers—customs that anthropologists know intimately through fieldwork.

Losing a few such systems will not threaten the ancient mammalian capacity for mothers to feed newborns with the specialized milk they produce for them—or will it? While lactation is an extraordinarily resilient evolutionary pattern, it is not hardwired or instinctive, and not unproblematic for all mother–infant pairs; there is a vulnerable uniqueness to every new breastfeeding dyad. There are few technical solutions for breastfeeding problems—a better latch, reducing women's stress and workloads, a nourishing meal, or a galactagogue (foods or medicines to increase milk supply); but mostly it comes down to time for mothers and newborns to be together, and well supported with food and care. Without such support, could chemical contaminants such as PCBs (or fears about chemical contaminants), new viruses such as HIV, and unfavorable working conditions push modern women over the threshold, creating conditions that make it difficult for women to breastfeed in the modern world, and at the same time, undermining women's confidence in their capacity to nurture the next generation? The postpartum customs that support mothers and newborns need to be actively defended and protected.

Such dangerous rhetorical questions about the possible collapse of human lactation have already been asked from an evolutionary perspective. The fear of that possibility among modern women has been used in the past to justify the unethical promotion of breastmilk substitutes, and even the reduction of support services for new mothers. Suggestions by physicians that modern urban women cannot breastfeed as well as their traditional rural sisters because of the stresses of civilization (cf. Martucci 2015: 67) provided the promotional context for breastmilk substitutes since the turn of the century in North America, and were obvious in a more crude form in much of the Global South. A huge billboard advertising infant formula observed in the early 1980s in downtown Nairobi displayed two women side by side: a frowning, droopy-breasted mother in traditional African dress breastfeeding, reluctantly, next to a "modern" woman in Afro hairdo, Western-style dress with a pushup bra, bottle-feeding with a wide smile on her face, and a caption above, "Which mother are you?"

Books on the rise and fall of empires, the collapse of civilizations have little to say about such things as child nurture. But the possible failure of child nurture should be just as scary as global warming. While environmental degradation and climate change could be catastrophic for human survival and life on earth because of the damage to natural resources, our capacity to solve such difficult complex problems requires functioning societies that nurture all their members. Questions about the loss of nurture are not even being asked in the centers of power. If they were asked, funding for maternity entitlements, breastfeeding clinics, child care, and school feeding programs would skyrocket.

Anthropology's Answers

Anthropologists have approaches and methods that would let us begin to answer these important questions about nurture, but lately, we have been frightened off from addressing the toughest issues, the big questions. In the early years of anthropology, Franz Boas and Ruth Benedict considered the tasks of anthropology as more urgent than other tasks. Like Margaret Mead, they were engaged with current debates of their time—debates about race and racism, eugenics, hunger, violence, and war. When anthropology ignored history to focus on present ethnographic facts, leaving behind Boasian historicism, it left an opposed biology and culture, politically correct identity politics, and postmodern meanings floating in space. Elements of past systems that influence present systems quickly became reduced to colonial and postcolonial histories, and questions of governmentality. Today the tasks of more and more anthropologists seem less and less urgent—at least to the public. And the gap between those who respond with enthusiasm to address urgent problems like racism, HIV, gender violence, or climate change, and those who prefer to explore narrower and narrower subject matter of importance to fewer and fewer people is growing larger. Humans are read (and often read themselves) as if the present moment is all there is. Postmodern anthropology fed into this tendency to ignore history. Even engaged anthropology is so concerned with the inequality that divides us that there is little notice of the commonalities like nurture that unite us. For better or worse, breastfeeding and nurture exist within systems of inequality and difference. To engage means to act within these systems of difference, or there can be no praxis.

Perhaps anthropologists feel inadequate to address the big questions because we speak with authority about the particular, the local. Speculative histories are not in vogue in the discipline, but they appeal to the public's desire for order and pattern, and for help in understanding how humans fit in to the world around them. These speculative histories make full use of ethnographic evidence without grounding them in disciplinary theory. If we do not reclaim this terrain in the area of infant feeding, we will be reduced to ranting against the extremes of paleo-parenting instead of suggesting how other groups effectively enable nurturing practices.

We have left other disciplines to tackle the big questions. Consider the work of those who manipulate huge data sets following the abundant "digital breadcrumbs" to find out that "social ties matter" (Pentland 2014). Observational fieldwork, not economic data sets, lead anthropologists to understand the importance of social ties and how humans interact. A world run by *datacrats* cannot address let alone solve the problem of nurture.

Because nurture is always open, always changing and negotiable, it cannot be easily manipulated by ideological positions, nor "improved." It is always about this case, this infant, this meal, this mother, this community. But humans are multilayered beings, with traditions beyond the consciousness of the moment, beyond the adaptation to current conditions. For anthropologists, breastfeeding provides another opportunity for considering political, moral, emotional, and sensual dimensions of human life in a holistic biocultural framework.

Nurturing practices are products of history and experience. This is why anthropologists can help explain why so many infants and young children die needlessly and too many adults suffer lifelong consequences from poor infant feeding. Why is this human tragedy happening? One explanation is that modernization has methodically undercut the embedded support that breastfeeding and new mothers once had. Postpartum customs related to what the British call "lying in," the Thai call *juu fai* (lying by the fire), or the Chinese, "doing the month" provided around forty days for women to recover from childbirth, establish a good milk supply, and be in intimate contact with their newborns. Institutional changes in industrial work patterns and modern medical care discouraged customary postpartum practices, undermining breastfeeding, often unwittingly.

Another explanation is intellectual. What Bateson called errors in thinking, the fragmenting logic of modern thought hides how breastfeeding works and why it is irreplaceable. Anthropologists have yet to come to grips with Bateson's (1972) fierce awareness of the unity of reality and the connectedness of all systems. The reductive, fragmenting logic of modern science that breaks wholes into bits that can be studied makes it difficult to see these connections. Bateson recognized the need to make thinking congruent with nature. Many of Bateson's arguments are compatible with feminist philosophy, although Bateson has not figured largely in feminist thinking. Nor have feminists used Bateson to advance their arguments. The prominent use of mechanistic, Newtonian metaphors such as power, force, and drive ring false to women's sense of lived experience, particularly with regard to relationships such as breastfeeding, and to the biological world of information, purpose, context, organization, and meaning. Bateson's work reflects the science of his day; our book builds on his approach and takes advantage of new approaches to epigenetics and neuroscience. Our approach to breastfeeding and child feeding also provides the space for feminists to reinsert nurture and care into the current equity and individual rights discourse, while avoiding biological essentialisms, an ongoing challenge.

The dualisms that remain embedded in Western discourses are both ethnocentric and pervasive across the social sciences. Bateson went so far as to blame these errors in thinking for most of the world's problems. More damaging, these ideas are exported to parts of the world where they may replace much more holistic approaches to gender, nurturance, and intimacy (cf. Descola 2013). For example, oppositions such as self/other, nurturance/sexuality, or subject/object cannot easily be applied to intersubjective activities such as breastfeeding or sexual relations. Both blur body boundaries, as people experience continuity with others. It is this continuity, this experience of other-as-self, self-as-other, that makes breastfeeding and sex both powerful transforming experiences for some, and a terrifying loss of personal autonomy for others (or more often, both at the same time). Processes such as commensality, nurturance, intimacy, and reciprocity emerge from human sentiments toward eating and feeding, and infant feeding creates the first contexts for these processes to develop.

What we call the infant-feeding complex is a tightly woven web of nurturing practices that are passed down the generations through women. The customs and logic guiding these practices relate closely to a group's food complex. Eating and feeding are morally charged activities. Like food, breastfeeding is "good to think" with and through. It is a metaphor for interdependence, nurturance, mutual support, and intimacy in an age dominated by metaphors for independence, greed, fear, and ambition. The process is an example of giving of oneself, literally and not just figuratively. It is evidence that humans feel sympathy for one another, and that humans, as social primates, are essentially moral creatures, regardless of how they act on occasion. Breastfeeding is about metaphor, pattern, and system, and requires an epistemology of relationships not an epistemology or epidemiology of cause and effect. Lineal causality is inappropriate to the world of living organisms that adapt, relate, and learn rather than react to laws. Mechanistic metaphors do not effectively explain relationships, holism, or synergy. Later in the chapter, we argue that dance is a more appropriate metaphor to capture the complexity of nurture.

Breastfeeding is the strongest reminder that we are not discrete beings; we emerge from other people, we merge into other people, our lives leak literally and figuratively into one another. We learn about the world through empathy; a mother learns about her infant, an infant learns about her mother through breastfeeding. This is not the only way to learn about another person, but physiological interdependence is the easiest and fastest way to learn; the mindful body does most of the work for you.

Today's discourse of autonomy, independence, and individualism is unsuitable for explaining breastfeeding, infant feeding, and feeding in general. While we know a great deal about the nutritional and immunological properties of breastmilk, relational factors provide the point of integration, the glue that binds the system together. The relational reality of nurture is under-theorized, made invisible by the reductive logic of both science and modernity, where the individual is defined as a discrete entity, an autonomous being. Autonomy has nothing to do with nurture; autonomy turns nurture into rational calculation; this is impossible for humans created by the nurturing acts of other humans and by society in general. Consider, for example, the corporate executive who was educated in the public school system and who uses public roads, but who insists that he (or more rarely, she) is a self-made individual who did it all on his (or her) own.

The dominant social science discourse marginalizes nurture. It takes competition and aggression as more basic to the human condition or at least more interesting to anthropologists than nurture. Those who have addressed nurture usually do so through an examination of food and eating, and often in order to intervene to "improve" situations that are themselves poorly understood. Consequently, despite libraries full of research reports on nutrient deficiencies and food security, we are still ill-prepared to deal with the vital problems posed by the failure of nurture, both at the policy level and at the individual level.

Nurture the next generation as you were nurtured is the heart of the message of breastfeeding, infant feeding, and of feeding in general; this is the crux of the life cycle approach we use here, which has all but disappeared in cultural anthropology. This approach stresses the need to consider nurture through multiple generations. The failure to nurture in one generation constrains the nurturing practices of the subsequent generations. Canada is learning this lesson in a painful way through the history of forcibly removing First Nations children from their families and confining them in distant residential schools where they were denied access to their own language and culture (cf. Mosby 2013). As a result, generations of these children were not adequately parented or nurtured, leaving them without the experience to parent and nurture their own children. This stripping away of the customary practices of nurture is destructive not only at the personal level, but also at the ideological level; it is possible that the relational logic of many indigenous peoples may provide a valuable way to view our relation to the planet, a point we return to in the conclusion.

Lactation as an adaptive complex is not exclusively human, but is lodged in our heritage as social primates. It is fundamental to the survival of all mammals and particularly other social primates. Society is built into our phylogeny (how we evolved as social primates), and is part of our ontogeny (how each of us developed as individuals) and ontology (how we all live day to day). To understand this infant-feeding complex, we must see it as the biocultural beginnings of personhood. This sense of personhood orients each of us to others and to the traditions our groups carry. Breastfeeding empowers an infant to harmonize with another person.

Within this universal grounding as social primates, and considering that human newborns generally have similar nutritional requirements, infant-feeding traditions vary culturally, locally, and personally. There are enormous differences in the way households and societies guide the feeding of their children, and even differences between children of the same mother. It is the way that local breastfeeding complexes fit with other complexes that makes it uniquely human—not just universal but a product of particular cultural and local traditions. However, by noting these primate commonalities, we run the risk of being misinterpreted as biological reductionists and reinforcing media-driven images of breastfeeding as animal-like behavior.

This book challenges these assumptions and provides new insights into theorizing breastfeeding from an anthropological perspective. It reframes questions about breastfeeding and young child feeding by considering nurture, and what practices, past and present, enhance or erode nurture, regardless of how an infant is fed. That is, we address nurture and not just breastfeeding, even though breastfeeding is the paradigmatic and ontological case for nurture.

We hope this book broadens the range of stories that can be associated with breastfeeding, and opens up both the metaphor and the activity to take us deeper into understanding the human condition. For the interpretive context for breastfeeding has been too narrow, too constrained by biomedical, patriarchal, and enlightenment thinking. What Ingold (2011: 160) calls storied knowledge enfolds within itself the history of relations that bind us up in other people's stories. Stories retrace a path through lived experience and leave traces that cut through classifications and ideologies; they should be respected, not only because they are more likely than academic analysis to engage the reader (including policy makers), but also because they make small truths jump out, to help connect the little and the large. For that reason, we have included a few of Penny's stories about the complexity of breastfeeding and breastfeeding activism in its social, cultural, and political context. These experiences in breastfeeding advocacy help identify some issues that motivated the arguments raised in this book, including the problems raised by the Cartesian dualisms pervading the subject. They also invite a life-cycle perspective and a way to explore change without creating backlash, a "we" vs "they" mentality that impedes both research and advocacy.

Breastfeeding has an unusual place in the life of North American mothers. It is something that matters a great deal to some of them for a very short period of their lives. In that period of intense focus on their infants, mothers are not likely to attend to the politics around breastfeeding, although they may be strongly influenced by those politics through public culture and media stories. But a discipline like anthropology, even engaged anthropology, has less impact on the North American public than social media; and the media has already defined breastfeeding as something trivial, heroic, bizarre, or humorous.

Cyberspace provides opportunities for endless personal storytelling through mommy blogs; some of these may be helpful to mothers, others harmful. Many North American mommy blogs include stories about what mothers consider their personal failures with breastfeeding and the inappropriate pressure or bad treatment they experienced at the hands of health professionals as they tried to solve breastfeeding problems or begin to bottle-feed under difficult circumstances. For breastfeeding mothers, the negative stories in mommy blogs may be discouraging. Barston's blog, FearlessFormulaFeeder.com, began in order to "frame breastfeeding as an empowering personal choice rather than as a government-mandated, fear induced act" (Barston 2012: 5). Breastfeeding critics such as Wolf (2010), Jung (2015), and Barston (2012) are quick to criticize these unanticipated consequence of the discourse of mastery whether it emerges in health care settings or breastfeeding promotion campaigns such as the National Breastfeeding Awareness Campaign of 2004 (cf. Hausman 2011).

Breastfeeding advocacy has also been treated critically in the media. Mommy blogs write constantly about the breastfeeding bullies who try to force new mothers to breastfeed against their wills. The distrust of breastfeeding and breastfeeding advocacy groups in Canada was reenforced in November 2006 when *Chatelaine,* a leading Canadian women's magazine published an article titled "Breastfeeding Sucks." The author refers to the "pro-breastfeeding tyrants," the "evangelism" of the "boob squad" who use "scare tactics" to stifle women's choices, and concludes, "We might have to suck up the pain of breastfeeding, but we can spit out the piety of the breastfeeding bullies" (Onstad 2006: 60). This attitude suggests there is something very wrong in the way breastfeeding is interpreted and promoted in North America.

The media loves inciting the mommy wars, where everyone loses except the industries that benefit from identity politics that pit mothers against each other. Usually, breastfeeding mothers are contrasted with bottle-feeding mothers, as if observers could tell what was in the bottle or why the mother was not breastfeeding at that moment. A video entitled the "Sisterhood of Motherhood" produced in 2015 by Abbott Nutrition, the makers of Similac infant formula, takes a satirical look at the personal judgments that fuel the North American mommy wars, disguising a manipulative marketing tool as a "we're all in this together" feel good message (www.youtube.com/watch?v=Kz4BUwaxj5c). The video frames infant-feeding decisions as trivial lifestyle choices embedded in the competitive parenting games of catty women. "We are all the same," the ad concludes, reinforcing the argument that formula and human milk are equivalent. But it is the actor playing the breastfeeding mother who is being mean and judgmental toward bottle-feeding parents, as she fumbles awkwardly under her breastfeeding "tent."

While the video purports to show the bonds between parents—bottle-feeding mothers and fathers, and breastfeeding mothers—it plays up people's fear of offending others because of the emotional and personal nature of breastfeeding, drawing attention to the wars themselves rather than working with the existing diversity of infant-feeding practices. Breastfeeding advocates criticize the quality of breastmilk substitutes and the promotional practices of the companies that market them, not the parents who use them.

Why are breastfeeding advocacy efforts perceived so negatively? Growing your own vegetables is not viewed as an attack on people who use canned vegetables. Making your own clothes does not challenge the fashion industry. Why should women who breastfeed, or people who research breastfeeding be viewed as attacking mothers who use infant formula? Why should every new discovery about the properties of human milk immediately trigger a debate and personal attacks? And why do North American women use so much creative energy to celebrate not breastfeeding and glorify second rate, unsafe substitutes? Part of the answer lies in the difficulty that mothers have in integrating infant feeding into their working lives. In WEIRD (Western, educated, industrial, rich, and democratic; Henrich et al. 2010) societies, this includes the modern bodily habitus of solitary sedentary work, and the lack of support new mothers receive, particularly mothers with no maternity entitlements. But the reasons are much more complex and take us deeper into the big questions.

We wanted to write a book that would address some of these questions but avoid the backlash, and would do for child feeding what Sally Merry (2006) does for violence against women—to show the potential of anthropology to address problems basic to improving the human condition—while at the same time critiquing the concept of "the human condition," and critiquing the urge to improve and reform. Using a wide repertoire of women's experiences, breastfeeding advocacy work, and secondary literature, we develop a theory of infant feeding, show how nurture is a highly developed capacity of humans, but rarely examined, and place interventions to improve infant feeding under the ethnographic gaze. These interventions are usually lodged in UN agencies such as the World Health Organization (WHO) and UNICEF, as well as activist networks such as the International Baby Food Action Network (IBFAN) and the World Alliance for Breastfeeding Action (WABA). This book is an opportunity to really go *Beyond the Breast-Bottle Controversy* (Van Esterik 1989: 211) with its expressed goal "not to have every woman breastfeed her infant, but to create conditions in individuals, households, communities and nations so that every woman could."

The Dance of Nurture

We started this book with a historically masculine competitive frame that ignores nurture. We proceed by showing how nurture shifts the frame from competition to complementarity. Dance is the metaphor we use to capture the complexity and complementarity of nurture. Minimally, we use dance to draw attention away from fights and wars as a way to talk about infant feeding, although war-like metaphors are still common in discussions of weaning practices. Mechanistic metaphors of drive and force, bullets and targets, do not enhance our understanding of the relationship between nurturer and nurtured. Another example, the gears model, was developed to express the coordination needed to support breastfeeding programs, with the master gear representing goal setting; "like a well-oiled engine, gears need to be co-ordinated and working in synchrony" (Perez-Escamilla et al. 2012: 798, 790). While the gear model may work at the policy level when institutions compete to master nurture, mechanistic metaphors are inappropriate for explaining nurture. Pump and dump, the practice of pumping and discarding breastmilk, often to relieve engorgement, is a particularly jarring mechanistic phrase.

Dance is more than just a metaphor for nurture. It is a creative principle, an embodied activity, a way of expressing complementarity. Dance integrates differences and encourages complementarity. Competitive dance undercuts the complementarity potential of dance (cf. Sandlos 2014). Working with diversity is a principle of nurturing, and dance is one way of working together. Even dance performances where the dancers do not get it perfect can be magical. Dance is a principle that organizes diversity, incorporating not excluding differences; there is not "one best way" to dance. Similarly, weaving differences into complementarity is a principle of human development. "If I could say it I wouldn't have to dance it," was the response attributed to Isadora Duncan and/or Martha Graham to a question about the meaning of a dance. Because dance is not text-based or obsessed with meaning, it is ideally suited for communicating about intuition, pattern and total systems—and nurture. The dancing body and the nurturing body are both instruments of expression and emotion. The movement patterns of work often inspire dance patterns, even when they do not mimic particular activities directly. For example, in the wet rice cultures of Southeast Asia, sowing, harvesting, and grinding rice reflect the fertility concerns of communities working to grow rice and children; the dances do not necessarily mimic the movements of agricultural work themselves.

Wrangham (2009) argues that cooking made us human. Cooking is a nurturing practice too, so perhaps we can agree that the dance of nurture also made us human. The dance of nurture has a rhythm and steps that exist before the dancers execute them. How do we separate the dancer from the dance, recognize the steps, and appreciate the music? The dance came before the dancer's knowledge of the steps, before learning how to dance the dance. Dance, like breastfeeding, is a cumulatively developed skilled activity; the more you do it, the better you get at it. How do past conditions (the steps) come to bear on present choreographies? The knowledge and practice of breastfeeding and infant feeding is a dance passed down from mothers and women of one generation to their daughters as a part of customary childrearing in local contexts. Breastfeeding is not a march nor a war nor a fight, but a dance. It is part of a tradition that is learned and shared in a group. Like music and dance, the knowledge is embodied, visceral, and passed on skin-to-skin. The dance of nurture has many variations, but they always include the dancers and the dance, inseparable and simultaneous. Every mother—infant couple has its own rhythm, its own breastfeeding style within the local breastfeeding style.

No first time mother anywhere in the world has had direct experience with how to lead the dance of nurture, or how to develop a breastfeeding relationship with her newborn. Most new mother–infant dyads are amateurs who may well need the help of a master dancer (an experienced parent who nurtures well or a lactation consultant). If mothers themselves were breastfed, they may have an indirect source of information, as they have already been socialized to know their part in the dance of nurture. Similarly, all children who have been parented know how to parent because they played the reciprocal role for their parents. To return to the dance metaphor, we learn coregulation from our partner's moves.

Dance forgives; get a move wrong, and a skilled partner can get you back in step, and the dance continues, assisted by the music and the rhythm. There is beauty in the way partners mesh together, feel self-in-other, other-in-self, and visible dissonance when the partners fail to mesh, and get so far out of step that the dance comes to a halt. The modern world has intruded on the dance of nurture, making mothering, nurturing, and breastfeeding more challenging. In some communities, the dance of nurture has been interrupted; more appealing partners have "cut-in" and taken over the dance. These intrusions often undercut the values that held infant-feeding complexes together. But nurturing practices are resilient and have adapted to many of these intrusions, transforming themselves in the process. Breastfeeding practices survive challenges such as HIV, poverty and malnutrition, chemical residues and toxins, and hospital practices, and almost have a life of their own. This mutually reinforcing resilience, the dance of nurture that persists against all odds, is the subject of this book.

CHAPTER 2

Studying Nurture

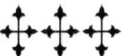

We live in the backwash of an infant-feeding revolution only half understood. Everyone knows roughly what happened: women chose bottle over breast. And some suppose they know why: they consider that using the bottle is easier and liberating. Yet this is far too simple, not to mention tautological and teleological.[1] It force-fits breastfeeding to the modern story—a tale where nurture never had any place anyway. A more realistic analysis would put breastfeeding in the human story—an epic where one generation nurtures the next. In this, breastfeeding's natural setting, the biocultural character of infant feeding explains the historical rupture whereby bottle beat breast.

What did happen historically? In the last decades of the nineteenth century, massive immigration, urbanization, and industrialization ripped millions of North American women out of breastfeeding-friendly surroundings. Stranded in cities and intimidated by progress, these vulnerable mothers listened to medical experts rather than older women (Apple 2006). In that historic shift, science killed custom. One snag: science does not breastfeed babies. Women do. And a breastfeeding woman is never just her biology but always also a social person who requires social support to pursue social activities such as nurturing as well as breastfeeding. What aligns these disparate realities? In group after group, custom (O'Connor and Van Esterik 2012) cobbles together compromises (Lévi-Strauss 1966) that get the job done. Take away how custom syncs person, body, and group, and breastfeeding becomes difficult for many, impossible for some. Witness the United Kingdom—90 percent of women stop breastfeeding earlier than they intended (Coloson, Meek, and Hawdon 2008). This shortfall is decidedly new, distinctively modern, and thoroughly entangled in marketing breastmilk substitutes.

Infant feeding is at an impasse. We cannot go back—the customs that once got mother, infant, and society dancing together are now long gone, never to return. Nor can we stay put, not when missing customs strand breastfeeding without vital support. Yet we can go forward: by seeing where modern thought errs we can begin to right its wrongs.

The Modern Episteme

> Modernity prides itself on the fragmentation of the world as its foremost achievement. Fragmentation is the prime source of its strength. The world that falls apart into plethora of problems is a manageable world. Or, rather, since the problems are manageable—the question of the manageability of the world may never appear on the agenda.
>
> —Zygmunt Bauman

Modernity advances by fragmenting. That breaking-apart style drives researchers to specialize in ever narrower pieces. So the breast-to-bottle shift is not studied as revolutionizing human relationships. That is what happens, but how we relate to infants is far too fluid, diverse, and complex to study reductively. So research details milk's composition instead. In this move, where studying parts (nutrition) replaces addressing the whole (relationship), we see how fragmenting works.

From Mother to Machine

Taken for granted today, this fragmenting mind-set is markedly modern and surprisingly new. Once Europeans saw Earth as a living organism, a place where nature was "a nurturing mother ... who provided for the needs of mankind in an ordered, planned universe" (Merchant 1980: xvii, 2). A baby at the breast was the way of the world, the life cycle shaping people as well as plants and seasons. Then the sixteenth century began to see nature as less a mother than a machine (Merchant 1980). In this new metaphor, where life unfolds by chance rather than Providence, biology's facts replace Creation's mysteries.

Seeing Earth as a machine strips away life's sanctity. Once nature loses its mystery, all life becomes mundane and manageable. Like a machine, you can vary inputs to learn how nature works. That is what experiments do. And experimenting assumes you can not only control the world, holding all but one element constant, but take life apart to study its elements one by one. Here, where a machine is never more than the sum of its parts, nurture has no place. In these features—seeing nature as tractable, knowable, and divisible—the machine metaphor gives science its laboratory logic and society its faith that fragmenting can answer all questions.

Cartesian Hegemony

Today's fragmenting owes its style to two thinkers. The older, Plato, puts truth behind appearances, fueling how fragmenting seeks underlying causes. In this logic, all breastfeeding is essentially the same everywhere. So how it varies in actuality—culture to culture, woman to woman, day to day—is incidental, even illusory. Its true form is the biology common to all cases. Here, in separating biology from all else, we see the thought of Rene Descartes, a sixteenth century French philosopher. In his epistemology, nature's oneness divides into two separately sovereign realms. One realm, the domain of matter, is an objective physical sphere where law-like regularities reign everywhere and always. The other realm, the domain of spirit, is a subjective mental sphere that differs from place to place and time to time. That division, Cartesian dualism, organizes modern science.

Descartes's mind–body dualism also organizes modern life. It is there when ordinary speech distinguishes "work" from "home" or we imagine a cruel "real world" apart from caring "friends and family." And it is built into how we separate our physical bodies from our social and moral selves. Lest anyone miss the message, our institutions enforce Cartesian distinctions: seeing the doctor gets your complaint put in your head or your body, just as going to school obliges you to divide art from math, English from biology, play from work. Indeed, dualism rules society, insisting that any clearheaded person divides mind from body, individual from society, nurture from nature, religion from science, love from sex, self from other, emotion from reason.

Yet there is an ironic catch: humans can think dualistically but not live that way. Dualism defies nature's oneness, its ongoing integration (Bateson 1972). Contrary to Descartes, reasoning *requires* emotions (Damasio 1994), our physical health *depends on* our social well-being (Marmot 2004), individuality *requires* societal support (Lee 1986), nurturing *implements* our nature (Goldschmidt 2006). Again and again, the modern mind-set imagines dualities that realities like breastfeeding mock.

Studying Breastfeeding Reductively

Breastfeeding evolved as an emergent system of lesser emergent systems, each with feedback loops that make its parts too interdependent to study separately. Although this feedback has parts continually changing each other, making part-by-part study tricky or even impossible, reductive research rushes ahead confidently nonetheless. That makes trouble. Consider five examples.

Fragmenting Wholes

Before Cartesian science, Europeans thought human milk had life-changing powers we would now call magical. It could cure the ill, revive the dying, seed a woman's character in an infant's body. Today, we credit the curing to antibodies and reject the idea that milk shapes character. We know this by analyzing the milk, by breaking the once magical whole into its constituent elements. In the pieces, we find antibodies but no character-carrying essence. This is sound and valuable knowledge. So far so good.

Do antibodies explain all the magic? Not likely. Skin-to-skin contact has its own curative powers and caring clearly speeds recovery. Although these intangibles (touch, caring) are not in the milk, they are built into breastfeeding as a physical act and a social and moral relationship. In these surroundings, where perhaps everything beyond the antibodies functions as a living whole, Cartesian dividing hides the dynamic feedback.

Fragmenting reduces infant feeding into debates about nutrients. Applying Descartes's spirit/matter split separates milk's nourishing (matter) from love's nurturing (spirit). So while nothing can replace the caregiver's love, chemical additives in infant formula can replace some of the nutrients in human milk. Of course, to get the chemistry right, one must isolate human milk (a physical substance) from humans, factoring out those variables (actual mothers nursing actual babies) to get at nature's constants. Cartesians do this unapologetically: we are, they would say, just separating what is naturally separate anyway. That is what the spirit/matter split wrongly presumes.

Where does this Cartesian logic err? It posits something that does not and cannot exist—generic human milk. Even if infant formula could be improved to match some hypothetical human average, no mother has ever produced and fed her baby generic human milk—it does not exist; and no baby fed from a human breast has ever imbibed matter (the milk) apart from spirit (touch, feelings). Nor can this ever change: human milk (a material product) and breastfeeding (a social process) coevolved into intricate interdependence. Here, only by functioning as a whole, can breastfeeding continuously adapt to life's ever-changing material and spiritual surroundings.

Divorcing Biology from Culture

In dividing spirit from matter, Descartes opposes nurture to nature, culture to biology. So while biologists study breastfeeding's physiology, anthropologists research its cultural meaning. Working separately, we have learned a lot. Yet kept as Cartesian halves, all we get is biology plus culture. What is missing, biocultural integration, is how infant feeding actually works.

Take the biochemical cues that release breastmilk so an infant can feed. While one might describe the physiology by itself, that biology serves many purposes. Far from being automatic, human lactation only occurs in the historically constituted body of an actual woman, someone immersed in surroundings she variously incarnates and resists. In this realm (her body) within a realm (her close surroundings), her biochemistry interacts with not just her infant but cultural cues, lifelong predispositions, feeding rituals, and more that all also interact with each other. Imagine a modern North American woman caught in a public place with a hungry infant. A sense of modesty built into her body since childhood may impede the let-down reflex needed to initiate breastfeeding. Or an onlooker's disapproval might bring the same biochemical response for a different reason—propriety. Or, with experienced breastfeeding couples, mother–infant interdependence may give her baby a control over her body that overwhelms her individual autonomy, not to mention modesty and propriety's counter-cues. In all these intricately interdependent loops, where does biology end and culture begin?

Reducing as Explaining

What we have just described (severing biology from culture) is a particular instance of fragmenting wholes. The problem is not the dividing itself. No, it is mistaking a useful method (breaking reality into its parts) that explains some phenomena (some underlying parts do determine the larger reality) for a timeless truth (all reality is the sum of its parts) that explains everything everywhere. That is how, whether it is apt or not, reducing becomes *the* explanation.

What does that do to breastfeeding? Take our earlier example of how nutrition dominates infant-feeding debates. We used it to show how fragmenting forgets the whole but it is also the end of a long reductive chain. Start with an indisputable truth—all infants need not just food but nurturing.

- Step 1: Reduce that larger truth (nurturing) to what is easier to study and, seemingly, most essential—feeding.
- Step 2: Reduce feeding, an act simultaneously social and physical, to its physical fraction—food.
- Step 3: Reduce this food to generic milk, forgetting that the substance varies woman to woman and changes adaptively over the course of breastfeeding.
- Step 4: Reduce generic milk to its nutrients as if it were not a veritable soup of living antimicrobial, anti-inflammatory, and immunoregulatory agents.

In four radically reductive leaps, the whole vanishes step by step. Talk about throwing the baby out with the bathwater! Or, to be specific, we might say baby, mother, milk, and the nursing relationship (all functioning wholes) get dissolved into bathwater (their various lifeless parts).

When nurturing (a flexible social relationship) turns into nutrients (fixed physical facts), we see biological reductionism at work. Social scientists rightly decry such crude biologism. That said, these researchers can reason reductively themselves. Take health surveys—they typically reduce breastfeeding's existential dilemmas to clear questions with check-off choices; or consider how "culture" homogenizes the way each mother–infant dyad creates a unique world with its own meanings and politics.

Neutering Gendered Wholes

Modern thought rightly challenges racial, class, and gender inequities. One step repudiates biologizing racial, class, and gender differences; and then a second step attributes these differences to culture. All this supposes a baseline human—someone who is neither black nor white, elite nor commoner, male nor female—whose culture assigns arbitrary racial, class, and gender characteristics anyway. Here modern fragmenting, by separating each person from his or her grouping by race, class, or gender, shatters prejudice brilliantly.

Does this separating work equally well for all aspects of gender? It does for race and class, where every distinction lost is a gain for equality and reason, but two gender distinctions are less easily dismissed because they are not just culturally constructed. First, each human has a unique constitution that is bioculturally gendered. Quite apart from x and y chromosomes, constitutional gendering begins in the womb and builds historical patterns that carry visceral weight and momentum quite apart from how the surrounding culture happens to define gender. Second, the human life cycle is bioculturally gendered because only women menstruate and have babies. In these two realms, each individual lives out a contingent yet cumulative gendered pattern. It can be fought but not avoided. A new mother who chooses not to breastfeed must fight how pregnancy prepared her body for lactation long before the baby arrived. And an adult who chooses not to parent silences a life cycle impetus to nurture as he or she was nurtured. Make no mistake—this impetus is neither biology (a drive to breed) nor culture (the meaning of having a baby) but biocultural; and while it need not be strong, it is constitutionally gendered and can neither be neutered nor wished away. Although contemporary culture can suppose otherwise, defining breastfeeding's cultural context as it chooses, it cannot freely remake how a woman's bodily context genders breastfeeding.

Erasing History

Although the modern episteme spotlights the present and forgets the past (Connerton 2009; Schorske 1998), breastfeeding is always historical, always a practice building on what came before. That holds not just for the nursing duo but for the mother's constitution as well as her group's passed-down practices. Consider, then, the modern malaise: every year millions of women start breastfeeding only to stop sooner than planned. Earlier we attributed this falling-off to an historic rupture: roughly a century ago, when "modern" women began listening to "scientific" doctors instead of their mothers, breastfeeding's enabling customs died. In Chapter 3, we explain why breastfeeding's biology evolved around historically contingent customs whose historic loss under conditions of modernity (Chapter 6) alienates women from their own bodies (cf. Martin 2001) and invites inner battles over "control" and "discipline" (Stearns 1999) that now bedevils twenty-first-century breastfeeding.

Contemporary research typically explains breastfeeding ahistorically. Surveys tally recent choices while interviews probe contemporary meanings. Both depict women who consciously calculate breastfeeding, adapting to current conditions. Added together, these individual decisions make the collective trend. And that is true—as far as this Cartesian logic goes. Yet suppose we do not pretend "individual" and "society" are separate entities. Suppose we recognize their thoroughgoing interdependence, a truth human phylogeny and ontogeny both teach. Then we must ask a hard historical question: where is the intimate mother-to-daughter knowledge that once embedded breastfeeding in the life cycle, that built a practice over generations? Textbook biology is no substitute and neither is romanticized mothering. In an earlier day, a new mother had seasoned advice suited to her locally grown body, her genes, her family, her community. So when today's breastfeeding gets cut short, is the mother choosing what she wants or just coping with impossible choices? Simply wanting to breastfeed does not equip a woman with the social and bodily tools she needs to succeed.

Studying Breastfeeding Realistically

The last section, in pitting the machine metaphor against breastfeeding's realities, made the classic matchup—reductionism versus holism. Once rabid reductionism advanced science against superstition. And as science specialized, reductionism legitimately set the standard that competing schools had to beat. Yet today's science increasingly favors short-term interdisciplinary projects, not the sustained programmatic schemes that built today's disciplines. In this emerging space, where researchers solve problems pragmatically and shift methodologies freely, holism and reductionism can become conversing complements, not stonewalling competitors.

How can breastfeeding research widen the conversation? Here we provide a vocabulary that is sensitive to breastfeeding's complexities:

- *Constitution:* Early in life, as the interacting mind and body interweave, each person develops a unique constitution. The result, a hybrid of biology and culture, begins epigenetically and progressively takes on a momentum that gives individuals their distinctive dispositions. In our usage, constitution is biography, character, habit, and body all rolled into one.
- *Life cycle:* The life cycle binds each generation to the next, to ancestors and successors. Breastfeeding enacts the life cycle: any woman who lives to nurture a baby was nurtured by others in her infancy, and in many cultures, she expects her children to care for her later in life.
- *Bioculturalism:* Humans are not "biology" plus "culture" but historically contingent biocultural hybrids that function holistically. Our constitutions are biocultural realities that begin in the womb. In breastfeeding, two constitutions intertwine in yet another biocultural reality.
- *Emergent systems:* The phrase "a whole is greater than the sum of its parts" captures how life organizes itself in complex systems that cannot be explained reductively. Known by various names (emergence in biology, Gestalt in psychology, metaphysical holism in philosophy), this principle is fundamental to anthropology's holism as well hermeneutics, systems theory, chaos theory, and ecology.
- *Social womb:* At birth and in the following weeks, neither mother nor baby can prosper without sustained and coherent support by family, friends, and neighbors. Human biology does not guarantee this vital support—it is not wired into our bodies—but well functioning groups provide it and, under stable conditions, integrate it into their customs and expectations. Integral to this nurturance is the womb-like protection that buffers the nursing duo from intrusions on their relationship.

Our five terms keep reductionism at bay long enough to weigh alternatives. Think of "constitution," for example, as holding off a hormonal explanation, the 900-pound gorilla in the room. Yes, breastfeeding involves hormones, but that biochemical constant cannot explain how women vary, how each has a unique hormone-mediating constitution. Our five terms thus hold reductionism accountable to breastfeeding realities that earlier science ignored or dismissed as derivative. Are we denying reductionism altogether? No, we do not even want gorilla-free space. Where biochemistry can enlighten us about mother or baby, that is all to the good. Besides, without reductionism's hard-won facts about oxytocin and placentas and much, much more, we could not understand how wholes like a constitution or life cycle work.

Can we have our facts and yet transcend their literalism too? Now that we have a vocabulary that captures breastfeeding's realities, we can open a still wider conversation between science's various fact-producing sites. Here the site that rules the roost is the Lab, capitalized to mark it as an ideal type and distinguish the physical place (a mere building) from the far more important process of research. While reductionism rules the Lab, our other three ideal types—Clinic, Field, and the New Ethnology—do science differently. All four ideal types are intellectually powerful sites that package facts, methods, theories, and values into distinctive combinations. By moving between these sites rather than choosing sides, research can develop a wider and more realistic conversation that supersedes the old disciplinary politics.

The Lab: Reductive Truths

The Lab discovers truth experimentally. It does that either physically by bringing life within the laboratory's four walls, or mentally by taking the lab's logic out into life as a way of thinking. Either way this is a powerful but limited strategy. One direct limit is an experiment's capacity to distinguish and then control variables. A second ultimate limit is the supposition that nature can be broken apart like a machine. Given these limits, the Lab's facts never stand alone. They are only true insofar as the Lab's reductive assumptions and fragmenting procedures hold. That said, findings from the other three sites are not freestanding truths either. All knowledge comes conditioned by the theories and methods that make knowing possible. That is the epistemology that keeps our interdisciplinary conversation going.

Where the Lab reduces reality artificially with no apologies, our three other sites—Field, Clinic, New Ethnology—pride themselves on capturing emergent systems naturalistically, in their own terms. Other than that common ground, each site's distinctive methods pursue a different truth.

The Clinic: The Truth of Healing

The Clinic cures. That is the measure of what all clinicians do. In their healing, they experiment on real people in real time, case by messy individual case. When they succeed, they cannot always know why: treating an actual person jumbles uncontrolled variables together. So the clinician's one-off results do not satisfy the Lab where truth is only what you can replicate. Not the Clinic. There each patient's well-being decides what is and is not true.

What truths can the Clinic's patient-by-patient particularizing discover that the Lab's generalizing loses? Consider this remarkable data: in Sweden, by methodically observing 506 infants over their first six months, clinicians found such wide "variations in breastfeeding frequency and suckling duration" that they concluded that "every mother–infant pair needs to be understood as a unique dyad throughout lactation" (Hörnell et al. 1999). Saying "unique" puts the Lab's universalizing in its place.

What place should human universals have in breastfeeding? Imagine a textbook-bound specialist working with those wide-ranging Swedish cases. Incidental and even apt variety would look dangerously abnormal. So any normative advice would be unhelpful, even harmful. Of course this opens the longstanding scientific controversy over lumping versus splitting. In this debate, the Swedish researchers are extreme splitters, seeing 506 types where lumpers would need but one (it is all human lactation). We might even attribute their splitting to how each patient is unique in the Clinic, whereas the Lab factors out all those particulars as confounding variables to find universals. Yet the Clinic captures a larger human truth: human lactation, it would seem, evolved around leaving mother–infant patterns open to personal decisions and highly local patterns. Certainly that adaptive flexibility would be superior to instinct-determined feeding. It is that openness—the room to roam creatively and ultimately adaptively—that the Swedish data records and the Lab's generic biology loses.

The Field: The Truth of Context

In the modern episteme, breastfeeding is largely biology. Of course, were it just that, breastfeeding would be the same across cultures and contexts. In fact, its practice is highly sensitive to its surroundings and varies widely culture to culture, place to place, person to person, even moment to moment. Reductive science, in supposing there is only one truth, dooms itself to perpetually rediscovering humanity's diversity and forever fighting its implications.

Now that science knows that context counts, research must factor in the surroundings it once so carefully factored out. Thus, the current question: how can we study breastfeeding naturalistically? The Lab will not do (an experiment is a context, an artificial one); taking lab logic out into life is tricky (how do you control variables you have yet to discover?); and the Clinic's context, the examining room, carefully separates people from their everyday lives (otherwise clinicians could not poke and prod half-naked bodies).

Where Lab and Clinic stumble, the Field excels. Its disciplinary home, anthropology, prides itself on doing the intensive, long-term fieldwork it takes to put humans in context. Here anthropology makes three defining moves. First and foremost, the discipline revolves around fieldwork—the longer and deeper the better. To know another culture you must live it, or live with it, firsthand. So truth-seeking leaves the Lab to enter everyday life. There real people trump abstract theory; you embrace serendipity since you cannot control variables; and you follow events as they unfold because you cannot stop time—all direct opposites of what the Lab does.

Second, as a field science, anthropology explains humans naturalistically. Taking an ecological approach, the discipline uses direct observation that focuses on life's surfaces to explain humans by their surroundings. All these defining features contrast with how the Lab constructs artificial experiments, cuts off natural surroundings, and infers underlying causes. So while the Field prides itself in looking at actual women nursing actual babies in real time in real places, the Lab prefers seeing through life's surfaces to find some one true and timeless form. For Cartesians, that is "biology" pure and simple—real life takes the hindmost. Anthropology flips that around, relating breastfeeding to everyday life, an endeavor neither pure nor simple.

Third, to stay close to how humans live whole lives, anthropology counters modern fragmenting with three rule-of-thumb correctives. First, look contextually. Give the surroundings a say before and after you focus in on a specific phenomenon. That is essential for studying breastfeeding—only by looking widely can research see how local life shapes biology. Second, reason holistically, not just reductively. Again breastfeeding makes that essential—nurturing an infant is a discourse of wholes (the activity of nursing, the mother–infant relationship, local support, and more) where each such emergent system is itself an irreducible reality with its own inner character, logic, and energy. Third, study comparatively. Insofar as a "person" or "culture" or "breastfeeding" functions as a whole, a single case leaves you guessing at its inner workings. Only by looking comparatively to find naturally occurring "experiments" that change one or another part can one discern how the whole works.

What does the Field teach that neither Lab nor Clinic knows? First lesson: breastfeeding is a cultural activity. Culture is an attribute of groups that neither Lab nor Clinic can effectively study. Second lesson: culture is a web of meaning. To understand breastfeeding, you relate it to the rest of life. That relatedness is the context that the Lab eliminates categorically, and the Clinic can only glimpse piecemeal. Third lesson: meaning is highly local. Against Lab-imagined generalities, a parade of ethnographies has shown breastfeeding varies much as the world's cultures do. Sometimes it is the essence of a culture as with Mandinka (Whittemore and Beverly 1996). Other times it is a practice that crosses cultures as in urban Mali (Dettwyler 1988) or divides ethnicities as in rural Cameroon (Yovsi and Keller 2003). And still other times, it echoes political restructuring as in Bolivia (Tapias 2006) or renegotiates social relations as in urban China (Gottschang 2007). All in all, naturalistic observation in the field tells us breastfeeding's character, meaning, and place vary widely across the globe.

The New Ethnology: Recurring Solutions as Human Truths

Giving Lab, Clinic, and Field separate yet equal voices widens the conversation. It lets us recognize breastfeeding's law-like unity (the Lab's biological regularities) as well as its riotous diversity (variety that Clinic and Field highlight). Once such incompatible findings would have compelled debates over who has breastfeeding right. Today, as epistemological pluralists, we can leave this unresolved. Indeed, what is there to resolve?—if you start with the Lab's universalizing assumptions and procedures, then you get law-like regularities; and if you start with the Clinic's personalizing and the Field's localizing, then the uniqueness in every case stands out. Breastfeeding can be "one way" and "almost any way"—it all depends on how you look (methodology) and what you ask. Recognizing unity and diversity becomes possible once we accept all science need not be reductive. Clinic and Field are worthy alternatives that should be in dialogue with the Lab.

While a wider conversation advances research, its postmodern openness is problematic. Once questioning science simply looked ignorant. Not anymore. Now that hardline biology is not the only truth, a scholar like Joan Wolf (2010)[2] can pick apart breastfeeding's scientific support to *The New York Times*'s applause; similarly, when Courtney Jung (2015) repeats these arguments, she too has space in *The New York Times* even before her book is published. As amateur voices grow strident, professionals fumble to engage antiscience. It is easy to see why: how does one set clear standards yet recognize diversity? When each of 506 breastfeeding couples does it their own way, it would seem anything goes. Yet public health cannot advocate for "whatever." An epistemological advance (the wider conversation) thus threatens health care (medicine needs clear norms) if not democracy (without science to referee, politics degrades to ideology).

Can we have a wider conversation yet not encourage antiscience? While most scholars rightly reject the specious rigor that denies the diversity of individuals and cultures, having no standards whatsoever opens infant feeding to anything-goes opinion. In fact, anything does not go. How infants are nurtured carries huge consequences, and breastfeeding can fail: some women try all sorts of things only to falter; and while most women do succeed, it does not always come easily or quickly. All of this tells us breastfeeding's causal chain has some missing additional link. So while taking Lab, Clinic, and Field together gives us a fuller picture, obviously it is not full enough.

The missing link is a social universal: to succeed, mother and infant must jointly develop a full and flexible social relationship. Anything less than full will not subordinate two individualities to one relationship; and anything without flexibility will not keep up with a rapidly developing infant in the mother's ever-changing world. Those are high standards demanded at a most difficult time: traumatized by birth, mother and baby must suddenly and rapidly replace the womb's biological relationship with a social relationship after birth. Were that not challenging enough, one party, the infant, is a socially incoherent creature. All this and the stakes are incredibly high: either the couple develops an effective nurturing relationship or the baby will not thrive and could die. With such life-deciding stakes, we might expect evolution to have wired in a perfect solution. But the relationship originates socially, not biologically; it develops interactively, not genetically; and it quickly takes on a negotiated rather than predetermined course.

While biology leaves this relationship-making to little more than chance, most human groups actively intervene. Certainly the physical act of breastfeeding never stands alone. Everywhere we look rituals, customs, and conventions surround the nursing couple. That is no accident: human groups embed the postpartum in surroundings that protect and promote the mother–infant relationship. That is what we see when we analyze postpartum customs across cultures. To be sure, we did not see this until we went back to how Ruth Benedict (1934: 1) characterized anthropology as "the science of customs." No anthropologist would say that today—we study whole cultures, not discrete customs; any custom is understood in relation to the whole, not in itself; and that whole, a web of meaning unique to each people and place, makes customs incomparable. But for Benedict (1934: 223–30), culture was integrated around history (it was an inheritance) and function (it was an adaptive tool), leaving meaning an optional extra. Were function and history our lens today, breastfeeding would look nowhere near as various as meaning now makes it seem. Were Benedict doing the analysis, breastfeeding's incredible diversity would be variations on a few widely diffused complexes that worked well enough (function) for the group to pass on (history) and neighbors to borrow (history again).[3]

Rebalancing the meaning/function/history equation revives ethnology. A century ago ethnography served ethnology. The former described cultures one by one to equip theorists to generalize about humankind. Were cultures alike because they were cousins, offspring of an earlier culture? That was diffusion—a historical explanation. Or were cultures similar because they independently arrived at similar solutions?—a functional explanation. That grand comparative project once organized anthropology as a comparative science. Then, as ethnographic fieldwork came to define anthropology (Stocking 1992), comparison itself seemed invidious. The discipline sought to understand each people in its own terms.

Our project restores the old questions but for a new reason. Unlike the old ethnology, we value the move to meaning as a true advance. Ethnography, then, is no longer comparison's servant but an end in itself—it helps us understand the depth of human diversity. This then gives ethnology a new role: to live together in a diverse world we need to negotiate differences that meaning alone renders absolute. In that negotiating, knowing humanity's recurring solutions to fundamentals like breastfeeding, can serve the common good in a realistic yet nonreductive manner.

The Social Womb: A Recurring Solution

Using custom as our lens, at first glance the postpartum shows grab-bag diversity: if one group sequesters mother and neonate for seven days, then another insists on forty; and if one culture isolates them lest birth pollute others, then yet another people worries others will pollute them! This enormous diversity shreds superficial generalizations. Indeed, read symbolically, each people is entirely unique and any cross-cultural commonalities are vapid (Geertz 2000: 135). Yet read functionally—focusing on what these particulars do rather than say—reveals two broad cross-cultural regularities: the new mother gets support; and the breastfeeding duo is sequestered from outsiders. That supportive-yet-separating mix takes up where the physical womb leaves off, organizing the postpartum world in ways that support the mother–infant relationship and otherwise meet the needs of infant, mother, and group.

While every culture construes pregnancy, birth, and the postpartum its own unique way, there are significant similarities in how groups handle the first few days and weeks after birth. People recognize mother and infant need special care and often protection. It is this package of symbols, practices, and understandings, what Jennings and Edmundson (1980) have characterized as a fourth trimester that we liken to a postpartum social womb. What does it look like across cultures? Supposing that what occurs together typically works together as a larger whole, we first describe the package overall before we isolate distinctive features to discuss one by one.

> *Breastfeeding [1] develops as a biocultural activity [2] where neonate and mother interact [3] opportunistically and ritually, [4] encapsulated within a historically constituted, [5] custom-structured and [6] symbolically weighty [7] womb-like cultural whole [8] where mother and group negotiate their differing interests.*

1. Breastfeeding develops as a biocultural activity: Pregnancy primes a woman's body to breastfeed. It initiates hormonal cues for lactation that steroids hold back until the placenta is delivered. While biology does this priming, what happens next is never just biological but always also social, cultural, and personal. Over the next few days, an able infant must establish lactation interactively (a social process), working with the mother's bodily past (her constitution—a biocultural hybrid) and her present intentions (individually yet culturally constituted). When these vectors work together, synergy establishes breastfeeding as a biocultural activity.

Characterizing breastfeeding as an "activity" spotlights four features. First, breastfeeding is creative. It does not simply implement a biological imperative or cultural code. Quite the contrary, the nursing couple innovates opportunistically and idiosyncratically as their joint efforts further the activity. Second, breastfeeding is cumulative. One act builds on another, scaffolding some developments while foreclosing others. Once made, those choices give each breastfeeding couple a unique history that neither "biology" nor "culture" can explain. Third, breastfeeding is world-making. Through their creative effort and cumulative growth, the nursing duo develops their own little world quite apart from the larger one. In this realm, feeding or getting fed changes from the means to an end into an end in itself (the pleasure of nurturing or being nurtured, of incarnating a relationship, of developing and exercising expertise). As this realm's sovereignty grows, it makes the rituals and rewards it needs to sustain itself. Fourth, breastfeeding is absorbing. As it is creative and cumulative, one can get lost in developing a skill and enjoying mastery. One follows the activity's unfolding cues not for the end result but to discover what is next and out of the pleasure of a practice. In these four closely connected features, the activity[4] develops as a biocultural hybrid that stands apart from its immediate surroundings and cannot be reduced to underlying conditions. In that separateness, the nursing couple develops a practice that outsiders cannot know, and externals like "biology" and "culture" cannot explain (Bourdieu 1990).

As an activity, breastfeeding is in tension with culture. In particular, culture pulls in three directions that the biocultural activity cannot readily go. First, in making meaning, the larger culture connects breastfeeding widely whereas the activity's inner logic isolates it narrowly around what works for the nursing couple. Here culture, by hitching breastfeeding to gender, status, or other such weighty and contested domains can only disrupt breastfeeding's practice. Second, where culture standardizes, breastfeeding individualizes. Each breastfeeding duo joins two biologically and bioculturally unique individuals who develop a unique relationship all their own. That activity-anchored individuality denies how culture constructs breastfeeding generically. Third, where culture is simultaneous (a web-like relation of parts), an activity is sequential (an unfolding). Breastfeeding on day one and a year later may look the same, but the activity changes over time.

In characterizing breastfeeding as an activity, we argue for cross-cultural similarities. Here a Cartesian would expect a biological explanation, but the regularities we have described are neither biology nor culture, neither in our genes nor our minds. Instead breastfeeding arises socially in the interaction between a human body seeking results and physical surroundings that yield in only certain ways. Here perhaps breastfeeding differs little from other culturally discrete interface-activities like, say, dancing or cooking. Each culture can define such activities its own unique way and yet, various as these definitions are, none can erase how an activity guides action and imposes constraints. Of course breastfeeding differs from these examples in that hormones initiate it, throwing mother and infant into the activity pell-mell. Yet once begun, if the activity does not take on a creative, cumulative, world-within-world absorbing life of its own, it will be hard to sustain after the postpartum priming fades.

2. where neonate and mother interact: Humans bear helpless infants. Uniquely helpless. Other primates bear newborns who have the physical capacity to act on feeding instincts that work hand-in-glove with the mother's instincts. While human newborns may have traces of such instincts, they are born weeks before they will have the neuro-musculature capacity to act on those urges. As a result, human newborns require active caregivers, people who not only do more than instincts ever could, but do it with a situational subtlety—a this-then-that variable responsiveness—that an instinct's one-best-way coding precludes.

Active caregivers interact with care-receiving newborns. That is two-sided, a give-and-take. Here infants do not just take but also give, offering visceral pleasures and moral gratification to caregivers as well as physical relief to a woman with engorged breasts. In this, infant care and especially breastfeeding are true exchanges, not one-way dealings, and the infant has a say in how the breastfeeding relationship develops and who he or she will become bioculturally.

In moving infant feeding out of instinct and into interaction, our species ensured every normal human would be a profoundly social creature. To be sure, Homo sapiens arose in a line of social primates, but the interactive character of early infant feeding develops the social sensibility that allows humans to keep up with an ever-changing society and to move between human groups.

As dyadic interaction, infant feeding is mutually determined and failure-prone. Either party can willfully frustrate the other, or mixed signals can accidentally frustrate both. When that happens in a skin-to-skin dyad, the feedback can be not just quick and clear but sweeping, filling multiple channels simultaneously. It is this richly responsive environment that turns the neonate's primitive reactions into the social game that babies learn to play.

3. opportunistically and ritually: Starting instinctually, breastfeeding builds opportunistically on whatever works. As mother and infant work together, routines quickly become rituals that coordinate their bodies and become gratifying in themselves. Then, too, whether a nascent ritual is followed, broken, or repurposed, it is an action that communicates. Ritual, we might say, is baby's first language.

4. encapsulated within a historically constituted ... cultural whole: Our species evolved around organizing breastfeeding culturally rather than instinctually. Where other primates preprogram more of lactation, human evolution moved toward culture's open-ended flexibility. Hugely adaptive as that was and is, breaking breastfeeding out of instinctual control exposes it to potential disruptions. Here culture cuts both ways. It is always necessary to breastfeeding and yet sometimes it can be disruptive.

Although the larger culture can disrupt breastfeeding, most groups have supportive traditions. In calling these "traditions," we recognize how what looks like a hodgepodge of customs and woman-to-woman advice and neighborly support can have integrity as well as longevity. To be sure, these are implicit traditions, worked out piecemeal over generations, and yet that is what keeps these quiet traditions grounded in nurturing practices that are richer and more nuanced than how any single person or generation can represent its actions to itself.

In saying breastfeeding references this tacit tradition, we stress how nurturing balances precedence against practicality. On the one hand, as no one breastfeeds "naturally," everyone can consider what others did and do. On the other hand, as these locally generated practices are not self-consciously systematized the way religion and law get codified, no one need choose to "keep" or "break" tradition. Customs can easily be adapted.

Breastfeeding builds heavily on the past. When a first-time mother first nurses her baby, she makes and lives history. She makes history in establishing a unique relationship with her child that takes on a life of its own and lasts at least another lifetime. And she lives histories shallow and deep. The shallowest is no older than her body and comes alive in how her nurturing builds on how her caregivers nurtured her. And the oldest may go back to how our species arose. In between, her breastfeeding style (Van Esterik 1989) and ecology will likely carry traditions that mark her group and region.

Calling all these traditions nesting within traditions "history" says each has a unique contingent character that the regularities of biology and culture can never fully explain. Here history best represents breastfeeding's enormous diversity. It varies not just culture to culture or just person to person or even just between the babies of one mother but from one episode to another for the same nursing couple.

5. *custom-structured ... cultural whole:* Everywhere custom structures breastfeeding. That is no accident. Custom is the medium whereby the breastfeeding mother and her community act on each other as well as themselves. For the community, custom orchestrates support and carries trade-offs that constitute breastfeeding culturally. For the mother, custom paves the way into the practice, and then, as a practitioner, it is how she develops her expertise.

From an evolutionary perspective, custom replaces what instinct governs in other animals. The less instincts determine our actions, the more humans can adapt to new conditions. Of course that adaptive openness allows maladaptive responses. In principle, custom moderates that risk, giving groups a vehicle to develop workable procedures over time. In practice, however, maladaptive breastfeeding customs are easy to find both in the premodern and the modern—particularly the modern world.

6. *symbolically weighty ... cultural whole:* Disparate meanings meet in breastfeeding. An infant at the breast enacts the life cycle, resonates creation, epitomizes nurture, polarizes gender, activates community, and evokes liminality—all richly symbolic domains that no group can take casually. So too breastmilk: mundane yet magical, it is not just food but a bodily secretion that crosses body boundaries and creates solidarities society can neither ignore nor control. All these highly charged symbols mean breastfeeding can never simply be the activity itself.

Are exogenous meanings always disruptive? Arguably every culture overloads breastfeeding with meanings but clearly some have more breastfeeding-friendly values than others. Take how modern life lionizes control and autonomy. Breastfeeding asks the opposite. As mother and baby become interdependent, she must share control and surrender autonomy. Has she embodied modern cultural values too deeply to give herself over to breastfeeding? And, if she has flexibility, how flexible is her group? Her social surroundings need not even be consistent: they can expect breastfeeding yet demean loss of control and autonomy nonetheless. Here these exogenous meanings create conflicts the mother can neither avoid nor easily resolve.

7. womb-like cultural whole: Here culture's pull is like the loose working coherence of Benedict's (1934) patterns, not the tight language-like coherence of a Geertzian web. Yet loose as it is, the more this inner gravity pulls mother away from her other demands and roles, the better for the mother–infant relationship.

8. where mother, group and infant all negotiate their immediate and life cycle interests: In modern societies, the incidence, length, and exclusivity of breastfeeding all adjust to what is practical. In effect how baby gets fed depends on what is workable for the woman and that in turns depends on her support and local conditions. Today, as biology specifies what is optimal, this contemporary compromising looks rather shabby, as if an earlier era's stronger customs and fewer options once did better by baby. In fact, negotiating infant feeding is nothing new. Ethnographies of nonmodern societies repeatedly show that groups adapt breastfeeding customs to local conditions just as modern women adjust infant feeding to what they and their household can comfortably manage.[5]

Can one understand breastfeeding apart from how it meets life-cycle interests? That is what biomedicine and social science regularly do. In stressing current conditions—be it the biology or practicality or meaning of the moment—they slight how any woman who lives to nurture her baby was nurtured by others in her infancy. The caring of others made her fully human. That is a biocultural fact: it shapes how her body functions as well as how she lives her life. Must she know this? No. Although some traditions recognize a human debt to nurture as you were nurtured, others like the modern ignore it altogether. Either way—whether a nurturing impetus is culturally marked or hidden—this life-cycle reality links breastfeeding to the mother's past, the group's present integrity, and the infant's future.

Conclusion

> *Where is the Life we have lost in living?*
> *Where is the wisdom we have lost in knowledge?*
> *Where is the knowledge we have lost in information?*
> —TS Eliot, *Choruses from The Rock*

The image of earth as a nurturing mother did not die quickly or easily in the West. While the machine metaphor rapidly revolutionized science, it only slowly colonized our bodily lives, taking centuries to invade infant feeding. Then, once established, it quickly devastated breastfeeding. Eliot's lines capture those losses cascading. One by one, breastfeeding's enabling partners fade way—the life cycle (Life), customs (wisdom), mother-to-mother mentoring (knowledge) all yield to the latest scientific information.

A century ago, assuming science and progress demanded change, experts wrongly biologized breastfeeding, naively lionized infant formula, and arrogantly shredded customs. All those mistakes, so typical of the twentieth century, plague us still. Now suddenly, twenty-first-century science is breastfeeding's best advocate. Going beyond the Lab's fragmenting, Clinic, Field, and New Ethnology all recognize the naturally occurring wholes whereby breastfeeding nurtures not just babies but meaning, custom, and well-being. And these deeply human truths nurture breastfeeding in turn.

Does custom still have truths to teach us? That is hard to ask when scholars take sides, casting custom as either handed-down ignorance (the Enlightenment view) or the wisdom of better and purer times (the Romantic Era's rejoinder). Both are nonsense. All human groups—ancient, modern, postmodern—live through their customs. Everywhere custom lets groups act on themselves over generations. What this social tool fashions piecemeal out of compromises may look like a Rube Goldberg contraption, yet this bricolage (Lévi-Strauss 1966) can develop emergent systems of great sophistication. The world's best example may well be Bali. Over centuries, by coordinating temple festivals to be good neighbors, rice farmers gradually wove the entire island into a vast irrigation behemoth whose efficiency, stability, and complexity humble anything modern irrigation engineers have proposed (Lansing 2007). Gracefully aligning humans with nature, it fed millions reliably over generations. Once postpartum customs did that too.

Notes

1. Supposing life comes down to straightforward choice is a theory (rational choice) wrapped in an ideology (society functions as a free market of individual decisions) saddled with a tautology (the argument supposes the free choice it then finds) built out of how Cartesian dualities (biology vs culture, individual vs society) arbitrarily halve breastfeeding's naturally occurring wholes.
2. Wolf turns the conditional character of good science against itself. Although all sound research recognizes its limitations, she collects these like clues to a crime. Adding them together appears to shred the scientific support for breastfeeding. But hers is a rhetorical move, not a scientific one. Science pulls an explanation apart to reach a better one. In contrast, Wolf disassembles the breastfeeding consensus as if unraveling science were intrinsically good.
3. Downplay how function and history shape culture, and suddenly meaning balloons by default. Then every culture looks completely unique and wild diversity paints the globe. That is not wrong—humanity *is* diverse—but meaning alone subordinates breastfeeding to a cultural logic it sometimes does not and often cannot obey. Against that outside rule, the mother–infant relationship has a sovereignty quite apart from how its surrounding culture constructs it. Like the Vatican in Italy, it is a polity unto itself. Getting at breastfeeding's truths thus calls for shrinking meaning so that function and history get a proportionate say.
4. Saying the activity creates its own rewards is not to say it is always rewarding. In fact, it can be painful and frustrating, especially if the couple does not get lost in the activity, and even when they do, the dance is not always graceful and happy.
5. Apparently that is not much of a compromise in the world's few remaining foraging societies. At least there the nature of women's work allows breastfeeding that is close to what biomedicine now finds optimal. Our fall from grace would thus seem to date from how agriculture changed women's work and human diets.

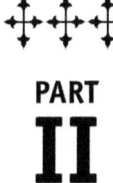

PART
II

Contexts

To meet the Challenges (Part I) of understanding and enabling nurture, we need to see humankind in the evolutionary, developmental, and commensal contexts that make us who we are. To that end, Chapter 3 shows how human phylogeny and ontogeny revolve around the way nurture unfolds bioculturally. Chapter 4 then shows how infants are drawn into culturally constituted commensal circles, with their foundations in the experience of breastfeeding. We explore nurturing others as part of the commensal core of humanity, and illustrate this using a life-cycle approach that begins with conception and ends at death.

II

Contexts

CHAPTER 3

Tracing the Human Story

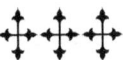

> *We learn to be human at our mother's breast.*
> —Ashley Montague

We no longer tell the human story as a grand Cartesian epic. There has been a historical shift away from dualistic approaches towards more integrated approaches to understanding the human condition, particularly in anthropology (cf. Fuentes 2015, 2016; Ingold and Palsson 2013; Parkin and Ulijaszek 2007). Lately two new fields, epigenetics and neuroscience, suggest a biocultural middle ground. We know epigenetics can adapt the phenotype to its surroundings and we also know breastfeeding is an interface with the wider world, starting with the mother's body that echoes her surroundings. Given the close, multi-channel communication between the mother's and the infant's body, it is not surprising that lactation became a tool of adaptation that made the most of the plasticity of human infants. The other field, neuroscience, shows how brain, mind, and culture are mutually constitutive, giving infants the opportunity to "learn to be human while their brains are experiencing growth" (Trevathan and Rosenberg 2016: 1). This vastly expands the significance of early infant care in the evolution of our species (cf. Hrdy 1999, 2009; Narvaez et al. 2014; Trevathan and Rosenberg 2016).

In this human story, where each person is a unique biocultural hybrid, our early upbringing gives us a constitution that shapes our lives ever after. That discovery, together with the growing evidence of infant plasticity, puts nurturing practices at center stage. Now two great dramas—how humans evolved and the way newborns develop into adults—turn on early infant care. Where the last chapter described how that was so empirically, this one explains why it is so historically, through the large history of human evolution as well as the little history of each lifetime.

Our chapter tells the human story as a biocultural tale where one generation's nurturing bids the next to nurture as they were nurtured. As parents we nurture our children because our parents nurtured us. That is how the life cycle turns. Many premodern cultures phrase that impetus as a moral debt—which it is—but we would add that it is also a biocultural imperative that lives in the individual as well as the group. To Cartesians, the link between generations was biological or cultural. While human nurturing is not simply genetic, that does not make all the rest cultural. If we focus on the immunological and nutritional properties of human milk, then we find extremely reliable, highly effective, and intricately nuanced processes that are essentially uniform across the species—all biomarkers of genetic adaptations that natural selection perfected over millions of years (cf. Quinn 2016). Breastfeeding's extraordinary immunological capacities date back twelve million years and its remarkable nutritional refinements, to seven million years (Sellen 2007).

On the other hand, if we look at the mother–infant relationship, it is a very different story. Anything but uniform, that relationship varies widely culture to culture, couple to couple, even day to day. Although we would not slight the cultural sources of nurturing, the strongest link between generations is biocultural. All humans develop a constitution shaped by their early child care. Humans, we would say, carry nurturing practices in the biocultural character of their bodies. The dance of nurture is where a mother and her supporters, in a long line of mothers and their supporters, work out the infant care practices that connect bodies across generations. To survive infancy, every human is constituted out of the caring of others. As a species, our capacity for culture grew from how local caring customs kept biologically immature newborns alive until, as adults, they can care for the next generation of infants. In that sense, all humans are biocultural hybrids genetically as well as developmentally, by phylogeny (how our species evolved) as well as ontogeny (how each individual matures).

Nurture as Biocultural Imperative

Strictly cultural or strictly biological models of infant feeding, care, and nurture have not been effective. In *Breastfeeding: Biocultural Perspectives* (Stuart-Macadam and Dettwyler 1995), Stuart-Macadam explains the biocultural perspective as "a cross-cultural and evolutionary perspective that acknowledges that there are both biological and cultural components to human behavior" (1995: 1). In this landmark volume, the authors treat bioculturalism broadly and avoid pitting strictly cultural models against exclusively biological ones. Most research on infant feeding focuses on either the biological or the cultural aspects, most often ignoring the biological in the biocultural (or the cultural in the biocultural). But that does not mean we should consider breastfeeding to be culturally constructed: "to fall into an unbounded cultural determinism represents a problematic advance from biological determinism" (Blum 1993: 297). The biological and cultural bits interact all the time; they cannot be separated because they are interdependent and determine each other. When we try to separate them, culture is no longer a factor; neither is biology. The separation between biological and cultural anthropology into mutually uncommunicative subfields without any shared overarching frameworks for understanding the human condition makes the search for holism difficult and suspect to contemporary anthropologists, and makes it impossible to explain biocultural hybrids like breastfeeding (cf. Ingold and Palsson 2013). Fuentes (2015, 2016) calls for an expanded toolkit to address what he calls integrated anthropology, and we call the new ethnology.

Walter Goldschmidt (1990, 2006) argues that affect hunger motivates humans to engage in social life. We agree. An infant constituted out of the caring of others, comes to care about others and to find pleasure in living with others. However, our approach to biocultural processes differs from his. His model defines the transformation of a biologically programmed neonate into a culturally programmed adult, from a genetically programmed biological entity into a socially programmed symbolic entity (1990). For him, first we are biological, and then by age three or so, we become enculturated and become cultural, symbolic beings. Fuentes (2013: 44) points out that this approach is still common among Darwinians and evolutionary psychologists. Like him, we stress the unfolding of nurture as a biocultural process that begins before birth. In this view, biology and culture interweave to create a biocultural hybrid that then takes on a life of its own—not either/or, but both/and. Hybrids are neither biological nor cultural, but simultaneously both. Our biocultural approach, like Fuentes' human niche (2016), explores how and why the pieces fit together.

As Geertz argues, the way to understand the relation between the biological and the cultural is

> not through arranging them into some sort of chain-of-being hierarchy stretching from the physical and biological to the social and semiotic, each level emergent from and dependent upon (and with luck, reducible to) the one beneath it. Nor is it through treating them as discontinuous, sovereign realities, enclosed, stand-alone domains externally connected ("interfaced," as the jargon has it) to one another by vague and adventitious forces, factors, quantities and causes. Constitutive of one another, reciprocally constructive, they must be treated as such—as complements, not levels; aspects, not entities; landscapes, not realms. (2000: 206)

Weak vs Strong Bioculturalism

For our purposes, we need to distinguish "weak" from "strong" bioculturalism. The weak version takes an ecumenical attitude toward scholarly disciplines. It recognizes the importance of both biology and culture yet treats them as separable; a biologist might study one and the cultural anthropologist the other, each in isolation. For example, consider oxytocin, a pleasure-giving hormone released in lactation as well as lovemaking (Uvnes-Moberg 2005). To biological reductionists, the hormone is the cause, and the effects can be studied in activities like breastfeeding. A biological exlanation might still acknowledge cultural triggers in its release. Yet bioculturalists recognize how onetime effects can later loop into causes. That aptly characterizes how breastfeeding's hormone-driven beginning meets the mother's bioculturally constituted body. Yet over time breastfeeding develops into an oxytocin-releasing relationship that comes to control both bodies. Here bioculturalism rejects the doctrinaire attitude that the explanation is *either* biochemical *or* cultural. To the contrary, it specifically allows for how the two can interact (cf. Fuentes 2015, 2016).

Or take the infant's immune system. Incomplete at birth, any child who survives eventually develops a complete immune system. That happens regardless of how the infant is fed Biology can explain the general character of every immune system. Yet suppose we want to know the specific character of one system? That differs person to person, even for identical twins. Indeed, each person's actual immune system reflects the chance particulars of early infancy. So happenstance gives one infant the flu, leaves a luckier one unexposed, and bolsters a third through antibodies in mother's milk. In the end, each child's immune system is a one-of-a-kind hybrid that integrates the regularities of biology and culture with the ecological landscape (cf. Fuentes 2016; Quinn 2016).

Two features distinguish strong bioculturalism. First, biological and cultural realities lose any prior separateness to function as a hybrid with a life of its own. Granted, one might still distinguish "biological" from "cultural" components, at least for analytical reasons, but in actuality feedback loops wrap "cause" into "effect." In that dynamic, where biology shapes culture and vice versa, an emergent system arises, coming to function as a whole that remakes the parts that first made it. What results is not, then, the simple sum of independent parts (what weak bioculturalism describes) but an organic whole born of the synergy of its newly interdependent parts.

Second, any strongly bicultural system has a one-of-a-kind character that must be understood in its own terms. It is a unique organic whole quite unlike a recurring mechanical composite. To be sure, that uniqueness is not always relevant. One might, for example, rightly recognize the uniqueness of each breastfeeding relationship yet still treat that truth as a human generality. Or one might legitimately background how breastfeeding varies person to person to play up biological or cultural commonalities. What breastfeeding actually does is create a particular human out of a long line of particular humans. These particularities are reflected in customs that are passed down and accumulate over generations. That is a truth we call the human story. It is a tale where breastfeeding becomes the mother-to-child link that makes this human chain and directs infant development adaptively. The maternal body buffers infant nutrition "while maintaining active intergenerational signaling through milk" (Quinn 2016: 106).

An adequate analysis of breastfeeding moves between weak and strong bioculturalism. Take a nervous first time mother whose disapproving father-in-law has her breastfeeding in the bathroom. When she does not let down, we might trace the problem to three interacting systems: her biology, the surrounding culture, and her constitution—a bioculturally created reality that mediates between the other two. Breastfeeding might go better or worse the next time around with the next child. In our analysis, we emphasize strong bioculturalism because it is the least studied and thus has the most to add to the discussion. Where weak bioculturalism is just the sum of its parts, the strong version creates an indivisible whole that is more than the sum of its parts.

The Breastfeeding Complex

The breastfeeding complex has web-like characteristics. To a Darwinian, the web has a biological core (lactation) surrounded by cultural realities. That framing gives a useful overview. It does, however, forget that our bodies live in history and it lives in us. After all, when no woman reaches her childbearing years until she has built a biocultural body first, that past enters how she bears, births, and cares for her child. One cannot then fully separate a tidy biological core from its messy lived-in surroundings. Fuentes's (2015, 2016) evolutionary approach to niche construction, proposes a synthesis of ecological, biological, and social landscapes. Stepping back an eon or two, lactation was well-established long before our species arose. This is our mammalian heritage. Now, however, this highly evolved biology must live with and within humankind's cultural and biocultural landscapes of history. In this, the biggest picture, the breastfeeding complex is where history meets biology.

The breastfeeding complex is a busy crossroads as well as an intimate school. As a crossroads, it is a place where history and genetics meet and send an infant down one developmental path or another. As a school, the web cues infants' bodily systems about the surroundings that await them. Here, by mediating those lessons through the mother's well-schooled bioculturally constituted body, the breastfed infant is entrained in time-tested adaptations. There, like it or not, mother and baby live in these historically created niches.

For well over a century, the central question of early infant care has been how breastfeeding and bottle feeding differ in their consequences. In recent decades, epidemiology has shown that, across a range of health indices, breastfed babies fare better than their formula-fed peers, including reductions in the incidence of type 2 diabetes, obesity, high blood pressure, and high cholesterol, for example (Rollins 2016; Victora et al. 2016; Quinn 2016). But the mechanisms are not always clear or simple to epidemiologists who need to be precise about correlations; causality is more difficult to establish. We know the inputs (human milk or infant formula) and the outputs (the measurable health differences) but not the causal links. We need to know causes, not just correlations. We may never know causation precisely - not without unethical experiments; but we can make better use of what we already know with better theories.

Current knowledge of infant development has moved past the model of "biology first, the rest later" that assumed wired-in biology determined human fundamentals (cf. Narvaez et al. 2014; Trevathan and Rosenberg 2016; Fuentes 2015, 2016). A biocultural model fits the currently known facts. It sees breastfeeding as shaping and not just sustaining the infant's development. Instead of only delivering raw material as commercial formula does, a biocultural model demonstrates how breastfeeding regulates the infant's growth adaptively. By this theory, breastfeeding is one of life's master choreographers. To test that out we look at human milk.

Is Milk Substance or System?

A little over a century ago, once health statistics showed substituting cow for human milk was killing babies, physicians scrambled to develop a healthier substitute (Wolf 2001; Apple 1987). Well-intentioned as they were, the mechanistic thinking of the day supposed human milk was a substance that a good chemist could duplicate—scientists just needed the right formula. That name stuck, giving a scientific aura to a long line of breastmilk substitutes.

Were milk composition uniform and preprogrammed, it would not have the flexibility to respond to the environment of the mother–infant dyad. But since human milk is integral to a larger adaptive system, then it should always be in flux; milk is the medium adjusting mother and a growing baby to each other and their ever-changing surroundings. For example, docosahexaenoic acid (DHA, an omega-3 fatty acid vital for brain and neural development) is highly variable within as well as across human populations (Milligan 2013: 225). In the Gambia the concentration of fat is highest in the early morning while that is when it is lowest for Euro-American women (Prentice 1996: 309). In spite of this variability, infant formula companies have manufactured and added DHA made from genetically altered marine algae and soil fungi (Minchin 2015: 116), but there is no evidence that the addition of DHA improves outcomes for formula fed infants (Cochrane Summaries 2009). Milk composition even differs according to the sex of the infant (Powe et al. 2010). Seasonality, maternal age and parity, and maternal diet also have an influence on milk composition. Not surprisingly then, even within the same community, milk composition and volume varies between mothers (Prentice 1996: 310; Quinn 2016). Human milk is never standardized but always personalized.

Output also varies. Australian mothers produce more milk than American mothers, and a mother of twins can produce more than double the average output of a one-baby mother (Riordan and Auerbach 1993: 107). A mother's right and left breasts may differ in milk production, perhaps because infants show "breastedness" in favoring one over the other (Hartmann et al. 1996: 304). Differences also exist in the rate of milk synthesis and the initial level of milk production (Hartmann et al. 1996: 317). Milk yield varies much more than milk energy density; it is the volume of milk and its energetic density (kilocalories per gram) that influences infant growth rates. The variation in milk synthesis among individual mothers is not trivial because it affects infant activity patterns (Hinde 2013: 189, 190) and regulates infant growth and development (Quinn 2016).

What explains all this variability? It is unlikely to be incidental, not considering the ancient evolutionary history of mammalian milk. It is far more likely that the variance shows milk doing its adaptive work. And indeed that is what the calibration process suggests. Although a demand-fed baby consumes "irregular quantities at irregular intervals" (Hartmann et al. 1996: 298), and so infant appetite has an apparent randomness, "the interplay between the mother and her infant" still manages to set "the broad limits on milk output ... to match the baby's needs" (Woolridge 1996: 317). Even the nutritional status of the mother does not affect the milk volume unless she is severely malnourished (Riordan and Auerbach 1993: 107).

This calibration occurring a few weeks after birth is part of the fine tuning that improves the fit between mother and infant, which is full of potential challenges. Both parties must learn bodily skills (handling, positioning, latching on, etc.) that dovetail with each other even as each is changing. Once on the breastfeeding path or trajectory, there are still potential problems to solve. For example, early top-up bottles may so upset this process of calibration and coregulation that the process of declining milk production may become irreversible (Prentice 1996: 317). It is a delicate dance, this dance of nurture. Dancing well together takes time and effort that pays rich rewards. It puts two bodies in sync with each other. And that, in turn, does not just strengthen their relationship. It makes the bodily lessons mother teaches all the more sensible and engaging for the baby. All these outward connections and far-reaching consequences make milk more than just a product. Milk, it would seem, is the material medium of a system that evolved around aligning mother and baby with each other and with their surroundings.

Filling in Fundamentals

How else does breastfeeding choreograph infant development? Milk is relatively easy to discuss because we can get it into the lab and under a microscope. For that reason, milk is the best studied facet of breastfeeding where the accumulated knowledge allows the greatest rigor. We consider other facets under separate headings; in fact, these are interlocking and overlapping processes. We begin with how breastfeeding sustains baby until the newborn's bodily systems are mature enough to function on their own.

All infants are born long before their bodily systems can keep them alive. Here breastfeeding fills in until the infant's own systems are mature enough to handle their tasks. First, as infants cannot digest solid food, they need a liquid nutrient. Breastmilk is the perfect food as it almost certainly coevolved with the newborn's digestive system. Second, an infant needs to be hydrated, but everyday sources of water can contain pathogens or parasites. Here the mother's body purifies the water that makes up 87 percent of breastmilk and, by producing about 850 ml a day, provides all the water a baby needs. Dilute high-water milks are adaptive in dry environments (Quinn 2016: 100); this reinforces the research that confirmed that breastfed infants have no need for extra water to keep hydrated (Almroth 1978).

Third, to meet the newborn's immunological needs, breastfeeding delivers unique antimicrobial, anti-inflammatory, immunoregulatory agents and living leukocytes through human milk and colostrum. Goldman (2012) argues that human milk evolved to compensate for the delay in the development of the newborn's immune system. That said, more than just filling in, it would seem mother's immune responses act as a tutor or template for an infant's developing immune system. Arguably the tutoring involves timing: when an immune system reacts too soon, the person can develop allergies that mistake one's self for an intruder. Here breastfeeding, rather than keeping the body pure, keeps the body negotiating self-other boundaries that divide mother from baby.

Fourth, breastfeeding keeps baby alive until its brain functions develop the capacity to awaken from a deep sleep. In most cultures, this is ensured by the custom of having baby sleep next to mother, a process McKenna and Gettler (2016) call breastsleeping. As mothers do not habituate to their cosleeping babies but remain semi-alert and responsive to their needs, breastfeeding episodes happen regularly (McKenna and Gettler 2007: 149). Given the "intertwined physiology of the sleeping human mother–infant dyad" (McKenna and Gettler 2007: 135), close body contact regulates infant respiration, muscle tension, acid-base balance, and temperature (Geddes et al. 2008). McKenna and Gettler (2007) argue that the cosleeping mother's carbon dioxide acts as a respiratory stimulant that decreases the infant's deep sleep, reducing the chances of sudden infant death syndrome (SIDS) as the newborn learns to breathe while sleeping. We began this book by contesting how today's ever-current crisis hides life's everyday nurturing. We now do the same for the past.

Breastfeeding and Human Evolution

Where does infant feeding fit in human evolution? As the biological anthropologists report (Hrdy 1999, 2009; Narvaez et al. 2014; Trevathan and Rosenberg 2016), breastfeeding has never stood static and alone, but is integral to how our species evolved, anatomically and socially. Nurturing is critical to how our primate ancestors evolved into humans. It deepens the individual's capacity to live in groups and strengthens the group's capacity to pass down successful practices as customs.

How did nurturing exert such leverage on human evolution? It was a uniquely malleable link in how our species evolved into the group-guided symbol-makers we are today. That epochal change rests on how sociality, plasticity, and neoteny all coevolved. Any increase in one fed an increase in the others. Over time, that had humans birthing ever more premature babies (neoteny) whose ever greater plasticity gave the sociality developed in and required by early infant care an ever greater influence on human development. To understand each feature better, we consider sociality, plasticity, and neoteny separately, although they are all interdependent.

Expanding Sociality

Humans are a successful species because, as highly evolved social primates, they are attuned to each other, and respond to each other. Our adaptive strategy requires living in groups to raise our immature young, protect them and ourselves from injury, enjoy life, and survive injury and illness. Humans evolved sympathetic and moral capacities that support group life. Cooperation is an important part of the human tool kit (cf. Fuentes 2014). Primates also get and give pleasure through grooming, a process dependent on sociality (Montague 1971; Goldschmidt 1990: 86). All primate groups do better if they cooperate and share.

Well-functioning humans have sympathy for others. We wince at another's pain, and smile at newborns. This feeling of human empathy is absent or suppressed in sociopaths, but we recognize sociopaths as deviant by labeling them inhuman, lacking in human feelings; even sociopaths are defined by reference to an underlying human capacity for empathy.

Sociality is not unique to humans—chimps, bonobos, and gorillas are also highly social primates (King and Shanker 2003). In primates, serotonin inhibits aggressive behavior and is high in socially attuned monkeys and low in noncooperative ones (Damasio 1994: 76–77; Gettler 2016). Feeding others—particularly the very young and the very old—is the most basic form of primate cooperation. Bonobos, unlike chimpanzees, share their food even with strangers, as long as the strangers interact with them (Tan and Hare 2013).

Humans are all born into custom-carrying groups, and remain in these groups for a long period of socialization. Like other primates, humans can also change groups, change customs, and adapt to new surroundings, although such changes can cause stress. Groups are smarter, stronger, more diversely talented, and, thanks to inherited knowledge, cumulatively smarter than any individual can ever be. We learn from the experience of the group, not just from our own experiences. Interaction with others is the primary, fundamental embodiment of sociality, the "primordial site of sociality" (Schegloff 2006). The longer and more open the nurturing process, the better a species can adapt to changing conditions.

Judging by what we share with our closest evolutionary cousins, our social nature dates back five million years or more (Ward 2003). Favored by natural selection (Silk 2002: 21), our sociality is "as much a product of evolution as is [our] ... bipedal posture and a larger brain" (Zihlman and Bolter 2004: 23). Indeed, it is so vital to our survival as a species and well-being as individuals that we might expect natural selection to have wired-in sociality as it did with social insects. We know, for example, that the offspring of more sociable female baboons are more likely to survive the first year of life than those born to less sociable females (Hinde 2013: 192). Yet if all primates have a built-in capacity for sociality, the form of the sociality that actually develops is not built in. Certainly sociality's salience and style differs widely across cultures as well as within groups where individuals range from gregarious to antisocial and everywhere between. That suggests sociality is culturally cued and bioculturally built one baby at a time.

What ensures the sociality our species needs to survive? Early infant care; all neonates are so biologically immature, so incapable of survival alone, that everyone who lives to reproduce has experienced intensely social caring at the very time that their biology is establishing parameters and patterns that will last a lifetime. Human ontogeny thus ensures the sociality that individual well-being requires (cf. Trevathan and Rosenberg 2016).

Breastfeeding develops an infant's social sensibility through two channels. One is interactive: to breastfeed, mother and infant must develop a give-and-take relationship that can change as they and their surroundings do. Arguably that develops a social sensibility that the infant needs in order to become a full member of an ever-changing society. The other channel is close bodily contact: to work with mother, an infant learns to read her body in order to better understand their intimate world (Chodorow 1999: 161). Through hormones in human milk, breastfeeding makes this reading easier and surer (Quinn 2016). Moreover, as the brain takes the body as a template of the world (Damasio 1994), mapping mother's body on one's own could develop the representational capacity that learning culture later requires. Of course enriching sociality is possible only if the infant's development is not already rigidly preprogrammed by instincts but is open to being shaped by its surroundings. That openness is plasticity.

Growing Plasticity

All humans are born long before their bodies are ready for postnatal life. Every infant arrives as a package of loosely coordinated and poorly differentiated bodily systems (Trevathan and Rosenberg 2016). Over the ensuing months and years, this raw material inevitably develops the specificities that set each of us on our life course. The more plastic this life stage is, the greater scope the environment has in shaping who we become. Although a person's genes are set at conception, the chemical processes of epigenetics can decide how some genes are expressed.

While this shaping begins in the womb (Nunez-de la Mora and Bentley 2008: 159), birth opens the floodgates. In the following months, a biologically ordered series of developmental windows open only to close. Although biology schedules the openings and sets their parameters, the environment cues the final outcome. In these prime moments, breastfeeding becomes a busy school whose lessons come through multiple channels (biochemically through the mother's milk; tactilely through skin-to-skin contact; behaviorally at the breast; analogically by mirroring caregivers). That opens the possibility for complex and nuanced environmental feedback. In any case, the infant's bodily systems mature largely following the biological clock. So the window opens and closes whether that educational moment is nurturing or harsh, finished or sketchy, adaptive or dysfunctional.

Neoteny and Its Causes

Once culture became our preeminent adaptation, larger brains became more advantageous. Since mature skull size increases in our evolutionary line, but size at birth remains relatively fixed (Dunsworth and Eccleson 2015), we can infer a selective advantage for mothers and groups whose sociality equips them to nurture these radically immature offspring as well as help mothers to recover from childbirth. In this loop, a larger brain supported a more complex culture and, as culture grew more complex, it called for an ever larger brain. That created what Washburn (1960) called the obstetrical dilemma: advantageous as a larger brain might have been, birthing large-headed babies endangered the mother. The timing of birth would be a tradeoff between neonatal and maternal mortality. The obstetrical hypothesis supposed adopting upright posture made a woman's hips a compromise between easy walking and difficult childbirth. That is now questioned, and recent research, following life history theory, proposes that individuals have a finite amount of energy that can be spent on either growth or reproduction, leading to a trade-off between fecundity and survival to maturity (Milligan 2013: 209). The tradeoff, Dunsworth and Eccleson (2015) propose, is between minimizing maternal cost of gestation and maximizing fetal growth to reduce infant mortality.

Whether the timing is set by the birth canal or energetics, the more immature an infant was at birth, the smaller the head would be but the less likely the newborn would survive. However, more sociality-inspired caring meant that more mothers and infants could survive the trauma of birth; and the more cultural our ancestors became, the more knowledgeable, skilled, and effective their caring would be. By providing reliable and extensive postpartum care, groups could increase the survival of both women and infants. This biocultural adaptation was so effective and reliable that human biology changed: our species has evolved so that what we call a full-term baby is actually born six-months premature, and fully 75 percent of brain growth occurs outside the womb (Trevanthan, Smith, and McKenna 2008: 26). In sum, our biological adaptation (premature birth) depends on a cultural practice (caring for the new mother and infant) that requires a social sensibility (caring for others) that the adaptation itself furthers. The more immature the birth, the more completely the individual is constituted out of the caring work of others.

Human infants are born with their neural, digestive, and muscular systems so unformed that they will be completed with—and thereby incorporate—their social surroundings. It is in this sense that every human is a biocultural hybrid, a being whose biology comes to function culturally. Here the loop wherein an earlier birth allowed an ever larger brain has a further payoff in birthing ever more plastic neonates whose early experience embodies a social world that they then support once grown. It is these multiple feedback loops that explain how humans developed the cultural and social capacities that set us apart from our nearest primate relatives.

Breastfeeding's Changing Practice

The more the coevolution we have just described hinged on sociality, the more important it became for newborns to be able to establish a relationship with their mothers. To be sure, lactation is an incredibly strong and stable process. Yet this one sure link interlocks with three tenuous ones: (1) mother and infant must develop a relationship that overcomes breastfeeding's ups and downs; (2) both parties must master the mechanics of breastfeeding; and, taken together, (3) the two prior steps must assert enough control over lactation that its biological processes become relatively independent of disruptive events (sickness, a marital dispute, etc.) that could otherwise impede breastfeeding. That is a tall order, particularly in the case of traumatic births.

Getting those three tenuous links to hold and interlock carries life-or-death weight. After all, until recently, babies died when breastfeeding failed. Given that selective pressure on human milk, we might have expected breastfeeding to be more instinctual. Yet it is not; mother and infant stumble along. At birth, mothers do not immediately and reliably bond with their offspring (Hrdy 2009). Each new mother must learn how to breastfeed an infant whose halting moves appear to favor dorsal feeding (Coloson et al. 2008) even though our ancestors adopted upright posture millions of years ago. Moreover, because women lactate as social creatures rather than automatic milk machines, the milk may not flow unless mother gets skilled help in supportive surroundings. Given those potential challenges, not every newborn or first-time mother can breastfeed successfully on their own without reliable and skilled help.

All mammals lactate, yet what sets lactation among social primates including humans apart from all other mammals is its vulnerability to failure. While some mother–infant pairs are resilient, others are easily stressed by abuse, neglect, hunger, and disruption of early attachment (Kinnally 2013: 156). We are just beginning to learn about the mechanism, causes, and consequences of variation in milk synthesis, and available milk energy and milk production in primates (Hinde and Capitanio 2010). The mechanisms underlying delayed onset of lactation, lactation failure, and low milk production in humans are poorly defined in part because such deficiencies are rarely investigated due to the ready availability of infant formula (Neville et al. 2012: 178), and the false assumption that it is roughly equivalent to human milk.

How has humankind arranged the help that new mothers need? The answer, Holman and Grimes (2003: 777) conclude, is culture: learned "maternal behavior in the immediate postpartum period has been successfully and continuously transmitted by cultural mechanisms over the course of human evolution." Our species could not have survived unless human behavior completed biology's breastfeeding script. Fuentes's human niche reinforces this point, stressing the important synthesis of ecological, biological, and social landscapes (2015: 305). The social womb passes nurturing practices from mother-to-child across the generations. That happens one bioculturally-constituted body at a time. Such nurturing is not—or not just—instinctual. We nurture as adults because we were nurtured as infants. And if we nurture as we were nurtured, then behavioral practices can become traditions that are passed down viscerally as unconscious embodied processes. What we call the social womb relies heavily on human sociality to provide the social support and cultural knowledge that breastfeeding requires. Our species survived the dilemma of the high cost of intensive infant care by competent caregivers through the transmission of these postpartum customs. Although the need for intensive infant care is costly for individuals and groups, it has been and remains effective, as Trevanthan, Rosenberg, and their colleagues demonstrate in *Costly and Cute* (2016). That is obvious today, when modern medicine keeps premature infants alive. But some solutions such as the social womb could date from the origins of humankind (Holman and Grimes 2003: 777). The traditions associated with the social womb would appear in all cultures by inheritance from our human beginnings. Over time they might diversify historically (as the social womb has), but whenever this behavioral adaptation fails, the immunological and nutritional benefits of lactation would be lost. It is this custom-dependent biology that has let our species adapt with a speed and over a range that genes cannot directly explain. In short, humans breastfeed by custom not by instinct.

If breastfeeding were instinctual, generations of mothers and newborns would not have to face the complex learning involved in breastfeeding and the risk of problems such as insufficient milk. That would have discouraged the development of the intense mother–infant relationship that mediates varied social and cultural realities, and simultaneously helps develop social capacity in infants. Instead, human infants have the plasticity necessary to adapt to changing social and ecological conditions.

Breastfeeding as a process is extremely sensitive to social and cultural context and to situation. Life intervenes with contingencies such as a grandfather's funeral (a dangerous place for Thai babies), the death of a mother in childbirth, an HIV-positive mother, a jealous sibling, a rigid work schedule, or an unplanned pregnancy. This interdependence between mothers and newborns makes new mothers vulnerable to some extent, but it leaves them open to absorbing information from their own infants and from others, particularly their mothers and grandmothers (and from health practitioners and baby milk companies' marketing materials and promotional practices). Without support, breastfeeding can falter for individual mother–infant pairs for cultural and emotional reasons. Yet, as we consider in Chapter 7, most breastfeeding policies and programs act as if the primary problem is to convince women that "breast is best" or to intervene to increase milk production.

Primate Lessons

Is there evidence for the capacity to nurture in our closest mammalian relatives, the other social primates? Biological anthropologists (Sellen 2007; Clancy, Hinde, and Rutherford 2013) have explored what primates can tell us about human lactation. Compared with other mammals, the length of lactation in primates is relatively long, and primate milk is relatively lower in volume; more dilute; lower in energy, fat, and protein; and higher in lactose. Humans wean earlier than other primates and have low postnatal growth rates and short birth intervals. This pattern of feeding a low-solute milk is consistent with constant carrying and suckling (Sellen 2007: 126). Compared with other primates, humans have slow maturation rates, long lifespans with slow aging, and postmenopausal longevity (Sellen 2007: 128). In addition to providing nutrients, the function of lactation in mammals is the transfer of the protective function of the fully developed immune system across the generations (Sellen 2007: 125).

Nonhuman primates, and indeed all mammals in the wild, have no alternatives to species-specific maternal milk for keeping their newborns alive. If a mother dies, the infant dies. An orphan primate who survives a mother's death will be marginalized, because both care and status depend on the mother. Humans are the only primates whose offspring can survive to adulthood even when they have not received any maternal milk (Sellen 2006: 186), a dubious honor. Humans are also the only primates that might have the opportunity or responsibility to have multiple juvenile dependents to care for at the same time (other than multiple births). This places a great strain on mothers. These two facts are interconnected, and have shaped the human niche for child care and nurture.

Lactation puts a metabolic strain on all mothers; primate females adapt to this by increasing their intake of high energy foods and spending more time foraging (Sellen 2007: 128). Maternal fat subsidizes human lactation. By providing their infants with complementary foods, including pre-chewed foods, mothers—both humans and other primates—can reduce the nutritional strain of lactation and keep infants alive before the young are able to feed independently. Some primate parents continue to provision juveniles after weaning (Sellen 2007: 126). Human infants cannot make efficient use of nonmilk foods before six months of age, and may suffer nutritional deficits and morbidity if they are fed earlier. Consequently, humans must actively feed their toddlers rather than encourage independent foraging as in other primate groups. "Humans are the only primates that wean juveniles before they can forage independently" (Sellen 2007: 131).

With humans, the accumulated knowledge about the interactive dimensions of breastfeeding persists through traditions that develop historically in groups. These interactive dimensions of breastfeeding, with their proclivity for ritual, helped to transform us into more social beings. In the short term, the fact that breastfeeding must be learned and is vulnerable may have contributed to many infant deaths throughout history. In the long term, breastfeeding's vulnerability is an intrinsic part of human adaptation.

Social and ethical conventions in addition to biological controls shape instinctive behavior and adapt it to changing environments (Damasio 1994: 124). Alone among the social primates, the ancestors of modern humans fully developed the capacity for culture as a means of adapting to the environment. Humans live in such diverse and unpredictable environments that they must rely on cultural survival strategies (Damasio 1994: 123). An added advantage, of course, is that cultural change occurs very quickly while genetically based biological change occurs at a slower pace. As our capacity for culture increased, individuals developed the ability to not just live in the world but to represent that world and share those representations with others. Arguably that developed out of ritual, and certainly it is closely connected to the emergence of language. Ritual and language set the stage for breastfeeding's contribution to person-making.

Person-Making and the Biocultural Individual

Person-making is a human universal, but it must be explained socially, not genetically. To survive, every human infant receives food and care from another human. That universal creates two social conditions. One is interaction. Here the infant plays a role with people who treat him or her as a person-to-be. The other is that the caring puts the infant in bodily contact with caregivers whose bodies move in purposeful ways that the infant feels and often follows. Here, as the human body serves as a template for the world, the infant enters a world of purposeful action. Every infant has access to biochemical and tactile models of how mothers manage to perform these functions. The lactating body acts as a cultural template (Cowley, Moodley, and Fiori-Cowley 2004: 109) for interacting with the world and lets the infant profit from past experience. While this begins in the womb, with the infant adjusting to the mother's sleep, waking, and dietary patterns, it continues after birth as the mother's body mediates cultural patterns that create a template on which the infant maps its ever-widening world. One inevitable consequence of the social womb is that every human becomes a unique biocultural hybrid with its own unique constitution. The group, as well as the individual, reaps great rewards because neonates, being so pliable, get shaped to fit their surroundings.

Just as no industrial product can replace breastmilk, nothing can fully replace breastfeeding when it comes to constituting the baby as a social being. Here, quite apart from how cultures differ, all humans face two critical developmental tasks. One is to awaken a desire for, and pleasure in, social life, including what Goldschmidt calls affect hunger. The other is to develop the social and ritual sensibility it takes to participate in social life everywhere in the world. Because these two traits appear across cultures and in all well-functioning people, one might explain their universality biologically. In spite of the need and capacity for social life among social primates, including humans, there is great variability within groups. Take a person's social sensibility—the intuitive capacity to understand what is going on with others. In any given group, some individuals are gifted and graceful, others slow and mechanistic, and still others in between. As these differences are apparent from early childhood, the simple explanation for such variety within universality is biocultural: every newborn has a biological capacity that gets awakened and shaped by early caregiving, becoming a foundation for later life. This is a biocultural universal, because all infants who survive have been nurtured; and yet it is variable because caregivers differ and so too does the infant-caregiver relationship. Here, until recent times, that relationship was established and structured through breastfeeding.

Although each culture defines personhood its own way (Geertz 2000), this sensibility is learned, we would argue, in the social womb where it arises from the relationship between the infant and one or a few caregivers who themselves embody their culture. How does this learning unfold? At birth the infant is not yet a person. All he or she has is a small repertoire of primitive responses, not enough to sustain a relationship, much less function as a person. Breastfeeding begins the interaction that eventually turns the neonate into a social being who, by getting treated as a person, becomes one. Or to be more precise, by being treated as a particular kind of person—a Lao, Zuni, or Chinese—becomes one. Whereas other biocultural processes adapt the infant to his or her immediate surroundings of the moment, becoming a culturally defined person also adapts a person for the future. As the infant begins to function as a person in relation to others, he or she has to develop the social, emotional, and ritual sensibility it takes to function in the ever-changing world of social groups.

Infant Development: From Coregulation to Self-Regulation

Another line of evidence comes from ontogeny, the development of the individual. Human infants develop bioculturally much as our species evolved bioculturally. Here we place breastfeeding in the context of the development of the mother–infant dyad where the local environment interacts with maternal and infant constitutions.

Because human infants are born immature and most of their critical cognitive development takes place after birth, they are both more adaptable and more vulnerable than other newborn mammals, including primates. The immaturity and plasticity of the human infant ensures the infant's sensitivity to social life. Breastfeeding mediates and encourages this coregulation between mothers and infants. In addition to providing unique antimicrobial, anti-inflammatory, immunoregulatory agents and living leukocytes through mother's milk, mother's immune system is itself a model or template for her infant's immune system. As we argued earlier, the close body contact required by breastfeeding regulates infant respiration, muscle tension, acid-base balance, and temperature.

Breastfeeding also influences facial and oral development. Palmer (2012) argues that breastfeeding for at least one year is critical for the proper development of the oral cavity, airway, and facial form. The palate takes shape early in life, orchestrated by the muscles used in breastfeeding, which differ from those used in bottle feeding. The different mechanisms of milk removal between bottle feeding and breastfeeding involve the integration of sucking, swallowing, and breathing.

Breastfeeding develops the peristaltic, rocker action of the tongue that moves the milk along, and teaches the infant how to breathe through the nose and swallow at the same time, a habit not continued into adult life. The intra-oral vacuum plays a major role in milk removal during breastfeeding (Geddes et al. 2008). Bottle feeding contributes to malocclusion, reduced facial muscle development, abnormal swallowing patterns, caries, and prevalence of nonnutritive sucking of fingers or thumb (Riordan and Auerbach 1993: 476; Geddes et al. 2008).

The World Health Organization (WHO) warns that use of pacifiers also increases the risk of dental abnormalities and ear infections. Psychologists have also explored the social and emotional consequences of pacifier use (Niedenthal et al. 2012). Infants get information on emotional states when they observe and mimic the facial expressions of those around them. This information is impeded by the use of pacifiers, because infants with mouths full of pacifiers cannot resonate with the facial expression of adults.

Another arena of interactive self-other boundaries is the ecology of the gut or microbiome. Recently, many authors have been writing about the importance of the microbial world we live in—the bacteria, viruses, fungi, and other microorganisms and their genes that live in us. Rather than being "at war" with these creatures inside us, we should be treating them with respect because they do things to our bodies that we cannot do for ourselves. Ninety percent of all cells in the human body are not human but bacterial (Martin and Sela 2013: 233). Most live in our intestinal tract with 1,000 trillion microbial cells and 1,000 microbial species. The varieties in the infant gut differ depending whether the infant was breastfed or formula fed, born vaginally or by cesarean section. Gut microbes coevolved with their hosts and facilitate brain–gut communication; they are sensitive to host diet and hygiene (Hinde 2013: 233, 240). Commensal gut bacteria that feed other bacteria also influence neural biological functioning (Hinde 2013: 198). Gut–brain signaling pathways are likely to be particularly sensitive during critical periods of neurodevelopment (Fairbanks and Hinde 2013; Machado 2013) when infants are reliant on mother's milk, becoming behaviorally active and establishing their gut microbiome (Martin and Sela 2013).

Infant gastrointestinal tracts are sterile at birth (Martin and Sela 2013: 244); however, the gut begins to be colonized within a few hours of birth. The infant microbiome goes from near sterility to adult levels of bacteria in three months (Hinde 2013). A newborn's gut ecology is established by the mother and her immediate environment, influenced by the mode of delivery and infant-feeding method. Infant microbiomes are populated either from the living cells in maternal milk or from industrially processed cow's milk or soy milk–based substitutes for breastmilk. Mothers set these initial microbiomes, as the neonate passes through the vaginal canal at birth, picking up appropriate microorganisms along the way. After vaginal delivery, infant guts are colonized by Lactobacillus and Streptococcus (Martin and Sela 2013: 239). Less sanitary conditions during birth and infancy may promote the colonization and growth of beneficial bacteria; home births encourage the growth of different bacteria (Martin and Sela 2013: 245). These bacteria provide the initial signals to activate the infant immune system.

Infants born by cesarean section are colonized by bacteria on the mother's skin rather than from the vaginal canal; infants born by cesarean section have higher rates of asthma and allergies, and are twice as likely to be obese at three years of age. Cesarean sections and hygienic hospital births interfere with the normal transfer of beneficial bacteria from mother to newborn, and transfer different bacteria into a newborn's gut, including Clostridium difficile, Klebsiella, and Enterobacter, environmental bacteria that persist in more sanitary conditions (Martin and Sela 2013: 244).

Since 2002, many different formula companies have added pre- and probiotics to their products in order to try and reproduce the complexity of the microbiome of a breastfed baby. Prebiotics include the Human Milk Oligosaccarides (HMOs), and are not digested by humans, but become food for the beneficial bacteria in the gut. Probiotics include the bifidus factor that supports the group of beneficial lactobacillus bacteria that inhibit the growth of harmful bacteria Although the baby food companies claim that these additives provide protection against digestive diseases and strengthen the infant's immune system, these health claims have not been supported (ESPGHAN 2011). Even company-funded trials show no differences in growth, and there is "insufficient evidence to recommend the addition of probiotics … for the prevention of allergic disease or food reactions" (Cochrane Summaries 2009).

From this initial foundation, our microbiome changes as we age; shifts in microbial composition change rapidly with the introduction of solid food and the end of breastfeeding. In fact, changes in the diet can trigger changes in gut bacteria within a day (David et al. 2014). No two people have the same microbiomes, because what people eat influences their gut ecology. These different diets result in cross-cultural variation in adult microbial profiles. Millions of pluripotent stem cells are ingested with breastmilk; these are used for tissue repair for the infant and the mother. Because only breastmilk, and not infant formula, passes mother's living cells (from her gut to her breasts and her breastmilk) to her newborn through colostrum and mature milk, many adult health conditions could be influenced by infant-feeding regimes, a fact seldom considered in modern research protocols that ignore or underestimate the importance of human milk.

Breastfeeding is the earliest and best example of personalized medicine. Understanding how human milk is personalized and how maternal gut bacteria translocate to the mammary gland to populate the infant gut through breastfeeding are key biocultural questions. For human infants, core constitution begins in utero and is set for life shortly after birth.

Mothers act as filters to mediate between their infants and their environments, beginning when the infants are still in the womb, and long after. Like other mammals, the human fetus uses cues from the uterine environment to monitor the conditions into which it is likely to be born and adjusts itself accordingly (Nunez-de la Mora and Bentley 2008: 159). This accommodation between mother and infant is not about perfecting regulation; it is about continually adjusting to each infant, each day. We are learning how past and present environments influence immunological factors in milk; as Quinn explains, milk memory cells "remember" mothers' and infants' past infections, and provide a rapid antibody-mediated immune response to repeat exposure (2015: 2). Some of this coregulation is accomplished with the assistance of hormones such as oxytocin and prolactin, products that unfold in the development of each infant.

The alignment between mother and infant can also be seen in the way an infant learns about taste, a subject explored further in Chapter 4. As a pregnant women eats, her food flavors the amniotic fluid, creating in the growing fetus a taste for flavors that will reappear in colostrum, breastmilk, and premasticated and other complementary foods. A mother who follows local, ethnic, or familial food customs thus prepares her child for the flavors it will likely encounter.

The relation between breastfeeding and obesity is part of a larger question about appetite control. How does an infant learn to self-regulate? Leptin, a hormone produced in the fat cells, stomach, and placenta, depresses appetite and encourages one to stop eating; leptin passes from mother to infant through breastmilk. After a meal, fat cells release leptin, which acts on the appetite control centers to create a sensation of fullness or satiety (Lieberman 2008: 76–78). Recent human and animal experiments have concluded that leptin is probably a key bioactive component that helps protect against obesity in childhood and adulthood. Leptin from the mother's milk gives moderate protection against excess weight gain in infancy and adulthood (Palou and Pico 2009: 251). Infants born to obese mothers are more likely to develop metabolic syndrome; breastfeeding prevents obesity in those infants who otherwise would have a tendency to those outcomes. The experimental evidence linking obesity and breastfeeding is mixed, even inconsistent, because there are many routes to obesity; breastfeeding advocates do not claim that breastfeeding protects all infants from obesity, only that formula-fed infants are more likely to be overweight (Smith 2007).

Nurturing practices set the stage for the messiness and uncertainty of everyday life, initiating an openness to change and plasticity. Anthropologists (and others) face challenges in conceptualizing this flow between bodies. To understand intersubjective, intercorporeal processes such as breastfeeding, we need to figure out how to theorize thinking and working across bodies in a scholarly landscape that works from the assumption of an autonomous individual body, a challenge for both biological and cultural anthropologists.

We have examined coregulation physiologically by identifying the biochemical component that accomplishes something in both bodies. Over time, as children grow, the process of coregulation between mother and infant becomes self-regulation. A biocultural model can simultaneously encompass both physiological processes and the social and cultural practices that provide feedback and continuity across the generations through local traditions (cf. Fuentes 2016).

Life Cycles: Regulating across Generations

Breastfeeding is part of the rhythm of life, resonating with other daily and seasonal rhythms (cf. Ingold 2000). It is a process with short-term, immediate aspects and long-term—very long-term aspects. It presents a temporal dilemma for both mothers and analysts. Phases that may be very fleeting and easily disrupted in women's lives in the Global North, stretch into years for women in communities in the Global South. Yet these moments of nurture reflect generations of past practices, and they have the potential for influencing generations to come, regardless of how long mothers breastfeed their children. Breastfeeding requires both an immediate present orientation and a future orientation, with human milk a fluid where human pasts, presents, and futures merge.

In North America, neither teenagers entering puberty nor women becoming breastfeeding mothers are likely to have experienced rites of passage that help them adopt new sets of values. In some societies, youth and new motherhood are times to reflect on how birth, growth, and death bind old to young, person to society, and human to nature. Modern Western emphasis on autonomous individuality discourages the linking across generations that custom emphasizes in rites of passage, as we show in the examples from Southeast Asia (Chapter 5). But continuity across the generations is not of great interest in the modern world, particularly in North America, nor of much interest to today's cultural anthropology.

Most transitions along a life course are gradual, one stage blurring into another until we realize we have become "the fragile elderly." Not so with birth and becoming a mother; the rupture of membranes, the transition stage of labor—these terms reinforce the dramatic disruptive nature of birth. Unlike adolescence where changes at puberty are gradual, and definitions of when the stage begins and ends vary across cultures and change over time, you know exactly when you have given birth.

Human milk also creates linkages through time, as milk flows through one generation to the next. Intergenerational information is exchanged through many interacting inheritance systems: genetic, epigenetic, behavioral, and symbolic (Jablonka and Lamb 2005: 319). For example, human milk can be envisioned as the accumulation of the long-term matrilineal experience in the form of grandmothers' nutritional history. A woman's nutritional history signals the past environments that her daughter and granddaughter have been born into (Ravelli et al. 1999).[1] Kuzawa and Quinn argue that these distant experiences are more significant than experiences during pregnancy in predicting future adaptation

(2009: 138). Other cues and signals about local ecology, a form of nongenomic information, are transferred between generations through human milk.

This places human milk (along with placentas and stem cells) at the juncture of the generations physiologically, just as nurturing practices supporting breastfeeding are passed across generations through local customs. For hundreds of generations, women who over- and underproduced milk helped each other, sharing milk within households and communities. Historically, concern with the characteristics of wet nurses provides evidence that people recognized the importance of what passes between lactating women and the infants they fed. This recognition is rare in the modern West, with the exception of personal memories of women who felt the need to breastfeed their children because their mothers had breastfed them, and among women who share breastfeeding or human milk with strangers.

However, links can be broken, cutting off one generation's knowledge of nurturing practices from the next. In many Euro-American families, knowledge of breastfeeding was lost for one or more generations, requiring the lost generation to turn to groups like La Leche League to bridge this knowledge and praxis gap (Ward 2000), although Martucci (2015) reminds us out that some American women continued to breastfeed even when rates of bottle feeding were highest. Residential schools accelerated this loss for Canadian First Nations, as traditions of parental nurture skipped a generation (cf. Mosby 2013). But even when women learn to breastfeed from books and blogs, they seldom have to "start from scratch." A new mother relies on what other mothers in her family and community have developed as a template for her own unique relation with her newborn. This customized and customizing template helps mothers respond to local conditions, socially, culturally, and materially. Were a phrase to sum up the modern era's unprecedented changes it would be "unintended consequences."

As mothers and infants coordinate their emotional states and develop empathy for each other, a mother's body becomes a model for learning other emotions. Children learn the meanings of emotions as they participate with the mother in constructing tiny cultural worlds and then expand these worlds to include other perspectives. The first tiny world constructed between infant and mother involves negotiating mutual expectations in the process of getting things (like breastfeeding) done, mutually reinforcing the correspondence between the child's world in the mother's world (Taggart 2012: 412). Yet mothers and newborns must still acquire the skills of breastfeeding for themselves—skills that are "grown through practice" (cf. Ingold 2000: 5).

Reading the Maternal Body

Breastfeeding teaches infants how to read the maternal body. The earliest readings by a newborn may be largely instinctual, but may be encoded into the human sensorium even before a child acquires language (Leys 2011: 797). Within an hour of birth, infants look into their mothers' eyes, and shortly thereafter, turn their heads toward their mothers' voices, attracted by her smell. Innate predispositions include the nuzzling-sucking response. Immediate access to mothers' breasts takes advantage of this innate capacity (Goldschmidt 1990: 87). A Swedish video of the *Breast Crawl* (described by Widstrom et al. 1987) shows a newborn infant crawling toward the breast, attracted by the familiar smell and ultimately taste recalled from the womb. A few hours after birth, infants begin to imitate the facial expressions of their caregivers, particularly the social expressions of emotion (unless a large plastic pacifier interferes).

These reading at birth rapidly develop into an awareness of others and efforts to compel others to respond cooperatively (Goldschmidt 1990: 87). At six to eight weeks, infants will track on human faces or masks, but not on bottles. Goldschmidt refers to the interaction between infant and mother as a dialogue because it exhibits the "turn-taking" of conversations, expressing mutuality and affect attachment (1990: 89). Affect refers to the capacity of a body to be open to other bodies. Affect is transpersonal, connecting bodies by flowing between them, emerging in encounters between bodies. Pile (2010) characterizes this flow between bodies as analogous to circulation (as in pipes), transmission (as in radio), or contagion (as in viruses). Instead of those material analogies, we use dance to characterize the emotional affect that connects bodies during breastfeeding.

Breastfeeding makes it easier and faster to develop this emotional intelligence because breastfeeding depends on the successful communication between mother and infant. This calibration of the social relation between mother and infant is critical for breastfeeding success, and explains why so much attention has been focused recently on the importance of breastfeeding in the first few minutes or hour after birth.[2]

Coordination of mother and infant is further strengthened by cosleeping, another important nurturing practice. Cosleeping is a way to reduce the distance between mother and infant and slow down the separation that begins with birth. It illustrates biocultural plasticity and the "intertwined physiology of the sleeping human mother–infant dyad" (McKenna and Gettler 2007: 135), a process now referred to as breastsleeping (McKenna and Gettler 2016).

Euro-American parents socialize their infants to encourage autonomy and independence rather than interdependence and connectedness, often against their own intuitions (cf. McKenna 2000). As a result, the medical model of solitary infant sleep has also become the popular model, and treated as a "moral good" (McKenna and Gettler 2007: 1370). Fueled by the Western ideal desire for parents to get a good night's sleep, the modern practices advocated by some experts such as prone sleeping, formula feeding, and separation of mothers and infants "have cost the lives of hundreds of thousands of babies in the Western world" (McKenna and Gettler 2007: 141), some through SIDS.

Research suggests that there is a close relationship between breastfeeding and maternal-infant sleep, and that bedsharing facilitates breastfeeding (McKenna, Ball and Gettler 2007; Ball and Volpe 2013; Ball et al. 2016). Longer bedsharing has been consistently associated with longer duration of breastfeeding in large trials (cf. Huang et al. 2013; Ball et al. 2016), although it is not clear how much of this association is due to breastfeeding intent (Ball et al. 2016). Ball and colleagues (1999) have highlighted that breastfeeding parents often end up bedsharing even when they have not planned to do so. There are numerous laboratory studies that have examined the physiological elements of the coordination between breastfeeding and bedsharing (cf. Ball and Volpe 2013 for a review). For instance, Gettler and McKenna (2011) and others have shown that infants have more frequent nighttime feedings when they are regularly bedsharing.

This relationship also has implications for Sudden Infant Death Syndrome (SIDS), since formula-fed babies have twice the odds of dying of SIDS compared with breastfed babies, with exclusivity and longer duration strengthening this relationship (Huack et al. 2011). While the exact mechanism for this is unknown, McKenna has suggested that infants need to learn to breathe, and mother's carbon dioxide acts as a respiratory stimulant to her infant by decreasing deep sleep. Mothers do not habituate to their babies when they sleep together, but remain semi-alert and responsive to them, increasing their breastfeeding episodes (McKenna, Ball and Gettler 2007: 149). Horne et al. (2004) has also shown that breastfed infants are more arousable than formula fed infants. Despite Euro-American cultural assumptions that breastfeeding is associated with less nighttime sleep (Rudzik and Ball 2016), breastfeeding mothers manage to get at least as much sleep as bottle-feeding mothers (Montgomery-Downs 2010; Doan et al. 2014; Doan et al. 2007). Nevertheless, the social womb often included customs mandating separation and rest for new mothers and newborns.

Mothers and infants have more interaction when they are in the same bed not just in the same room. McKenna's, Ball's and colleagues' research confirms that breastfeeding and bed sharing are mutually reinforcing (2007: 150–51). Tomori's ground-breaking research on *Nighttime Breastfeeding* (2014) expands on these arguments ethnographically, teasing out the moral complexity of breastfeeding and cosleeping among middle-class Americans, who struggle with dominant cultural ideologies that encourage separation and independence and their unexpected findings that bringing babies into bed facilitates breastfeeding and sleep.

Cosleeping in the context of breastfeeding helps the infant to regulate bodily functions; breastfeeding creates the physiological interdependence of the mother–infant dyad. While breastfeeding confers an evolutionary advantage for the dyad and for human evolution, social support is necessary to confer the personal advantages of breastfeeding for an individual mother. When mothers move along the mixed feeding trajectory, combining breastfeeding with bottle feeding, bottle feeding quickly becomes a necessity, leaving the family dependent on finding financial resources to purchase a regular supply of their preferred brand. In turn, bottle feeding with commercial milks leaves mothers independent of the emotional, psychological, and bodily entanglements that are entailed with breastfeeding.

Adapting to Current Conditions

Never on Thursdays

I taught a double set of tutorials in anthropology every Thursday from the time Chandra was two weeks old. Every Thursday, she was sent to a babysitter with the ready-to-feed formula samples and the supply my mother purchased with the Similac coupons included in the hospital gift pack. I had never been told about expressing breastmilk. Chandra was never breastfed on Thursdays until late at night.

One weekend, Chandra took a fall, injured her lip and stopped breastfeeding. My supportive pediatrician insisted that she return to the breast because of our plans to travel to Thailand for fieldwork. After a short battle of wills, she began to nurse again. She continued breastfeeding in Thailand; at thirteen months, we tried to give her a bottle with the popular Dumex full cream milk powder mixed with bottled water, but she would have none of it. Soon she began to eat more Thai food—soup, chicken legs, rice, noodles, fish balls, and fried bananas. Just before her second birthday, I recall pouring water over myself in a Thai bath and looking down at my flattening breasts, tearfully aware that we had just had our last breastfeed. But she survived my teaching schedule, doctoral exams, formula on Thursdays, and Thai street food. (PVE)

Mothers make do. That is the nature of mothering babies. It is neither new nor avoidable. It is, however, getting harder for contemporary mothers to accept. One reason is the way today's intensive mothering shuns compromises. Another reason is society's ever-increasing demand for cleanliness, control, and perfection (Stearns 1999). These pressures can push some women into breastfeeding, drive others away, and make caring for baby less gratifying for everyone. We need to put these distinctively modern pressures in historical perspective.

We need to go back roughly 10,000 years to find a time when most women did not have to make compromises in feeding infants. That is what contemporary studies of hunters and gatherers suggest (Fouts et al. 2012). A woman could take her breastfeeding baby along while foraging. The advent of agriculture changed all that. Women who went to work in the fields could not always take baby along, and everyone had to put more time and effort into feeding the family (cf. Van Esterik 2011). Agriculture led to states whose impositions and population pressures often made matters worse. Then as now, mothers bring babies into households that must make compromises to meet everyone's needs.

The modern era has made some unprecedented compromises. The most obvious and controversial is replacing human milk with formula. Increasing rates of food allergies, food sensitivities, food intolerances, and specific inappropriate immune response to a food can be linked to the early introduction of alien milks to infants. These products skew the immune system toward reactivity rather than tolerance (Minchin 2015: 75). Maureen Minchin provides convincing evidence to explain that "what will become you began in your maternal grandmother's womb" (2015: 77). The immune system is inherited across generations, and the newborn gut has evolved to be uniquely receptive to, and dependent upon, both breastmilk and microbial colonization (Minchin 2015: 83). Infant formula companies acknowledge that their products will always lag behind human milk, but they seldom reveal the extent to which the nonhuman proteins in the formula trigger immune responses in the infant (Minchin 2015: 84).

Harder to measure is how bottles alter the nurturing relationship. For better or worse, they make both mother and child more autonomous, if a caregiver other than the mother bottle feeds the baby. That said, if reading mother is a means for understanding the world, breastfeeding's feedback loops and biochemical cues would seem to give baby a surer early reading of the world. There are no feedback loops to feeding bottles, even with responsive bottle feeding.

Ritual Dance

Breastfeeding has been redefined, repositioned, and reinterpreted through time and across cultures; its plasticity has allowed it to fit into new niches, respond to new stresses, and meet modern challenges. Consider breastfeeding and postpartum infant care as a ritual dance consisting of actions that coordinate the minds, bodies, and emotions of mother and infant. Rossano writes:

> Ritual plays a critical role in ontogeny. All of the elements of ritual (attention-grabbing, formalization, rule-governance, invariant sequencing) are present in the social exchanges between mothers and their infants. ... These social exchanges, including such things as protoconversations and "social games"

(e.g., peek-a-boo), have proven to be crucial to an infant's social and cognitive development. (2009: 251)

Mother–infant social interaction includes all these elements of ritual, including the very basic ritual of taking turns. In 1979, Trevarthen wrote that "infants invite mothers to share a dance of expressions and excitements. The infant needs a partner but knows the principles of the dance well enough" (347). Seligman and his colleagues (2008) argue that ritual is about doing things, not about texts or meanings; the doing of ritual becomes encoded in procedural memory, carried out as entrenched embodied habits (cf. Whitehouse 2007: 226). "Ritual continually renegotiates boundaries" (Seligman et al. 2008: 11). Children receive cues as to how they are supposed to feel in a given situation particularly in ritual situations ... if child fails to pick up on cues he is punished by a breach in attunement (Bruner 1986: 116). While anthropologists and other observers stressed the strangeness of postpartum practices (particularly "food taboos"), they neglected to observe the effectiveness of this ritual framing in strengthening the mother–infant bond through postpartum customs. When the dance of nurture goes well, breastfeeding has the potential to choreograph infant development.

Breastfeeding and dance illustrate what Ingold calls the "essential complementarity of the biogenetic and the sociocultural dimensions of human existence" (2000: 2). Both are also reciprocal activities that have the potential to benefit both the giver and the receiver (cf. Van Esterik 1995: 379). Although not all women experience breastfeeding as a pleasurable activity, the activity provides the potential for visceral well-being, as Parkin notes, "well-being occurs through laughing, running, swimming, cycling, eating, and breastfeeding" (2007: 240). It is rare to see breastfeeding included in such lists.

Dance is rooted in bodily physiology, dependent on individual constitution and habitus, and shaped by past and present customs. Pleasure and discipline, play and creativity, collide in the dance; the joy is encouraged hormonally by oxytocin and serotonin. In couples' dances, someone has to lead, but good dancers develop their partners. Dancing, like breastfeeding, involves visceral entrainment through the body of a teacher, as the couple moves between closure and openness, interdependence and independence.

The cradle of our humanity is contingent on early infant care. It is there, at a mother's breast, that the impetus to nurture passes between generations, and infants develop the desire and capacity for group life. That happens bioculturally; the important relational function unfolds variously, not uniformly, and must be understood historically and culturally.

Breastfeeding and human milk has the potential to choreograph infant development. We stress potential because this is too sweeping to be a testable hypothesis. It is, like evolution, a theory for making sense of otherwise disparate evidence. Breastfeeding as a master choreographer fits the evidence that we examined in this chapter. Studying the dance of nurture realistically is a task that anthropologists can undertake. In the following chapters, we take on some of this work, beginning with nurturing practices around food, eating, and feeding, adding the concept of the commensal circle to the social womb to illustrate the powerful role custom plays in the human story.

Notes

1. A First Nations woman who attended residential schools learned about the nutritional experiments done on children from Mosby's research (2013); she told him, "now I understand why I always miscarried." (PVE)
2. Several global health campaigns including the Baby Friendly Hospital Initiative (BFHI) stress the importance of breastfeeding in the first hour after birth.

CHAPTER 4

Entering the Commensal Circle

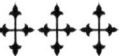

The dance of nurture operates throughout the life cycle, through sharing food, eating together, and the relations created through food and eating. In this chapter, we consider breastmilk, breastmilk substitutes, and complementary foods as separate but linked parts of infant-feeding complexes, the systems of provisioning infants, each with their distinct histories and linkages to the moral core of human sociality. The commensal circles formed by these activities have their own logics that have relevance for infant and child feeding in general and breastfeeding in particular. Commensality— the act of eating together and sharing food is a special kind of consumption that affirms social relations, a long-standing interest of anthropologists and sociologists such as Robertson Smith (1889) and Weber (1963), and more recently, Kerner, Chow, and Warmind (2015). While people relate to each other through eating and feeding, commensality always includes some people and excludes others from the circle. But it is a process seldom explored by economists or nutritionists.

Commensality is one way to understand relatedness. We discuss it here in a linear life-cycle narrative, aware that there are nonlinear aspects to what flows through, including the transfer of young cells into old bodies in embryonic stem cell research (Kaufman and Morgan 2005: 320), and the transfer of stem cells between mother and newborn. The commensal relation created by food sharing involves intimacy, nurturance, and reciprocity. As we defined in the first chapter, nurture involves building social relations to ensure the empathetic provision of food and care that encourages something or someone's growth and development to full potential. Nurture has a commensal component—food sharing, and a person-making component, encompassing processes of intimacy and reciprocity. Intimacy requires being totally open to another. Because of the embodied individual nature of breastmilk production, breastfeeding is considered a very intimate activity.

Food sharing is a contemporary practice that begins in utero and stretches back to our evolutionary and ontogenetic pasts. Martin Jones points out that meals, like sex and reproduction, "resist attempts to distance the person and the organism" (2007: 12). But there is a domain that necessitates taking the next analytical step—putting meals, sex, and reproduction together; they come together ontologically in feeding the fetus in utero and breastfeeding, the most intimate act of nurture.

Social reciprocity is a basic part of what makes us human. For example, meals that are shared insure that invitations to share future meals will follow. Reciprocity is not without calculation, as with dinner parties where households decide who to invite and how elaborate the meal should be, sharing the cost of rounds of drinks or food, and, of course, the business lunch. This process can become competitive or exclusionary, as competitive feasts such as potlatches on Canada's west coast illustrate.

Most studies of commensality consider the food sharing practices of adults, where the social obligations created by food sharing are usually reciprocal. Breastfed infants and young children are seldom included in discussions of commensality, because the youngest members of society have no independent agency and are passive eaters, having to be fed what others offer them. Babies can of course refuse to eat what is offered.

Breastfeeding is not technically food sharing between mother and child. Rather food taken in by one is transformed and given to another, creating a unique precommensal relationship. As nonmilk foods are introduced into the infant's diet—ideally around six months of age—they may not always be shared. In North America, baby foods are usually made for one baby, sometimes for only a single meal, which is often thrown out if not finished. Infant feeding is more directly connected to adult meals in the Global South where mothers may premasticate their own food for an infant, share a bowl with them, or finish their leftovers, a practice not uncommon in Euro-American kitchens.

But by drawing attention to infant and young child feeding, new dimensions of commensality emerge, including the contrast between dependent and independent eating, feeding and eating, and feeding self and others. Michael Pollan, in *The Omnivore's Dilemma* argues that the perfect meal is one that you make yourself, and that does not incur reciprocal debt (2006: 409). Using this definition, breastmilk might be defined as the perfect food since women do make it themselves, but in many parts of the world, it puts children in their mother's debt. With infant feeding in Southeast Asia, for example, this debt is made explicit.

Breastfeeding is the paradigmatic precultural core of human commensality, preceding cultural systems of food sharing. This commensal core is set in infancy and sets the stage for future culturally patterned commensality and food sharing. Without being fed by someone, a newborn dies; the act of feeding a newborn sets up a social relationship that can last a lifetime and beyond. In his work on *Feasts: How Humans Came to Share Food* (2007), Jones asks how we came to eat together face to face; the answer must begin with the mammalian moments of eating face to breast, the first experience of social meals around the breast/hearth.

Of course, the fact that bottle feeding using infant formula provided the commensal core for millions of healthy North American adults today complicates the argument about breastfeeding as *the* commensal core of human food sharing. Caregivers can buffer the nutritional and immunological limitations of breastmilk substitutes, including soy- and milk-based formulas. However, bottle feeding can be accomplished without the relational component; breastfeeding cannot. Breastfeeding requires the relational, but the relational is backed up by redundant biocultural and biochemical processes in both mother and infant, as we showed in Chapter 3. Bottle-fed babies (and mothers) have no biochemical backup.

Bottle feeding with infant formula, the most common commercial product used in North America, is clearly modeled on breastfeeding—hence the common phrase, breastmilk substitute. All infant-feeding complexes are ultimately modeled on breastfeeding as the standard, from the nipple on feeding bottles, to the efforts to "humanize" cow's milk formula; both men and women usually bottle-feed in the breastfeeding body position. Still, breastfeeding is normal for humans, and not breastfeeding, an in vivo experiment with significant but unacknowledged consequences. North American mothers dependent on expert advice books such as those by Dr. Spock are reassured that if mothers make the infant formula carefully and cuddle when bottle feeding their infants, they show their devotion to their babies. "This great build up of importance of nursing is not justified by the facts," Spock concluded in 1968, in his influential advice book, *The Common Sense Book of Baby and Child Care*; decades later Wolf (2010), Barston (2012), and Jung (2015) followed suit, cherry-picking evidence to argue that breastfeeding is no better than formula feeding.

Commensality has a life course component through its influence on a newborn's developing constitution. The mechanisms are becoming increasingly clear with respect to breastfeeding, but we know less about how infants' constitutions are shaped by bottle feeding after their constitutions are cut off from the maternal body at birth. Chapter 3 reviewed some of the routes to constitution building with regard to dental systems, immunity, and the microbiome of the breastfed baby. A breastfed baby shares maternal substance for a longer period of time than a baby that is not breastfed; what the mother eats and attends to shapes infant development in a much more profound way than we previously thought. A colleague once explained in jest that in Scottish cities, people go from the baby bottle to the pop bottle to the whiskey bottle, with the subtle suggestion that pleasure in the former sets up the pleasure in the latter.

Feeding on demand, scheduled feeding, and forced feeding all shape the developing individual's relation to food. Food practices in infancy have long-range effects on food practices later in life. Hence, the policy focuses on the importance of the first 1,000 days of life. But while adults in some parts of the world survive very poor diets, what a baby consumes during the first year of life shapes subsequent adult health. Unlike adults who expect and thrive on food diversity and varied diets, infants thrive on a single food—breastmilk or an inferior substitute. It is adults who try and force diversity on infants and toddlers, bringing them to the commensal table before they are ready. Unlike adult diets that are so culturally shaped that it is difficult to establish what could be considered an ideal diet, there are agreed upon biomedical standards about the ideal diet for infants and young children. Although cultural factors do affect breastfeeding and young child feeding, there are clear policy guidelines for meeting this agreed upon universal standard. Problems arise in the implementation; only in Scandinavian countries have policies been implemented to successfully support exclusive breastfeeding.

We illustrate our argument by reference to the commensal circle, a conceptual tool that has developmental, structural, ontological, and cross-cultural implications (Van Esterik 2015).[1] The commensal circle is a space where people share food, eat together, and feed each other. These circles are preconstituted culturally before any individual guest or newborn enters them, and may include ancestors or spirits who are fed along with human family members.

The levels of the commensal circle include:

1. in utero
2. breastfeeding or breastmilk substitutes
3. shared breastfeeding/premasticated food
4. ritual prelacteal feeds such as honey
5. sharing food with siblings and other household members
6. sharing food with community members
7. feasts and political commensality
8. sharing food with strangers, food aid.

Participation in these circles can be simultaneous or sequential for an individual; consider for example a breastfeeding infant (level 2) who is ritually presented with a taste of honey (level 4) during a special feast (level 7). Commensal circles expand from feeding in utero, to include breastfeeding and practices such as wet nursing and premastication. The first act of feeding sets up a social relation between a mother and infant, or whoever has the primary responsibility for feeding a newborn. All children move from a period of being fed milk in the form of breastmilk or substitutes, to the ability to eat a range of foods independently and eventually to feed others. The period from pregnancy to sevrage, when breastfeeding ends, is a period of embodied commensality, when all or most of the nutrients an infant consumes are produced within the mother's body.

Embodied commensality accomplishes several things: it socializes infants and children into the taste regimes of their households. It is where and when they shift from coregulation of appetite to self-regulation. Embodied commensality sets the emotional tone for eating; is it a time for pleasure? fear? abuse? It attunes infants to recognize social and relational cues. It is the period that shapes the new person's constitution through participation in socially constituted commensal acts.

With the first introduction of food produced outside the body, we shift to a period of enculturated commensality where the foods selected (prelacteal feeds, ritual food offerings such as honey) and the mode of sharing (shared breastfeeding, eating premasticated foods) are culturally determined. While embodied commensality is driven by custom and by the postpartum practices of women, culture increasingly comes to shape the rules that govern commensal circles—the foods served, the order served, and the etiquette of eating. When women are gatekeepers of the commensal system, they still adhere to cultural rules that may have them eating least and last (as in much of South Asia).

Religious practices shape commensal circles, influencing the food served, who eats with whom, and the meaning of individual food items. Orthodox Jews' and Muslims' disgust reaction to pork, for example, links them to everyone else in their commensal circles who also reject pork. This religious-based shared response differs from disgust for a food as an expression of individual preferences.

It is in these transitions from embodied to enculturated commensality, from internal to external food source, from mother to other as feeder, from custom to culture—where child-feeding problems develop. As commensal circles expand and contract to include or exclude siblings, other household members, community members and strangers, infants and young children face increased risk.

Breastfeeding is the paradigmatic act of embodied nurture. Food sharing becomes more complex as older infants begin to eat household foods, and toddlers enter already established commensal circles. Enculturated commensality may take place in gender or age segregated circles. Modernity with its notions of progress and reform has had a dramatic effect on commensality, both through the provision of new foods and through the development of ideas of self-improvement through healthy eating, encouraging new forms of relatedness. The effects of modernity, further explored in Chapter 6, will be visible in each stage in the life cycle, as eating and feeding others reveals the mutual interdependence of nurture. We begin with commensality in the womb.

Eating in pregnancy, like breastfeeding, unfolds within the universals of human reproduction, in individualized, yet enculturated ways, building on every woman's unique constitution. During the embodied commensality of fetal and neonatal nutrition, women come to have sympathy for their fetuses and nurture them as future people with food likes and dislikes. The experience of nurturing the unborn conditions the nurturing of the newborn. The relation between mother and child unfolds from the moment of conception, through pregnancy and breastfeeding. Commensality begins in utero where maternal food provides the nutrients for infant growth in the placenta, the umbilical cord, and the nutrients in the amniotic fluid. As food passes from outside to inside the pregnant woman's body, it also moves into the fetus, embedded inside the inside. Food that is external to the body becomes internal, and is incorporated into the body—first by the mother, and then by the fetus, and finally by the breastfed child.

Flavors from the pregnant mother's diet enter the amniotic fluid and are swallowed by the fetus throughout the pregnancy. Thus, the types of food, spices, and drinks ingested by women during pregnancy, guided by the flavor principles of their cuisines, are experienced by their babies long before their exposure through breastfeeding or eating foods. Taste preferences develop in cultural contexts, shaped by ethnicity and food customs. The flavors from foods ingested by pregnant women, including garlic, mint, vanilla, carrot, anise, and alcohol are present in amniotic fluid and breastmilk, another example of alignment between maternal and infant bodies. Research shows that infants whose mothers consumed anise when pregnant showed a preference for anise (Shepherd 2012: 234). Similarly, in a study where pregnant women drink water or carrot juice in late pregnancy, the children of moms who drank water had more negative reactions to carrots than children of women who drank carrot juice (Mennella, Jagnow, and Beauchamp 2001).

For pregnant women in Euro-American societies, food choices are imbued with new meanings and tensions. Research in the UK concluded that "Women's diet modifications during pregnancy are constantly under negotiation" (Markens, Browner, and Press 1997: 361), as women experienced the tension between their indulgences and cravings and what they think the baby likes and wants. Women made degrees of accommodation and modified their diet by changing degrees of intake (cutting back on some foods) or kind of intake (cutting out certain foods entirely). Clearly, pregnant women are aware that their food choices are affecting their unborn children, and many are prepared to alter their diets accordingly. This food negotiation during pregnancy begins the process of coregulation between mothers and their children that develops into self-regulation.

Murphy, Parker, and Phipps (1998) examined how women in the UK who say they intend to breastfeed end up bottle feeding, and how they talk about these decisions. Her study mothers were acutely aware of the importance of these decisions before the babies were born: "'you suddenly think,' it's a new little life … if you start it off on the wrong feed, on the wrong foot, giving it the wrong foods, I mean, you're going to have rotten teeth and bad health and what's going to go wrong with them if you don't feed them right." They worried about eating a healthy diet during pregnancy, fearing that they would produce poor milk. They also felt that their babies colonized their bodies: "I'm just dying to get my own body back and know that I can eat that and not worry about it or drink that and not worry about it" (Murphy 2004: 144). Here, the needs of mother and baby were viewed as in conflict during both pregnancy and breastfeeding.

In Euro-American communities, pregnant women are encouraged to avoid additives, not gain too much weight, and get enough protein and fiber. In the Global North, pregnant women are expected to have food cravings. In the Global South, food prescriptions and proscriptions during pregnancy may push women out of the commensal circle for a short time by specifying what they can and cannot eat. Often commensality serves the household and community better than it serves the pregnant or new mother and newborn, particularly when postpartum customs have eroded. For example, in parts of the Middle East, customs where women brought food to the new mother have shifted subtly; now new mothers are pressured to get up and cook for guests, as cultural changes erode custom. Reintegration into the commensal circle comes later after food prescriptions end. Such rules can be advantageous to or a problem for pregnant women. Rules could give them access to more or less food, better quality or poorer quality food, depending on the society's view of women and their reproductive work. But, as anthropologists have noted, food rules are more often stated than followed (cf. Laderman 1983).

Biocultural practices handed down as customs are not reasoned out or rational, but nor should they be dismissed as ignorant. Some cultural food rules might turn out to be adaptive, such as providing extra food for pregnant or lactating women; others might deny pregnant and lactating women key dietary items. If adaptation were the only reason for customs about food proscriptions and prescriptions, then it would be hard to understand food restrictions that denied extra food resources to women when their needs were greatest. However, sometimes science catches up with custom, as some researchers argue that eating too much meat may be harmful to the fetus. Eating less meat and more fruit during pregnancy might be beneficial, but that is not all that customs accomplish.

There is often a relation between the food proscriptions and prescriptions for pregnant women and those for lactating women, particularly if the rules are derived from the humoral system or other culturally validated medical system. Still, there are often inconsistencies, since even systems of humoral medicine are not fully coherent, but more like guidelines tested through the experiences of generations of women. As a rural Thai woman explained, "I followed the rules for the first baby; now, I test them out with each baby." This observation resonates with the research on Malaysian women (cf. Laderman 1983) and women research subjects in the UK. More likely, food prescriptions and proscriptions embedded in postpartum customs are followed or not, based on the experience of generations of pregnant women and new mothers, with elders providing advice and exercising oversight regarding their consumption practices and general behavior.

When pregnant or breastfeeding, women have a double responsibility; they are responsible for their own eating as well as for feeding their infants. They may need to exercise restraint on their consumption of food and drink, or be restrained by others. Modern Euro-American observers feel they have the right to advise a pregnant or lactating woman what she should and should not eat or drink. Pregnant women in the Global North are discouraged from consuming alcohol, because alcohol alters the sensory properties of milk (Mennella and Beauchamp 1991). Although the public may be concerned about a mother's occasional alcoholic drink, they are ignorant about or choose to ignore the alcohol produced from formula in the infant gut (Minchin 2015: 350).

Birth to Breast

The experience of a first pregnancy and birth shapes a woman's constitution and conditions it to continue her nurturing work through breastfeeding. Just as maternal food shaped the constitution of the growing fetus, as the infant moves from inside to outside the mother's body, it continues to take its food from the maternal body in the form of colostrum and breastmilk. Birth also shapes the constitution of newborns, as they experience the world outside the womb directly for the first time. At the moment of birth, iron stores in mothers move through the pulsing cord into the newborn. Waiting a few minutes for the umbilical cord to stop pulsing provides more iron stores for the newborn. As discussed in Chapter 3, vaginal and cesarean births each set up different flora in the newborn's gut.

The hormonal environment of pregnant mothers prepares the breasts for nourishing infants after birth. In fact, maternal breasts are capable of lactation from about sixteen weeks of pregnancy when they can secrete milk proteins, but are kept in check by high levels of steroids circulating in the mother until the infant is born. With the birth of the placenta, these hormones no longer hold back and the increase in prolactin stimulates the production of colostrum and later, mature milk.

At birth, the maternal body is ready to nurture a newborn with human milk, and someone must deliberately intervene to stop this from happening by preventing the newborn from suckling, binding the new mother's breasts, or providing a drug to suppress lactation. Drugs used in the past to suppress lactation such as DES, (diethylstilbestrol) a known carcinogen, are considered dangerous today, and there are no FDA-approved drugs to accomplish this suppression. When mothers do not give their milk to their newborns, prolactin levels drop to pre-pregnancy rates around two weeks postpartum, and lactation ceases.

After working hard, we get hungry.

Postpartum Hunger

I have never been as hungry as I was after the hard work of labor and giving birth, particularly after fasting for hours the day before the birth. Yet I was left in my hospital room for several hours with no food or drink after the birth of my daughter, while my mother and husband went out and celebrated with steak and wine, and my newborn was stuffed with infant formula in a distant nursery. (PVE)

It is natural to assume that the newborn who has also worked hard to be born would be hungry. But this is not the case. Yet most North American institutions rush to feed the newborn infant not the mother; the new mother needs to be fed; the newborn infant does not need to be fed. Newborns have enough nutrients to last until their digestive systems are working. They need skin-to-skin contact and the opportunity to lick small amounts of colostrum from their mothers' nipples. About 100 ml of colostrum is secreted daily for about two days after birth. In addition to providing special anti-infective properties, colostrum contains the scents and flavors from the maternal diet and acts as a "flavor bridge" between the maternal diet, breastfeeding, and the flavors of household foods such as vanilla, garlic, or coffee. Postpartum customs that encourage providing food for new mothers not newborn infants are particularly beneficial for both.

Copious milk secretion begins between thirty and seventy-two hours after the delivery of the placenta. If any placenta is left in the mother, there is no milk production, a point that makes customs in Southeast Asia that focus attention on the placenta make perfect sense. To produce and secrete a copious milk supply, prolactin needs to be released; but it is the infant's direct stimulation of the nipple/areola that releases the prolactin in the mother.

The first embodied lesson from breastfeeding is responsiveness, as both mothers' and infants' bodies are given over to a shared activity. Infants latch on to feed from a mother who has already learned her society's embodiment patterns. If mothers have never experienced these embodied patterns of being nurtured, the activities must be learned by both parties. The embodied intimacy of breastfeeding can be disturbing to some mothers, particularly those who were not breastfed themselves or who lack adequate social support. All social life involves negotiating such boundaries between self and other, inside and outside. This play between inside and outside is often disrupted first in North American hospitals, and later in North American households when parents decide that there will be no more maternal embodied contact after the birth, and that commercial foods, originating totally outside the maternal body, will be used to build the new infant's constitution.

Breastmilk is the reference food for all human infants. It meets all nutritional, health, and care needs of the infant for the first six months of life. Phrases such as "breast is best" and "decision to breastfeed" make little sense biologically, as pregnant women already produce milk proteins long before their babies are born. "Breast is best" also suggests an inappropriate comparison; but there is no comparable product. Rather, breastfeeding sets an infant on a different trajectory with implications for infant, child, and adult health. In short, breastfeeding builds a different constitution, and thus a different person. As a recent American Academy of Pediatrics policy statement confirmed, breastfeeding is not a lifestyle choice but a critical health decision with impacts on infants and mothers (2012: 837).

The composition of human milk is not constant. Fats are the most variable compound in breastmilk, lactose, the most constant and invariable. The fat content of mature milk is related to the relative fullness or emptiness of the breast, and it changes during each feed, increasing from the foremilk to the hindmilk. As a breast is emptied during a feed and over a day, the proportion of fat increases, depending on the length of time between feedings. The foremilk is more like a soup to satisfy immediate thirst followed by a rich dessert to ensure satiety (Labbok 2012: 38), on an analogy with a common Euro-American meal format.

All milk starts out as concentrated hindmilk, and as it remains in the breast, it draws in water and becomes more dilute foremilk. This is a particularly important part of the interdependence of mothers and infants. Because breastmilk is composed of about 87 percent water, there is no need for another source of water for breastfed infants, a critical advantage where water supplies are unclean or insecure. Variation in milk composition occurs within a feed—from start to finish, and over twenty-four hours. It also changes through the lactation cycle as the infant grows. Even mothers of twins note differences in the breastfeeding experiences between their children. A Swedish study quantified the incredible variability among breastfeeding dyads (Hörnell et al. 1999).

Breastmilk is predominately sweet and contains volatile food odors that vary from mother to mother. Newborns have an inborn dislike of sour and bitter tastes in high concentration, as do many children. Human food choices are not hard-wired; rather, food preferences depend on learning and social context. There is no "wisdom of the body" other than seeking out a diet that makes us feel good and avoiding foods that cause discomfort. Even our innate aversion to irritants such as chili peppers or coffee can be overcome.

Infants' first experience with food flavors occurs long before they are given solid foods, as they experience the flavor of their mothers' food through the amniotic fluid. Taste memories from pregnancy and breastfeeding provide the foundation for cultural differences in cuisine (Mennella et al. 2009: 780s). Mennella's research has shown that

> Early flavor experiences gained through breastfeeding enhance the acceptance of a wider range of foods during the weaning period and throughout childhood. It has been argued that breastfed babies, whose mothers regularly eat a wide variety of foods, are exposed to a diversity of flavors that are absent from formula milk and this early exposure augments the acceptance of various flavors. (Burnier, Dubois, and Girard 2011: 200)

There is extraordinary variation in the rate of transfer of flavor compounds into breastmilk, as well as variation between women and even variation in individual women. Ingested flavor compounds are eliminated from mother's body quickly, but enter mother's milk selectively and in relatively low amounts, resulting in "continuous flavor changes in mother's milk" (Hausner et al. 2008: 123). The first six months of life is a sensitive learning period for the flavor image (Shepherd 2012: 235); as Mennella's extensive research demonstrates, children live in a different sensory world than adults.

The symbiotic relationship between mother and newborn infant is also illustrated by considering the relation between a hungry baby and its mother's engorged breast. The more milk an infant removes during a feed from its mother's breast, the greater the amount of milk the mother produces for the next feed. The rate of milk synthesis speeds up as the infant removes milk from the breast. Milk synthesis is controlled independently in each breast with the result that one breast may produce more than the other. The less productive breast may produce 65 percent of the volume of the other breast. This physiological fact is reflected in local customs where one breast is considered to produce food, the other, drink, or when one breast is used to feed during the day, and the other at night, as in parts of rural Java. North American mothers are often concerned that their babies prefer one breast over another. This might be due to nipple shape, over or under supply, comfort from the heart beat, habit, or discomfort when the infant lies on one side. This example of infant individuation adds another layer to the development of the infant's unique constitution.

Breastfed infants cannot be overfed; their appetites are held in check by the leptin that passes through maternal breastmilk. Breastfed infants just stop working when they are full, a powerful example of coregulation becoming self-regulation. Breastfeeding is after all the first "work for food" project an infant experiences, and requires focus, concentration, and effort on the part of the infant. Breastfeeding also requires self-regulation on the part of mothers; women may stop breastfeeding when they are unable to self-regulate any longer, particularly if they are without social support and under pressure to resume their other roles. At some point, they may be unwilling to restrict their eating, drinking, sexual life, or mobility any longer. But the period of coregulation that we refer to as the social womb is self-limiting and most intense in the first six months after each birth.

Because breastfeeding mothers and infants are not constrained by the need to be close to a kitchen for a heat source or water supply, breastfeeding can occur anywhere. In practice, social constraints limit breastfeeding in public in the Global North, in spite of health messages proclaiming "Breastfeeding Anytime! Anywhere!"

The end of milk production or involution occurs about forty days after the last breastfeeding, or longer if mothers have been producing milk for many children for a very long time; this helps explain the ease with which many African grandmothers can relactate to feed their grandchildren orphaned by HIV/AIDS.

Mother's Milk Plus

Triple nipple feeding refers to mixed feeding where breastfeeding is combined with the use of breastmilk substitutes, usually fed by bottle. Triple nipple feeding offers the possibility of confusion between nipples; while not recommended, it is widely practiced around the world. In some places, this results in the decline in frequency and duration of breastfeeding and consequently a decline in lactation amenorrhea and child spacing; in other places, the practice results in the long duration of partial breastfeeding. Often mothers believe that adding infant formula in addition to breastmilk would make infants healthier (Latham, Agunda, and Elliot 1988). This idea of topping up breastmilk feedings has a long history in the hospitals of industrialized countries such as Australia (cf. Minchin 2015).

In spite of studies that compare breastfed babies and those fed with infant formula, we have no idea how the combination of breastmilk and infant formula or other substitutes affects the resistance of infants to infections and other aspects of development (Neville et al. 2012: 171). In fact, we have almost no research on exclusive breastfeeding from birth or exclusive bottle feeding from birth, a reminder of the uselessness of categories like ever breastfed for researching health outcomes (Minchin 2015: 162).

Throughout human history, some women have sought alternatives to maternal breastfeeding. In the absence of adequate breastmilk substitutes, the commensal circle may expand to include other female relatives who may offer their breastmilk informally on occasion to help the mother, or more formally and strategically, on a regular basis, creating very special relations such as wet nursing and milk siblingship through sharing breastmilk.

Wet-nursing was so common in Paris in the 1780s that it was estimated that of the 21,000 babies born in 1780, only 700 were nursed by their own mothers (DeLoache and Gottlieb 2000: 8). Kertzer (2008) examines an interesting case of wet-nursing from late nineteenth-century Italy where the wet nurse took on an infant from a nearby foundling hospital and then contracted syphilis from the infant. Much attention was given to the choice of the wet nurse, because parents assumed that important characteristics pass through the milk of the wet nurse to the child.

Today, shared breastfeeding raises similar concerns with regard to knowing the character of the woman who breastfeeds your child or provides donor milk. Mothers usually prefer close friends or relatives whose habits are well known, because of the possibility of the transmission of diseases such as HIV. Today, as in the past, the need for trust is paramount.

It has been estimated that over 55,000 North American women sell or donate their breastmilk online (Keim et al. 2013). Milk sharing has expanded and become more public since "milky matches" can now be made over the internet. This is part of the process of demedicalizing and commodifying breastmilk (Palmquist 2015), as the product is often pooled and pasteurized for sale. Donor milk banks discourage community-based milk sharing since the latter are not concerned with screening or pasteurization. Sharing networks such as *Eats on Feets* and *Human Milk for Human Babies* stress the noncommercial altruistic exchange of a product that is priceless (Gribble 2014).

In the Global North, mothers are advised to trust donations from milk banks more than milk that is sold over the internet. Women selling milk online may be tempted to over dilute their milk, mix it with cow's milk, or not disclose health problems. Keim et al. (2013) found that 75 percent of milk sold online was contaminated with "the same kind of bacteria found in human waste." Human milk always contains these bacteria—the good bacteria that jump-start the infant's immune system. But the information is enough to repulse the reader who knows little about the microbiome, human milk, or milk sharing. Strangely enough, there is no comparable concern about the bacteria that commercial breastmilk substitutes deposit or encourage in the infant's microbiome.

When the poor wet-nurse the infants of the rich, class and economic status may separate the wet nurse from her charge, but the taste continuities through milk still operate, which might explain why wet nurses were sometimes provided with special foods from the estates of the nobles whose children they fed (Fildes 1986). The amount of contact between wet nurses and the parents of their charges vary in time and space, from absent to constant supervision in the family home, as when the wet nurse becomes almost a member of the family.

Substances like breastmilk serve to create special relations between mothers and infants. But these relationships formed may go beyond the mother–infant bond. There is no more intimate act than consuming milk from someone's breast. In the past, some Muslim societies built on this intimacy to acknowledge the power of relatedness through milk—milk siblingship. Islamic sharia law recognizes three ways to establish relationships—through blood, affinity, and milk. Through the act of breastfeeding another child, strangers can be turned into relatives, enemies into allies, marriageable relatives into ineligible relatives. In the next chapter, we consider some Southeast Asian examples where relatedness through milk is elaborated.

Another intimate act of commensality, premastication, or pre-chewing food for infants, has recently been reexamined (Pelto, Zhang, and Habicht 2010). In a review of research on pre-chewed foods cross-culturally (based on ethnographic reports in the Human Relation Area Files), the authors found that pre-chewing of foods was referred to in nearly one third of the cultures that had entries on infant feeding. Most entries referred to premastication as a way for mothers to prepare food for infants, with occasional mention of medicinal or religious use. A wide range of food was offered in this way: meat, fish, nuts, seeds, roots, and legumes—most with a relatively high iron content. The authors argue that before the availability of cereals and iron-fortified foods that could be cooked into paps and gruels, premastication of meat and seeds might have provided extra iron to infants and young children. Iron stores are high enough in breastfed infants until about six months of age when the infant needs to get iron from complementary foods. When mothers pre-chew food for their infants, the process of taste socialization is further strengthened.

Colonialism and new definitions of modernity disparaged pre-chewing food as an unhygienic "yucky" practice, so that reports on the subject are likely to be biased and its extent, underestimated. This is obvious in Thailand where several decades of nutrition education have all but eradicated the practice. In contrast, in Lao PDR where there have been fewer nutrition interventions, mothers in food insecure households and in upland hunting and gathering groups often pre-chew food for their infants. In the margins of Southeast Asia where premastication is useful for getting seeds and meat products into infants, it is not valued as an ideal way to feed an infant, but practiced in households who have no access to "better" or more modern infant foods. Premastication is not as deeply embedded in the cultural repertoire as breastfeeding. Analysts view the process as a rather backward traditional custom. Modern aversion to pre-chewing has to be considered within changing ideas of hygiene, body boundaries, and intimacy.

Nurturing Without the Breast

There are only a few generations of infants who have survived to reproduce without having ever consumed human milk; the consequences for future generations are yet to be fully explored, although Minchin (2015) has provided evidence backing some powerful arguments. Meanwhile, there have been significant historical changes in the production of commercial baby milks and complementary foods; in spite of improved products, infants everywhere have adapted to very inappropriate products and continue to survive on industrially processed foods.

Millions of infants in developing and developed countries thrive without human milk, and grow up to be healthy adults, well nurtured and nurturing of others. But they are biologically different (cf. Minchin 2015: 242), and have very different constitutions from breastfed infants; they experience and learn nurturing practices through a different route. Millions more, primarily in the Global

South, do not thrive without human milk. The composition of infant formula has changed over time, and the damage done to infant development caused by errors in industrial processing and excess or deficiency of key nutrients only become obvious decades later when it is more difficult to trace back to infant-feeding practices, demonstrating "proof of humankind's astonishing omnivore adaptability" (Minchin 2015: 315, 400). While bottle feeding may be viewed as a modern high status way to feed a newborn among the elite of the Global South, the morbidity and mortality rates confirm the dangers to other infants in the Global South (World Health Organization 2000) and the wealthier more industrialized Global North (cf. Stuebe 2009; Rollins et al. 2016). Jim Grant, the director of UNICEF from 1980 to 1995, estimated that at least one million infant lives were lost every year through not breastfeeding or premature weaning (Fifield 2015: 26).

Infant formula is available in powdered or liquid form, as well as more expensive options such as fast dissolving cubes and ready to feed bottles. The products are constantly being updated and improved in response to publicity about industrial accidents and new evidence concerning the constituents in human milk. For example, companies like Prolacta and Medolac now process human milk to extract and sell proteins, fats, and sugars to the infant formula industry to replace genetically engineered components. There is little evidence to date as to whether these extracted components keep any of the properties of live human milk cells. These components and resulting products are not equivalent to human milk and do not begin to substitute for breastfeeding, as even the formula companies acknowledge.

Infant formula is not a sterile product but is rated as GRAS (generally recognized as safe), in spite of the constant recalls that receive minimum publicity (Walker 1993; Minchin 2015). Additives to infant formula are exempted from safety testing (Minchin 2015: 397). Minchin refers to infant formula as a non-sterile dehydrated soup powder (2015: 176). It is a standardized product with a constant flavor. Mothers usually stay with the same brand of infant formula if possible. Thus, the infant is exposed to an industrial food product offering no taste variation or continuities with the flavors infants encountered in the womb.

The private sector became more involved in the very lucrative baby food market in the 1960s, with the development of specialized products such as hypoallergenic formula and preterm infant formula. Mothers' own milk is now the standard of care for preterm infants, with pasteurized or fresh donor human milk used when mothers' milk is not available. Since the 1960s, soy-based infant formulas have come onto the market, although the first recorded use of soy for infant feeding was in 1909 (Minchin 2015: 295). Other specialized baby foods include lactose-free, thickened, and follow-on formula as well as toddler milks for older infants. This is now considered the fastest growing part of the baby food market (Bandy 2014).

Modern replacement feeds include suitable milk- or soy-based commercial products like infant formula, as well as riskier, inappropriate replacement feeds such as unpasteurized animal milks, herbal teas, or coffee creamers. For example, Bear Brand coffee creamer was widely used in Lao PDR to feed infants and young children. Although not advertised as a breastmilk substitute, it was chosen by women based on the logo of the baby bear cradled by a mother bear in the breastfeeding position (Barennes et al. 2008). Nestlé, owner of Bear Brand, made a sign on the can label—a cross through a baby feeding bottle in a red circle—as a way to discourage use of the coffee creamer as a baby food. Because infant formulas are not financially available to most Lao women, coffee creamer was the most similar-looking product available in rural markets (until small cheap packets of Chinese infant formula began crossing the border).

Bottle feeding with commercial substitutes solves some of the problems mothers face with modern scheduling and the coordination of high periodicity tasks, tasks that are high frequency and nonpostponable (Douglas and Isherwood 1996: 86); bottle feeding avoids the need for close coregulation between mothers and infants. This method of infant feeding also has great appeal to women who are personally disgusted by breastfeeding, and is chosen by women who have found breastfeeding difficult, often because of lack of social support or help with solving problems.

A UK study concluded that bottle feeding met the needs of mothers and babies simultaneously and independently, without putting one at odds with another. If women breastfed, they put the baby first. "In contrast, formula feeding was seen as bringing flexibility, freedom, and particularly among those intending to formula feed, relief from an embarrassing and even distasteful responsibility" (Murphy et al. 1998: 258). Until we learn precisely what problems bottles and breastmilk substitutes solve for women, and then turn our attention to offering better ways to solve those problems, ideally, through making breastfeeding more appealing and convenient, breastfeeding rates are unlikely to improve.

Complementary Feeding

The introduction of complementary foods draws infants more directly into the larger culturally constructed commensal circle of the household. Complementary feeding refers to the regular addition of food and liquids to an infant's diet to complement breastmilk. Infants consume a wider range of foods as they move to these expanded commensal circles. The introduction of foods produced outside the maternal body marks the beginning of the shift to enculturated commensality, ideally along with the continuation of the embodied commensality of breastfeeding (Van Esterik 2015).

Historically, the difference between breastmilk substitutes and complementary foods has not been clearly defined. Semisolid mixtures of grains, often mixed with animal milk or water, were given to infants to replace or supplement breastmilk using feeding devices made from horn, ceramic, or glass. In many parts of the world, an infant's complementary food is prepared from food that is consumed by other family members. Generally, infants move from liquid to semi-solid to solid foods.

After much research and deliberation, WHO and its expert consultants concluded that complementary food was neither useful nor necessary for infants before six months, and could indeed be harmful (World Health Organization 1979). However, the global recommendation from WHO did not fit with patterns of infant feeding in most parts of the world, where complementary foods are often introduced either too early or too late. Too early introduction of nonmilk solids increases the chance of contamination and puts a strain on immature kidneys; introducing foods too late may leave infants short of nutrients and calories.

Nutritionists, therapists, and psychologists in the UK who deal with feeding problems in children assume that complementary foods are added around fourteen weeks, noting that during the period from four to six months, infants are unusually receptive to new tastes (Harris 2000: 79). Bentley shows how advice about when to introduce complementary foods kept changing in North America (2014: 10). Breastfed infants in North America are typically introduced to foods at a later age than infants fed infant formula. Breastfeeding mothers typically exert less control over feeding than mothers of formula-fed babies (Mennella et al. 2009: 787s). Of course, breastfed babies have been exposed to a wide range of taste combinations even before they are introduced to table foods. Breastfed babies generally prefer to feed themselves as they retain control over their own intake. Our model suggests that breastfed infants seem to be better able to self-regulate their intake and recognize their appetite cues, as they develop from maternal-infant coregulation to self-regulation.

Foods given to infants include homemade or commercially produced baby foods or family foods used for household meals. Family foods may be modified for infants and young children by pre-chewing, diluting, or mashing. Some food items such as bread, maize porridge, or sticky rice are given to infants without modification. Other mixtures are made at home from family foods but prepared specifically for children, such as *bubur* (rice porridge made from rice flour, fruit, beans, and vegetables) in Indonesia. With policy makers' increasing attention on micronutrients, the Indonesian government began distributing fortified baby food in 2001, arguing that homemade foods like *bubur* could not meet the nutritional needs of infants, as they were "sub optimal in micronutrients" (Kimura 2013: 111).

For much of the developing world, family meals are based around a cereal staple such as rice, wheat, or maize, with the addition of vegetables, legumes, and only occasionally meat or fish. This presents a problem for infants who adopt their family's meal format around six months of age, because breastmilk may constitute their only animal-based food, a fact that vegetarians who insist their breastfed children are vegetarian may overlook. Vegetarian mothers can breastfeed their children but they cannot claim to be feeding their children a diet based solely on plant products. To maximize the benefits of breastmilk, mothers are encouraged to breastfeed before meals, that is, before offering any other foods to their infants. But of course, because meals are defined and structured differently in all societies, we need to know more about local meal cycles and meal formats before making recommendations on breastfeeding in relation to meals. (It would also be interesting to know if mothers consider a breastfeeding episode to be an infant's meal.) In short, an infant needs to be breastfed and fed complementary foods more often than adults have meals.

According to WHO guidelines (2003), diets that do not contain animal source foods (meat, poultry, fish or eggs, plus milk products) cannot meet nutrient needs unless fortified products or nutrient supplements are used. Even small amounts of breastmilk increase the bioavailability of nutrients in complementary foods. This is one reason why breastmilk is so important to infant diets even after the addition of complementary foods. Without breastmilk, complementary foods available in poor households may well be inadequate. The non-breastfed child is considered to be in need of fortified complementary foods that baby food companies are ready to provide. Increasingly, breastfed infants are also considered to be in need of these special foods. This is not the case, according to Michael Latham, one of the most knowledgeable nutritionists concerned with infant feeding. He calculated that if a one-year-old consumed around 750 ml of breastmilk a day, he or she would meet 123 percent of their daily protein requirements, 113 percent of their vitamin A requirements, 60 percent of vitamin C, 83.3 percent of calcium, and 70.6 percent of their energy requirements. With moderate breastfeeding after the first year, a child might only need an extra 200 kcal from family foods to remain well-nourished (Latham 2008).

Sometimes adults or older siblings force an unwilling infant to swallow food that they do not want to eat or that they refuse to eat when offered. Force feeding is not limited to the Global South. The practice is not uncommon in North America among women who adhere rigidly to guidelines in advice books concerning the order and amount of foods that infants should eat at various ages. UK therapists dealing with children with feeding problems argue that coercive feeding is never helpful. In their efforts to conform to expert advice, mothers or caregivers may be unwilling to give up control over the infant's food intake or to tolerate messy inefficient self-feeding (cf. Southall and Schwartz 2000).

In some societies, adults and children eat together; in others, children eat first or after adults; in others, women and girls eat in a separate commensal circle from men and boys. These are part of culturally defined food systems and local customs. Infants everywhere love experimenting with the new foods available to them as they enter new commensal circles and learn to manipulate and taste the most valued foods (and nonfoods) within their reach. For the first year or two of life, babies put everything in their mouths rather indiscriminately. This experimental play with new tastes does not lead to immediate adoption of a new food. It takes around twenty-eight days or ten to fifteen tries from first taste to eating new foods. But by the end of the first year of life, infants have formed taste preferences that soon develop into very clear food preferences (Harris 2000: 79).

By three years of age, toddlers who previously enjoyed experimenting with new foods may suddenly begin refusing food and become picky eaters; neophiles may become neophobes. While their need for food increases, toddlers may meet those needs by consuming more food from a narrower selection of preferred foods (Nicklaus 2009: 254). In households where meals are both bland and monotonous and where children feed children, these universal facts of child development may not be so obvious. In such cases, imitation may play a more significant role. In the Global North, parental food and vegetable intake predicts child fruit and vegetable intake (Burnier et al. 2011: 200). But with no observations made at the commensal table the mechanisms are not clear; do toddlers imitate their parents and siblings or take foods from their hands or plates? In parts of the Global South such as Bogota, infants are expected to be able to eat anything by seven months of age (Castle et al. 1988: 51). In pre-revolutionary France, the "alimentary repertoire of early childhood was very limited." Historian, Ferrieres asked if the late introduction of complementary foods resulted in a rejection of or a greater sensitivity to "the strangeness of foods that lacked the scent of childhood" (2006: 85). Of course, for breastfed children, no family foods consumed by a mother and offered to her child would lack the scent (and taste) of childhood.

Biomedical research suggests the importance of introducing a wide variety of foods to infants early in life, as this predicts future food variety in adult diets, and food variety adds to the pleasure of eating (Nicklaus 2009: 254). Burnier et al. (2011) explored how exclusive breastfeeding influenced the range of food that children accept as they grow older, particularly vegetables. Euro-American children often fall well below recommendations for vegetable and fruit consumption. In an experiment with Canadian four-year-olds, the authors found that children who had been exclusively breastfed three months or more consumed more vegetables than four-year-olds who were formula-fed or not exclusively breastfed. Children who were sensitive to bitter taste rejected broccoli and cauliflower (Burnier et al. 2011: 198–200).

Commercial Baby Foods

Modern scientifically developed baby foods are a commercial form of transitional foods designed to meet the specific needs of infants six months of age and older. Commercially produced complementary foods are more expensive than traditional local foods and inaccessible to families in localities distant from markets. Amy Bentley's book, *Inventing Baby Food* (2014) documents the development of the industry in North America. The development of mass-produced baby foods in the 1930s had an enormous impact on North American infant-feeding patterns, and through development projects, in the Global South as well. Criticized as expensive industrially processed convenience food in small jars laden with sugar, salt, and preservatives, consumer critics pounced on every food safety violation, industrial accident, and misrepresentations in labeling and publicized them widely.

In Euro-American communities, commercial baby foods are available, relatively affordable, and heavily advertised and promoted. The first milk-based commercial infant formula was developed by Nestlé in 1867. Early infant formulas often included cereals and were marketed as foods not liquid breastmilk substitutes. These proprietary milk products competed alongside condensed and evaporated milks and custom-made preparations around the end of the century. In 1928, Gerber developed and marketed specialty foods for babies such as strained vegetables including peas, carrots, and spinach, and this successful innovation was emulated in the next decade by products developed by Heinz, Beech-Nut, and Libby's in North America. In 1931, Beech-Nut developed thirteen varieties of strained baby foods and sold them in patented vacuum-sealed clear glass jars, replacing lead-soldered metal cans. Over the next twenty years, the use of commercial baby food increased in middle- and upper-income North American homes (Bentley 2014: 50).

When these complementary foods were given to breastfed infants before six months old, they replaced more nutritious breastmilk. In the 1950s, when breastfeeding rates were lowest, commercial baby foods were given as early as two weeks (Bentley 2014: 64). North American doctors believed that breastmilk alone was inadequate. Mothers were proud when their babies ate solids early, taking it as a sign of rapid development. More likely, these baby foods supplemented infant formula, because only few women breastfed; in 1969, 73 percent of American infants used infant formula (Bentley 2014: 183).

In the 1970s, baby food companies began to promote age-specific baby foods including products for toddlers such as first dinners and junior foods. In July 2015, a range of organic mixtures in 4.5-oz. pouches were available at reasonable prices (four for $5.00) even in small towns in Ontario. These gourmet pouches included flavors such as peach maple cobbler, banana, apple and carrot; sweet potato and carrot; and banana, apple, apricot, and rice. Baby Gourmet offered meals of roasted squash and fruit medley; vanilla, banana, and berry risotto;

and apple crisp. Many mixtures advertised the addition of vanilla or cinnamon.[2] Pouches indicated whether they were suitable for babies seven, eight, or twelve months of age.

Food as medicine is part of the discourse that fragments the food system, making more room for commercial foods. Interventions to improve infant and young child feeding are part of this food as medicine trend. Nutritionism views food as a vehicle for the delivery of nutrients, creating profitable marketing opportunities for food companies, as we show in Chapter 7. In the process, it depoliticizes the food problem, reducing it to a technical problem to be solved by experts (Kimura 2013: 4, 5). In the case of baby food, experts were particularly fond of fortification, the addition of micronutrients to food products to increase their value.

Fortified foods for adults and children are neither new nor controversial. Iodized salt and fortified milk and flour have a long history in improving the nutritional status of populations. The search for protein-rich weaning foods with a flour base such as Incaparina in the 1960s and 1970s made profits for many NGOs as well as for food corporations, but failed to solve the problems of infant malnutrition. The search for these silver bullets ignores the fact that the causes of malnutrition are complex and include inequitable food and resource distribution. To succeed, fortified foods need to taste like familiar foods. That is, they need to be a source of pleasure as well as micronutrients. They should not be considered a medicine to be "well-tolerated" but a means of improving a diversified diet and enhancing the experience of eating.

Just as some adults survive on diets of soda pop and potato chips, so too some infants survive on dilute animal milks, herbal teas, and contaminated gruels—evidence of the adaptability of omnivores. But the cost of inadequate diets is much greater for infants and young children whose adult health will be compromised in ways we are just beginning to understand.

Modernity brought in the idea that individuals are responsible for eating a healthy diet in the face of increasingly complicated food choices. These ideas soon spread to diets of infants and young children. Individual responsibility for eating culminated in the idea that given time and no interference, infants would choose a healthy diet on their own. However, the experiments where infants selected their own diets that Clara Davis conducted in the 1920s and 1930s provided no junk food or foods with sugar (Bentley 2014: 48). The knowing infant contrasted with the idea of babies as born tabula rasa. Young children can regulate their diet to achieve an appropriate calorie load—even infants consuming infant formula; those who fail to thrive are often those who are unable to regulate their diet, and do not show compensatory feeding (Harris 2000: 80–82).

The study of infant and young child feeding cannot be isolated from family meals within the local food tradition. But research rarely explores how breastfeeding habits contribute to the eating styles of children or even adults. In fact, we seldom examine the relation between child feeding and adult eating, either through the life course of one individual, or the examination of child feeding within the context of household meals. But practitioners who deal with feeding problems of children have provided some hints, noting that active cooperation between mother and baby in breastfeeding sets the tone for later encounters with food with regard to the timing of meals and appetite control by infant. Breastfed babies later prefer self-feeding with spoons and finger foods, rather than being fed (Smale 2000: 129).

Early on, breastfeeding mothers recognize their children as guzzlers, nibblers, or as slow and steady feeders not easily disrupted from their meals. Their personal food identities, their eaters' careers begin early (cf. Rouch and O'Neil 2000: 182). How early are patterns such as picky eating or food refusal in order to control others established? Breastfed babies exhibit early infant responsibility for food intake, a pattern associated with less food pickiness in toddlers. Highly controlled feeding discourages children from adjusting their food intakes, with clear implications for childhood obesity (Fisher et al. 2000). Infant food preferences have been shown to persist well into childhood (Nicklaus et al. 2004). The practices of commensal eating also involve regulating of meal times, and we have yet to explore how child eating relates to learned mealtime hunger.

Weaning

Weaning or sevrage (the end of breastfeeding) can be a difficult and even dangerous time for children. Recall that humans wean their infants earlier than other primates, leaving them dependent on others for food for a longer time period (Sellen 2007: 124). Weaning is used in several senses to refer both to the end of breastfeeding and the introduction of nonmilk complementary foods. Because these processes may overlap over a long stretch of time, we refer here to the weaning interval as the time between the first introduction of solid foods and the last breastfeeding episode. The term, sevrage, reduces this ambiguity and refers to the end of breastfeeding. An infant who was never breastfed and introduced immediately to gruels, for example, might be said to be weaned onto gruels. In the English Oxford dictionary, the word weaning suggests the struggle to remove oneself from a valued activity.

The definitional problems are compounded by the fact that "human adults are never completely socially or nutritionally independent of others" (Sellen 2001: 3). In this sense, humans are never fully weaned. Anthropologists and others have tried to determine the ideal time for human infants to be weaned from the breast. Some have used primate models. But primate age of weaning models are poorly predictive for human populations (Sellen 2002a: 20) partly because of the flexibility and variation built in to the process. Ethnographic evidence reflects that variability, with weaning either gradual or abrupt taking place when children were around thirty months of age (Sellen 2007: 132). Based on primate models, Dettwyler (2004) predicted five to seven years for human age of weaning. But there is no upper age limit at which breastfeeding ceases to be of benefit to children (Sellen 2007: 131).

The WHO set standards based on biomedical evidence; weaning should begin when breastfeeding alone can no longer meet an infant's nutritional needs, at six months of age, when complementary foods should be added to the diet (World Health Organization 1979). The age of weaning emerges from the interactions of mothers and infants and should be "exquisitely sensitive to local feeding and disease ecology" (Sellen 2006: 160). The timing of weaning depends on the individual constitutions of mothers and infants, and their local food system, influenced by seasonality and resource distribution. Some communities identify cues such as walking, talking, teeth eruption, or a new pregnancy that changes the taste of the breastmilk; an event like carrying a food dish to father marked both the end of breastfeeding and the resumption of sexual activity among Tanzanian groups like the Chagga (Raum 1940).

When we focus attention on the mother–infant dyad, we move away from looking exclusively at the nutritional impact of sevrage on infants and consider, too, the costs and benefits to mothers. Sellen points out the potential for conflicts of interest in the trade-offs between mothers, infants, and siblings (2006: 161), reminding us that "assumptions that the interests of the mother usually coincide with those of the child remain untested" (Sellen 2002b: 226). His research on pastoral groups in Tanzania shows that weaning stress does not necessarily reflect maternal-infant conflict of interest but rather ecological constraints on both (Sellen 2006: 183). By focusing on the mother–infant dyad, we avoid the problem of measuring to what extent the interests of mothers and children coincide or conflict. North American popular culture presents weaning as a battle that mothers must win as they battle for control over their infants.

When a child no longer depends on its mother's body for sustenance, profound changes occur—in the food consumed, the process of eating, the relation between eater and feeder, and even where and when the meal is consumed. Sevrage can be a dramatic activity change for infants. Breastfeeding, an activity the infant was very skilled at, and derived emotional and sensual pleasure from, ends. Rage, depression, and a feeling of rejection are some of the emotional responses of infants when the end of the activity of breastfeeding also marks (or is interpreted as marking) the end of a special relationship with the mother. This is compounded when the mother is pregnant or breastfeeding a new baby.

Sevrage represents an activity change for mothers also. An activity that has defined and organized much of their mothering work has ended, requiring women to reconnect with their pre-breastfeeding bodies and lives. This transition may be formally marked by a return to sexual relations, a change in sleeping arrangements, and a rearrangement of clothes, completing the bodily separation from her infant. The transition may be easy for mothers who may be filled with relief at getting their bodies back, or quite difficult.

Sevrage defines a change in the nurturing relationship; a special bond is ending, incurring a loss for both, regardless of who began the process; it is always a negotiation for every mother–infant dyad, even when it appears to be easily accomplished. Mothers may have to remove themselves entirely from the commensal table until a toddler is content to forego breastmilk. It is possible that before sevrage, mothers and infants have had special access to each other and to special foods, and that access may be lost after breastfeeding ends, when, for example, siblings may be assigned to feed or oversee the feeding of a toddler. The health consequences for the baby displaced from the breast may be quite severe in locations where breastmilk was the major protein source. The process of weaning can be gradual or abrupt, initiated by the infant or the mother, and shaped by customs on how to ease the transition. Common in the literature is the tactic to smear hot pepper on nipples to discourage nursing.[3]

Some North American women look back at the experience with pride and humor; as a mother who planned to nurse for six months, but ended up nursing for "two and a half unforgettable years," prepares to "close up shop," she writes: "As that time approaches, I treasure this magical milk as if it were the last sweet drops of my youth. When Sydney Rose nurses, I savour the silence, and her slumber, and the warmth of her little hand against my arm" (Scott 2009: 14). These sentimental mothering experiences could not be further removed from the dangers of kwashiorkor, the malnutrition caused by being displaced from the breast.

To return to the dance metaphor, weaning should not be a march or a battle, but more like that awkward moment when the dance ends and the partners do not quite know what to do. Should they walk away? Continue to hold hands? Mumble a thank you? Or look around for someone new, a better more interesting partner for the next dance?

Sevrage marks the end of embodied commensality. After sevrage, mothers and their children are no longer bodily linked, but young children remain dependent on others to meet their food needs. They now share household foods with other family members, whether these households are food secure or food insecure. They may have special dishes prepared for them or simply consume the dishes prepared for other household members; either way, they experience a wider range of tastes and textures as their food universe expands.

Families and Child Feeding

All human societies develop distinct food traditions that help balance our craving for flavorful food and the amount of food we consume before we experience food aversion (Shepherd 2012: 239).[4] In fact, cooking, along with language, may have emerged together in our human evolution, as we bonded around the pleasures of sharing and preparing cooked food (cf. Shepherd 2012: 231). We experience contemporary food systems through inherited customs and traditions, and then live within these traditions, preparing, producing, and distributing food, planning meals, and eating them—the common bowl of rice with side dishes, the bread to soak up thick soup, the wild greens eaten with game or fish, or pizza from a fast-food outlet. Each food item and meal format has a history and a place in a broader culinary system. Each new generation shapes old recipes, introduces unfamiliar food items, and creates new recipes. Food systems, cooking, and cuisine are constantly evolving in all societies, making it impossible or foolish to identify an authentic or traditional dish as an unchanging signifier of group identity. Institutional meals, as well, are never left to chance. For example, prisons and monasteries provided meal regimes that encouraged the formation of self-reflecting, self-regulating individuals (Coveney 2000: 87).

During family meals, age and gender differences may be reflected in spatial differentiation (eating in different places), temporal differences (eating more or less often or at different times), as well as qualitative and quantitative differences in the foods served (cf. Dietler 2001: 91). For example, research on intrafamily food distribution suggests that women may compensate for reduced access to food at meal times by finishing up the food remnants on their children's plates, snacking while preparing food or nibbling tidbits from kitchen leftovers.

A Canadian mother and food writer notes: "They say you learn a lot from your children. Mine have taught me how to eat." She recalls that her breastfed twins eat everything, "sometimes combining foods in unexpected ways." As she finished the honey-garlic chicken wings on their plates along with bits of apricots for dessert, she appreciated their messy mixture: "It was a delicious combination, the tartness of the fruit complementing the sweet chicken" (Pataki 2006).

Infant-feeding complexes are embedded in food traditions, not separate from them. Thus, information on such seemingly esoteric details as meal format (how dishes are combined and presented to make a typical meal) is critically important for understanding infant and young child feeding. For example, simultaneous common bowl formats and formats where all dishes are served at once create different modes of food sharing from meals where courses are served sequentially. Different meal formats offer different rules of commensality, with potential consequences for feeding infants and children. With this perspective in mind, we could determine what meal formats give children an advantage, common bowl or their own plate, for example.

Breastfeeding and young child feeding develop out of household practices including kitchen activities, and are shaped by conditions such as poverty, family traditions, and adult food preferences. If there are fortified foods such as salt or flour in the kitchens, these ingredients will likely be used for infant and child feeding. But if fruits and vegetables are considered unhealthy food items for adults, they will unlikely be served to children. That is, beliefs and resources that guide adult eating also shape infant and young child feeding. As North American urbanites became more enamored with organic foods, commercial baby food companies began to provide gourmet organic baby and toddler food using ingredients such as brown rice, quinoa, and roasted squash.

Children also use meals as opportunities for independence: "When a parent tries to spoon up food for her, she snatches the utensil away, for she would rather do something poorly all by herself than have someone else do it well" (Wolf 1993: 319). Wolf refers to this childish desire to feed herself as the expression of her "inner bad girl," calling to mind the conversations of recovered anorexics (cf. O'Connor and Van Esterik 2015).

The differences between French and American approaches to child feeding are instructive. In a comparison of American and French family meals, American parents allowed children more control over their food intake and used energy-dense nonnutritive foods as rewards, all the while teaching their children about nutrition. In contrast, French parents monitored and restricted their children's food intake, but served them fresh, high-quality food items; these observations reflect very different approaches to food, meals, and the body (Musher-Eizenman et al. 2009). Toddlers in day care in France are served three-course meals, where they learn to appreciate the taste of good food and the pleasure of mealtimes. This pattern continues in elementary schools where collective eating of school lunches provides an opportunity to further teach children the patterns and pleasures of commensality in shared public spaces.[5]

French food culture challenges the "food liberalism" associated with North American practices of undisciplined eating—eating to excess at any time of the day. But rarely have the links between adult and infant feeding been clearly shown. In a powerful innovative study of infant feeding in France, Gervaise Debucquet and Valerie Adt (2015) explore how French mothers use different medical and naturalist discourses about infant-feeding methods. Feeding infants involves teaching them how to eat in the French way, including learning about taste and the rules of eating a balanced diet. Both mothers who breastfed and mothers who bottle-fed believed that their chosen method was the quickest, most efficient way to transmit these norms of French cuisine to the next generation.

The research was part of larger efforts to understand the nutritional footprint that might predispose adults to diseases later in life. In addition to observing mothers breastfeeding or bottle feeding their infants, the researchers asked about the perceived risks of breastfeeding and formula feeding. Their sample selected for women at two extremes of a spectrum of infant-feeding practices, those strongly supportive of breastfeeding and those who favor artificial feeding, noting in particular their diametrically different views of the maternal body.

Women who bottle-feed by choice not by default generally lack confidence in their bodies; when pregnant, they used vitamins and supplements to enhance their pregnant bodies. Their preference for infant formula is an extension of their confidence that the product is scientifically controlled, carefully monitored, consistent, pure, and standardized. They are concerned that human milk is not always clean, because it is dependent on the lifestyle and hygiene of the mother.

Breastfeeding mothers held a more symbiotic body image, recognizing that everything is interconnected, including morality. They valued eating well, balanced their meals, and considered the origin of every food item. They recognize that human milk is a living substance, constantly changing and adapting to the infant's needs. Even the risk of chemical contamination is interpreted differently by mothers who breastfeed. They trust their bodies to do the work of purifying the breastmilk as it passes through the maternal body.

Mothers trust that their breastfed infants can self-regulate their food intake; they know when they are hungry and know when to stop eating; they cannot eat too much. In contrast, bottle-feeding mothers assume that breastfed infants are indulged, cannot self-regulate, and will become obese, because their mothers cannot control or measure the amount of breastmilk consumed at a feed. To these mothers, the bottle itself imposes healthy rhythms and correct rules on the child. However, the bottle-fed baby can be force-fed or encouraged to finish the bottle or bowl and thus does not learn to self-regulate.

Mothers of breastfed infants aimed to expand the taste and sensory experiences of their children. As one breastfeeding mother explained, "When you breastfeed, from an early age the child is already 'at the family table.' They taste everything the mother eats. The milk never tastes the same" (Debucquet and Adt 2015: 93). In this explanatory model, there is no need for early introduction of solids or family foods because breastfed infants have already tasted family foods. On the other hand, bottle-fed infants need solids earlier than four months in order to learn to eat the full taste range of family foods.

Commensality is not a singular process but is open to many levels of individualization from collective to individual. Collective eating is the commensal ideal—family and friends sitting at the same table, eating the same food, at the same time. But for many Euro-American individuals and families, that is a fantasy, a nostalgic memory of shared meals that never were. A study of family meals in the UK identified two strategies families use to incorporate children's tastes into the family meals. The first strategy, "what we fancy," stressed the continuous negotiation between parents and children around the content of meals, with the result that parents often served individualized meals to suit their children's tastes. Another familial strategy focused on creating a repertoire of set meals that the whole family could share, and discouraged the preparation of separate meals to cater to their children's individual tastes. The study hinted at the importance of embedded practices around commensality and how these reflect and respond to individual taste preferences of family members (Thompson et al. 2016).

While Europeans value meals as bonding moments, North Americans have difficulty sustaining the myth of the bonding aspect of family meals. Michael, an American teenager, was always berated during family meals; he shoveled food in and dreaded family meals, creating great stress associated with eating that played out in other aspects of his adult life as emotional and health problems (Taylor 2002: 53, 66). Scheduling conflicts compromise family meals. In North America, commensality as food sharing and eating together is changing form. Microwaving a precooked stew or grabbing a frozen muffin, and eating it alone after school or work suggests that eating is just an act of fueling the body-machine and should be done quickly and alone.

Does commensality require consuming the same foods at the same time? Is it strengthened by meal formats that allow for some individuation—a little more of this, a little less of that as French school children learn? Meal formats in Southeast Asia use condiments to make it easy to have individualized tastes in a collective setting, as we show in Chapter 5. Individual taste preferences in these meal formats do not break down commensality. This pattern of individualization of tastes is replicated in North America in the elaboration of processed foods such as Ramen instant noodles and Kraft dinners (in Canada, macaroni and cheese in the United States). Certainly shared tastes strengthen commensality, as the French socialization of tastes in toddlers and school children indicates.

The Challenge of Choice

Commensal circles expand and contract, shaped by explicit and implicit boundaries of similarities and differences, including class, caste, age, ethnicity, gender, and state of health. Individuals move in and out of these circles throughout the life cycle. Commensality presents many tensions, but when the will to eat together and share food is strong, accommodations can be made in the kitchen or at the table, and commensality of a sort can be maintained. The gatekeepers of family meals, usually women, may go out of their way to cater to the preferences of their children and spouses, regardless of the extra work involved (cf. DeVault 1991). A North American professional woman might have to adjust meals to meet the needs of a diabetic family member, a dieting teenager, and her visiting kosher Jewish friend. A rural Kenyan woman might have to consider the food needs of a pregnant daughter, an elder with missing teeth, a breastfed toddler, and a cousin with AIDS.

Commensality is under challenge, often glossed as the decline in family meals. This may reflect the lack of shared food ideology; food is fuel for some and cultural identity within the commensal group for others—and they may be eating at the same table. Fewer people follow group-defining commensal restrictions such as caste, halal, or kosher rules. In North America, the situation of the vegan in the meat-eating household, the kosher wife with a nonkosher spouse, the health nut on a perpetual search for the perfect diet for losing weight, for increasing energy, for recovering from the flu, might be solved by eating out.

Eating out facilitates eating together without necessarily eating the same food and solves certain problems associated with family meals, such as avoiding conflict over items to be served, particularly as eating in North America becomes more individualized. Buffets also solve some of the problems of individual food preferences, allowing people to eat together while choosing their own combination of foods. But buffets offer even greater potential for excess consumption and excess waste. They also offer an excess of choice, and choices can complicate our lives, adding to stress and depression. "Suddenly, everything was too difficult: too many glasses, utensils, and waiters. Choices needed to be made" (Weiss 1997: 133).

In industrialized urban settings, bottle feeding may be perceived as solving problems for some women and some infants (but causing problems for most). To start with, parents must choose between a wide range of bottles and brands of infant formula. For a trip to a restaurant, a bottle-fed baby needs more equipment, and may require the services of a restaurant to heat up the meal. Yet many stories recounted by mothers who breastfeed in public involve being asked to leave restaurants.

The myths of the harmony, intimacy, and commensal pleasure of family meals makes it hard to talk about picky eating, both as a development phase that toddlers go through and an identity marker of some teenagers and adults in Euro-American communities. Picky eaters consistently reject large groups of food or preparation methods and refuse to sample new foods, limiting the variety of foods they consume. A recent study confirmed that breastfeeding and delaying the introduction of complementary foods until six months reduced the chances of picky eating during childhood; exclusive breastfeeding for six months reduced the odds of developing a preference for specific food preparation methods by 78 percent, food rejection by 81 percent, and food neophobia by 75 percent (Shim et al. 2011). As we have shown earlier, breastfeeding broadens the palate, encouraging children to appreciate a wider variety of flavors. When infants are exposed to a wide variety of tastes in utero and then through colostrum and breastmilk, they are less likely to be picky eaters and more likely to enjoy trying new tastes. But if complementary food is added too early, the gut is not yet ready to receive the food and eating may cause pain or an allergic reaction.

For picky eaters of any age, meals can be unbearable, food tastes awful, and the fear of gagging or throwing up might trigger eating disorders such as bulimia later in life. When we think that a food has made us sick once, we lose our taste for it, and avoid it; perhaps this lies behind the food phobias that develop in childhood and may last a lifetime. It is hard to change aversions to foods (Shepherd 2012: 127, 236).

However, UK therapists argue that there is no direct causal relation between childhood feeding problems (including picky eating) and eating disorders; in their framing, feeding implies a relationship, while eating does not (Southall and Schwartz 2000: v). We have argued that eating disorders are also embedded in social relations and cannot be considered as simply individual pathologies (cf. O'Connor and Van Esterik 2015). Eating disorders may be one consequence of an abundance of food, where eating more than your share, or the fear of eating more than your share are both realistic possibilities. Certainly, disordered eating brings out the tensions between commensality and choice. We have yet to fully explore the relation between picky eating, commensality, and food security.

Anorexia in North America is a rejection of commensality, intimacy, reciprocity, and nurturance, characterized by the refusal to nurture self and join commensal events. Even after treatment, anorexics can relapse if they go back into same toxic food environments with the same relationships to food (O'Connor and Van Esterik 2015).

Goody (1982) argues that eating is a way of placing ourselves in relation to others. And Probyn develops the argument that food and its relation to bodies is fundamentally about power, that eating is an alternative way to look at power (2000: 7). Eating and hunger connects us to other humans, but not to anorexics, most of whom have food and cannot or will not eat it. To Probyn, the anorexic body engenders disgust (2000: 9). Probyn situates the moral dilemma of anorexics: "One half of the world sits eating their evening meal in front of the set watching the other half starve to death" (2000: 40), or worse, sits eating nothing when food is available to them. Do anorexics make us feel shame because we have eaten their share of the food (Probyn 2000: 130)? Or is our sense of shame because their asceticism makes us feel weak and indulgent? In Thailand, ascetic monks restrict their food intake so that laity can be indulgent. It is not only people who are anorexic who avoid sharing food. Some institutions refuse to share excess food, including restaurant workers who mix garbage in with leftover food to make leftovers inedible for hungry dumpster divers.

Some of us stay too long at the commensal table, overindulging in the pleasure of the table. Or perhaps it is not time at the table, as Italians and French may spend two to three hours at the table, compared with Americans' fifteen minutes. It is more likely that what is consumed at the table that causes the problems. Modern diets with sugars, salt, and fats in abundant supply contribute to the rise in obesity (Moss 2013). Many people are attracted by the smell of fast foods and the appeal of salt and sugar, as human brains respond to multiple sensory inputs (Shepherd 2012: 185, 186). The high content of salt and sugar in some baby foods sets the stage for the demand for salty or sweet processed foods later in life, contributing to the development of the industrial palate, the taste preference or craving for salt and sugar.

Infant feeding has important links to obesity. Generally, breastfeeding advocates have been very balanced about claiming that breastfeeding reduced the chances of obesity later in life. In fact, the evidence is mixed, because the routes to obesity are varied. Breastfeeding and healthy eating early in life is the first strategy for combatting obesity. On the other hand, the mechanisms as to how breastfeeding might protect against obesity are quite well understood; these include appetite control, portion size, and the fact that breastfeeding requires work on the part of the infant. How does bottle feeding disrupt an infant's capacity to self-regulate? According to Joan Wolf, the evidence that breastfeeding reduces later obesity is not compelling, the protective effect, small or inconclusive (Wolf 2010: 25, 142). Yet research clearly shows that use of infant formula links to obesity in later childhood and adulthood (von Kries et al. 1999; Bergmann et al. 2003). Smith (2007) documents the links between rising rates of obesity and poor infant-feeding practices in Australia, particularly the increasing use of artificial baby milks.

Childhood obesity is also linked to the genetic make-up of parents along with the eating environment they provide. Efforts to control or restrict a child's access to foods—especially appealing foods—appears to promote the development of overweight in children; the mechanisms may be through increasing the child's desire for those foods, or by increased eating in the absence of hunger (Faith and Kerns 2005: 165). Neurogastronomical research suggests that eating dull boring food stimulates craving for more flavorful foods (Shepherd 2012: 166). Bored with one flavor, a new flavor stimulates renewed eating (Shepherd 2012: 189). This could be one route to the obesity associated with infant formula use. Infants may be bored by monotonous tasting food such as the standardized taste of soy or cow's milk-based infant formula, and seek out new tastes. Does that child then lose its "taste" for flavors or find new foods unappealing? How long do they remember the tastes they experienced in utero? How long do taste memories from "eating in" last?

Exposure to food shortages or famine in early gestation programmed obesity in later life, as Ravelli et al. (1999) showed using the data from the Dutch famine of 1944. Human rights advocates go so far as to argue that socioeconomic disadvantage is perpetuated across the generations by the channel of overweight or obesity (de Schutter 2011: 16).

An American policy maker asks why breastfeeding is invisible in the conversation about increasing rates of obesity and chronic disease, recognizing breastfeeding as a natural method of getting baby to regulate appetite and understand portion control (McTeer 2012: 325). Once again, we find the inability to see or acknowledge the risks of infant formula use in North America.

Much like other eating disorders, attempts to deal with obesity have not been successful because eating is deeply embedded in commensality and social relations as well as the political economy of poverty. Fat activism and Overeaters Anonymous are not like Alcoholics Anonymous where abstention is required. We still need to eat every day (but not to drink alcohol every day); thus an overweight person must self-regulate at every meal, every day, putting an extra strain on them, particularly if they occupy a toxic food environment. The self-regulation that is set in infancy through breastfeeding is very different from the self-regulation demanded of an obese adult trying to lose weight.

Leaving the Commensal Circle

Like infants, the frail elderly thrive only if someone nurtures them in their last days. Those with dental or digestive problems may return to the soft bland foods of infancy. The elderly may lose their appetites, and take themselves out of the commensal circle to eat alone or be fed. The elderly, like infants and young children, may be categorized as "failure to thrive" on the basis of loss of sensory abilities including smell, suggesting the need to "reactivate the cravings of childhood, enhancing the senses that contribute to flavor with strong smells, strong tastes, crunchy texture, bright colors, pleasant music—and talking pleasantly together as you eat the shared meal" (Shepherd 2012: 241). Such nurturing practices are still active in many parts of the world where the elderly, particularly elder women, have a special role to play in nurturing the next generation.

Modernity brings new problems of isolation in North America where elderly widows or widowers may be eating alone, refusing food, as appetites and capacities diminish. Stories of widows who did not know what they liked to eat after their husbands died or the widows who only began eating what they liked after their husbands died attest to the degree to which women who spend their life preparing food for others may find they are unable to nurture themselves.

Other communities may form a new commensal circle of and for the elderly. Thai elders often become Buddhist precept keepers, restricting their eating to one meal a day eaten before noon, emulating the monks. Often their grandchildren accompany them to the temple and consume some of the snacks that have been donated to the monks and shared with the precept keepers. In South Asia, elderly widows may be pushed out of the commensal circle and have difficulty feeding themselves.

The end of life, the process of dying, occurs in an orderly progression when it is not medicalized. Part of the process of shutting down includes a decrease in appetite and the reduced intake of food and fluids, as the body reduces its need for energy. At the end of life, particularly in North America, decisions may be made to enforce nurture by attempting to pressure a dying person to eat or drink or to resort to tube feeding. Force feeding, in infancy and old age, takes control away from the person fed. This removal of agency is harder to explain for competent elders who may simply not wish to have commensality imposed on them.

End of life decisions in North America often concern inserting or withdrawing feeding tubes. In extreme cases, withdrawing nourishment or deciding not to use a feeding tube may be the last act of nurture. Although such decisions usually involve the elderly, end of life decisions are particularly poignant when a child is dying. Catherine Porter documented the death of Stella, a redheaded three-year-old in Toronto, writing of the last days and hours as Stella took ten steps toward the dark and a step back into the light. In Stella's step back, she ate her favorite foods—porridge, applesauce, chocolate donut holes (timbits), macaroni and cheese, washed down by milk. But this honeymoon did not last long, and she declined into a state where she could not eat or drink. Her palliative care doctor explained that eating less is a symptom of dying, not its cause. Even if others force people to eat, they do not gain weight, feel better, or have more energy. Her parents decided not to subject Stella to tube feeding. Feeding tubes are for the benefit of the survivors, not the dying, and may cause painful complications. "Dying is a physically hard process … It's parallel to giving birth," her palliative care doctor explained. Her family made a death plan much as they had made a birth plan (Porter 2012).

Humans come in and out of life by way of nurture not hunger. We come into the world without hunger and leave without hunger, in spite of the desire of others to feed us. A medicalized birth makes it difficult to start feeding; a medicalized death makes it difficult to stop feeding. Either way, the dance of nurture choreographs the first and last moments of person-making. Death is also a dance—danse macabre—as artists have known for centuries.

Food Fights vs the Dance of Nurture

The dance of nurture is not without its food fights. But these are ongoing negotiations, a taken-for-granted part of nurture. Even weaning should be a dance based on mutuality and coregulation, not a battle for control. But today breastfeeding problems are often addressed as if they represent the first food fight, a pattern that sets the stage for later food fights in the family and beyond. Food fights are local and personal experiences reflecting embodied tensions around food.

This chapter orients us back to the life cycle and how breastfeeding fits in to wider food systems. Here commensality or food sharing epitomizes nurture, as culture and custom shape who eats what, and how much with whom. By placing breastfeeding within the broader context of the life cycle, we show that it is more than a method of feeding and not an isolated activity but a larger biocultural practice that links generations.

What does commensality teach us about the dance of nurture? It might suggest we replace the phrase, "You are what you eat," with "You are how you were fed," or "how you feed others," putting the stress not on the food consumed but the social relations of eating and feeding. Commensal circles ensure that people eat and feed each other regularly. Collective cooking and eating is one way to solve the problem of making sure that everyone is adequately fed. There are many different ways to do this, from church potluck suppers to soup kitchens to potlatches and feasts of merit. While individuals move in and out of commensal circles, the circles themselves never end; new people are always brought in as others leave. We examine these circles as they operate in Southeast Asia in the next chapter.

Notes

1. An earlier draft version of this argument was published in Van Esterik (2015).
2. Mixtures like these make it difficult for parents to identify food sensitivities.
3. Would this be uncomfortable for the mother? I tried it on my own nonlactating nipple but felt only a mild warmth (PVE).
4. Shepherd does not discuss the role of breastfeeding in creating this balance.
5. Wendy Leynse discussed food socialization of school children in France at the meetings of the Association for the Study of Food and Society held at the University of Vermont, June 2014.

PART III

Diversities

Part III explores in two chapters how and why context matters. Regional patterns exist within the wide range of cultural styles of infant feeding in households, communities, and societies around the world. Chapter 5 illustrates the diversity of infant feeding styles in Southeast Asia, a region where nurture is highly valued. Chapter 6 examines how modern life disrupts the contexts that make nurture possible, including the intimate act of breastfeeding. Modernity alters the way we experience nurture, often by terrorizing our bodies and beings. Modern logic complicates nurturing practices, denying their evolutionary and biological roots. But modernity does not erase the fact that we exist by virtue of the nurture of others, and most families successfully nurture their children, but at an increasing cost.

CHAPTER 5

Customizing Nurture in Southeast Asia

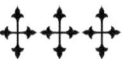

This chapter looks at regional solutions to the universal problem of how to feed and nurture a newborn (cf. Goldschmidt 1990: 120). Because breastfeeding is embedded in regional contexts, we turn to one region of the world, Southeast Asia where, by comparing cultures that are cousins, we can begin to tease apart biology, culture, history, and chance to better understand nurture and breastfeeding. Breastfeeding, a highly evolved biological universal, joins with deeply felt cultural particulars to create biocultural hybrids that take on contingent lives of their own. That hybridization typically unfolds in culturally protected space, the social womb (Chapter 2). Ontogenetically breastfeeding develops a social sensibility that equips the infant to enter the commensal circle (Chapter 4) where the newcomer learns the wider culture's ways. How do these customs play out in Southeast Asia? Are customs surrounding the social womb and the commensal circle stable legacies or ever-changing adaptations to local conditions? Or both?

What is a possible entry point for examining diverse patterns of nurture in Southeast Asia? Would religion or seasonality make a better starting point? Do subsistence patterns account for some of the variation in infant-feeding practices? How do these relate to meal formats and food-sharing practices? Everyday religion across Southeast Asia is probably so well adapted to subsistence and seasonality that it may not matter where we begin. The way infants are nurtured in Southeast Asia is entangled with cropping patterns and gender systems, for example. Although we want to avoid an unproductive materialist evolutionary approach based on subsistence patterns (cf. Huber 2007),¹ different crops create different worlds (cf. O'Connor 2011). Many of the commonalities in the Southeast Asian worlds we explore here are shaped by an underlying adaptation to rice agriculture; in brief, you nurture people as you nurture rice. Even in the root crop economies of Southeast Asia, rice is still the prestige food (cf. Janowski and Kerlogue 2007). If different crops create different worlds, surely the first food given to a human newborn—either food produced by another human or food produced by a cow—also create different worlds. These different worlds also exist inside infant bodies in the form of distinct gut ecologies or microbiomes, as discussed in Chapter 3.

Ethnographic evidence from this region illustrates the incredible local diversity in nurturing practices among mothers and infants across the region, among mothers and infants in the same society, and even between any two children of the same birth mother. We try to look beyond the clichés about the nation-states of Southeast Asia to the legacies of the Southeast Asian core, where we find contingencies and continuities, and not simply the contrasts between mainland and island, upland and lowland, and bounded ethnic groups. Although we would like to get beyond ethnic groups into themes, the evidence we have to work with is coded by ethnicity.

We use the term, infant-feeding style, to describe some of these patterned continuities. Breastfeeding style is a conceptual tool that is useful for addressing patterned variation within traditions. The term breastfeeding style and infant-feeding style refer to the systematic manner of feeding an infant characteristic of members of a group, in a particular time and place.[2] Like typing, riding a bicycle or blacksmithing (cf. Dougherty and Keller 1982), breastfeeding is an activity learned through practice until it feels natural. If it never feels natural, it may never fit in to a woman's everyday life and be abandoned. Every mother–infant pair develops their own personal breastfeeding style within a local style of infant feeding. A woman's personal style reflects her own constitution and that of her newborn, as well as the continuity of a breastfeeding style shared among related women and passed down through the generations in the form of customs and even memories. Each infant-feeding style touches a truth about the human condition and reflects back to our shared primate and human heritage. But as we explored in Chapter 3, this heritage did not produce a fixed template for feeding or raising infants, nor even a guarantee of problem-free milk production and milk ejection among all women all the time.

Using Ethnography

Women give birth and breastfeed in highly local life worlds in very specific local niches. These local regimens occupy the middle ground between the uniqueness of every mother–infant pair and inherited customs, framed within biocultural universals. Ethnographic work provides the local contexts that fill the conceptual gap between individuals as actors and population groups as defined by epidemiologists (cf. Sellen 2002b: 224). But it is epidemiological models, not ethnography, that inform health and nutrition policy around infant feeding, a topic we explore further in Chapter 7.

Our ethnographic examples are not introduced to suggest how our distant ancestors fed their children (cf. Hausman 2003) nor as guides for paleo-parenting, following the style of contemporary hunters and gatherers. Nor are they reminders of how other people's traditional customs so often get it wrong, thus identifying what needs to be changed through modern interventions. Nor is ethnographic evidence presented in order to train health workers how to show cultural sensitivity to different clients in order to improve compliance. Health educators use ethnographic examples to predict how health messages and interventions are likely to be received. When messages and policies about infant feeding fail, then "cultural factors" can be blamed for the mismatch between global policy and local practice (cf. Nichter 2008).

Ethnography does show the plasticity and variation in infant-feeding patterns in time and space—information that anthropologists have been supplying to health professionals for more than a century. But ethnographic evidence does more than provide positivist provision of anecdotal evidence to spice up bio-medical reports and demonstrate cultural awareness. How can we make the best use of ethnographic information and get beyond the "culture box" included in health education materials?

Cultural sensitivity plus lab logic does not produce answers about nurturing practices such as breastfeeding. These practices are wholes that cannot be reduced to the sum of their parts. Breastfeeding in Southeast Asia, as in other regions, is always a product of different historical heritages. Individual ethnographers cannot always see these patterns in the field; they can only be seen comparatively. For us, they are glimpses into pieces of larger puzzles about nurture that we have yet to fully recognize. Hence our call for the New Ethnology, when fieldwork alone is not enough.

Using the logic of the New Ethnology, we can take these surface observations, these ethnographic tidbits, and use them to look for patterns based on deeper historical causes. These might include the movement of Austronesian and Austroasiatic speakers into the region, the fact that Tai groups are latecomers to the mainland, and the Hmong, later still, each bringing their distinct heritages to the region. The mosque built on top of the cockfight pit in Bali is a reminder that Bali is not as Islamicized as the rest of Indonesia.

We use these ethnographic examples to illustrate nurturing practices not to define culturally normative patterns throughout Southeast Asia. We show that breastfeeding in the region is itself a product of different historical heritages that are not obvious to the ethnographer in the field, but to the ethnologist comparing cases. We provide evidence about how local regimens fit breastfeeding and child feeding with other activities. Local ethnographic contexts provide the conditions that personal breastfeeding styles must adapt to or react against, providing the raw materials for mothers as bricoleurs to use, as they make do with the available material and social resources at their disposal.

This wide variation in infant-feeding practices is not surprising, given that breastfeeding is one way that mothers embody and pre-adapt infants to their widely varied social and ecological surroundings. Clearly, not all of these feeding and nurturing practices are ideal "best practices" from a biomedical perspective, but they illustrate the importance of social relations in nurturing a child. For example, they show us how postpartum customs often separate the mother–infant pair and relieve the mother from daily work responsibilities.

Ethnographies may unintentionally contribute to stereotyping other ways of life. Just as there is no generic human milk, there is no generic Southeast Asia. While we cringe at creating "the pastoral mother," "the hunting and gathering mother," "the urban industrial mother," all ethnographies contribute to the creation of categories, as much as we might try to avoid the abuses of generalization. We aim to look for regional patterns, the commonalities within horticultural, pastoral, agricultural, and industrial societies. While we recognize that terms like Thai or Canadian or Navajo or Egyptian are too broad, we argue that there is a coherence to Thai child-rearing that resonates with Malay or Burmese child-rearing, and differs from Navajo child-rearing, for example.

Southeast Asia consists of the mainland countries of Burma, Thailand, Lao PDR, Vietnam, and Cambodia, and the island countries of Malaysia,[3] Indonesia, Singapore, Brunei, East Timor, and the Philippines. It is perhaps risky to invoke a regional pattern based on a definition coined in World War II to define a military operation, but there are commonalities that give an integrity to the region. Traditional scholarship defines its coherence partly from a series of contrasts—between mainland and island, upland and lowland, palace and village, rice and root crops, dry rice and irrigated rice—contrasts that help organize the incredible diversity of ethnic groups and languages in the region. Here we try to move beyond these contrasts to identify a Southeast Asian core of continuities and shared legacies.

An underlying feature that exists in contrast to surrounding east and south Asia is the importance of gender complementarity in the region, glossed as the high status of women, a concept that has also been critiqued. The centrality of women in the production, preparation, and marketing of food is near universal in the region. The title of Barbara Andaya's book on women in Southeast Asian history, *The Flaming Womb* (2006) draws attention to women's reproductive power in premodern Southeast Asia. She cites a Javanese myth that describes a woman's glowing secret part, the gleam of light visible between her thighs (Andaya 2006: 1). This sacred power was not framed as impurity until the world religions layered more patriarchal ideology over indigenous Southeast Asian concepts of feminine nurturing power. Nurturing power included the skilled use of medicinal plants, healing, assisting at births, and wet nursing. Andaya points out that Islam reinforced indigenous ideas of a special relationship between individuals breastfed by the same woman (2006: 129).

Differently constructed food systems and meal formats manage the work of care and nurture differently. A common meal format in Southeast Asia consists of rice in a common bowl and dishes that go with the rice—soups, stews, steamed or stir-fried vegetables, sauces, and condiments. Sharing rice and rice wine creates community while dividing meat imposes hierarchy, as we see in the Torajan example, among others. Female rice with male meat emphasizes the complementarity of meals and gender throughout the region.

The patterns around nurture and care flow through different levels of analysis and across linguistic and ethnic divides in the region. Southeast Asian examples are of special interest because some groups are in the process of leaping from local traditions of fertility or ancestor worship to operating within modern bureaucratic capitalism and public health systems in a single generation. Customs can change quickly; within one generation, women in Northeast Thailand chose to give birth in hospitals rather than at home (Whitaker 1999: 221). How will these rapid changes affect nurturing practices, encoded in local customs?

For much of the world, nurture is embedded in traditions much deeper than the textually traceable dictates of world religions like Christianity, Islam, and Buddhism. The former are deeply patriarchal, but they are often preceded by life-cycle fertility religions—agricultural cults that respect nurture in its feminine form. In much of Southeast Asia, mother rice and mother earth are honored in the form of a pregnant woman who make plants and children grow. Rice and humans both have spirits that must be nurtured (cf. Hanks 1964). Coding the spirit protectors of rice, rivers, and earth as female is not a simple form of earth-mother ecofeminism, but a crop-based understanding of what makes things grow. It is not only the souls of rice that need to be nurtured. Wa women from northern Burma participate in agricultural rituals honoring the soul of maize, buckwheat, sorghum, and millet—"you who feed us," and act as spirit mediums to insure good harvests (Andaya 2006: 19). The Black Tai of Vietnam view earth spirits and the spirit of rice as male, whereas other Tai groups consider them female, a reflection of the Chinese influence on Vietnam (Andaya 2006: 24).

In the margins of Southeast Asian modernity, local life-cycle rituals still exhibit the habitus of nurture. That is why the evidence from small-scale upland minority communities is so valuable. These upland communities, identified as zoomia, are considered peripheral to the state (Scott 2009). But even among groups shaped by local traditions, few people remain unaffected by the state and by dominant world religions through processes such as colonialism, missionization, imperialism, and globalization.

Our working definition of nurture draws attention to the building of empathetic social relationships to ensure the provision of food and care that encourages someone or something to grow and develop to its full potential. This definition owes much to the Thai concept of *liang,* but can be applied beyond the region. In Thai, the verb *liang* means to support or make something or someone grow by feeding them. The English and Thai dictionary meanings of the word nurture are both intimately connected with food. But they differ in the extent to which they are also about power relations. Although there are parallels in the meaning and use of the terms in English and Thai, the differences are more instructive. The word *liang* is probably of great antiquity because its cognates are widespread among groups of Tai speakers, including those in South China. Vietnamese separates the debt of birth (*sinh*) from the debt of feeding (*duong*)—both debts owed to parents, while *nuoi* refers to the kind of nurture and care implied by the English word, nourish. *Con nuio* refers to bringing up an adopted child, as opposed to a birth child (*con sinh*). The Thai/Tai term, *liang*, would not make this distinction.[4]

Southeast Asian regional traditions value skilled nurturing—the ability to breastfeed an infant, raise children, feed families, feast others, and grow rice and orchids. The power to control life forms through feeding is also deeply political; it is certainly not a female personality trait. Throughout Southeast Asia, nurturing power is exercised through food. For example, all Southeast Asian languages have separate words for cooked and uncooked rice, probably because they enter differently into ritual food exchanges.

In Southeast Asia, while nurture matters at the local level, it is respected all the way to the top. Guardian spirits at the northeast corner of a bedroom in a Thai village must be fed, just as the guardian spirit of the city, *lak muang* in Bangkok (cf. Van Esterik 1982). It is efficient, valued, and can be modern to *liang* others. Nurture supersedes formal religion, nation, and ethnicity, providing the commonalities that allow symbolic and literal communication throughout the region. Nurture, modeled on growing rice, allows easy movement across many borders: "A Malay marries into a Tai village, Tai into Mon, Mon into Burmese—crossing four language families" (O'Connor 2011: 188). Nurturing rice and nurturing children have an integrity across the region. Common idioms show the sophistication of Southeast Asian forms of communicating about nurture, so that nurture makes sense even to contemporary politicians, who cook for or feed their supporters (Van Esterik 2000).

For example, the cultural logic of Malay commensality is similar to the Thai in many ways. However, Thai and Malay cultural identity are both intimately linked to very different religious traditions—Theravada Buddhism and Islam, respectively. Thai and Malay also speak different languages from unrelated language families; Thai belongs to the Tai-Kadai family, Malay to Austronesian. This supports the argument that the customs that support person-making through breastfeeding and feeding others are even more fundamental than religious identity; nurturing practices glossed as custom trumps culture glossed as religion throughout Southeast Asia.

Customizing Nurture: Nurturing Custom

What are the distinguishing patterns of nurturing practices in the region? We suggest a few possible directions here, although no feature is independent of the others, in spite of the linear list that follows; the reality is more like a Mobius strip where the life force flows through human bodies nurtured by milk and rice. The logic of nurture has most coherence in rice-growing villages and least in urban factories, but nurturing practices continue to have resilience in the region, even as global flows blur ethnic and national boundaries.

Theme 1: Separation and Containment

In Southeast Asia, postpartum seclusion fits as part of the container logic that roots a newborn in place, in its household and village. Container logic stressed life-holding closure. This core idiom makes sense of customs surrounding houses, rice growing, raising children, and rituals that tie souls into bodies. Container logic models the social womb; the container protects vulnerable infants. These rituals align nurturing "life" (souls, infants, relationships) by holding it in containers (body, house, village, granary, paddy field) with growing rice as an agro-cultural complex (O'Connor 1995). Breastfeeding in Theravada Buddhist villages thrives in the essentially pre-Buddhist system dominated by spirits where individuals struggle to nurture rice as well as infants, and fear the death of a pregnant woman, knowing her capacity to produce the most feared and dangerous ghosts. Following birth, mothers drink warming soups to increase their breastmilk and rest by a heat source to dry out the uterus (Thai, lying by the fire, *juu fai*). Until the uterus is dry, the milk is not considered fit to drink. This is why colostrum was thrown out. But mothers, past and present, often only throw out the first drops of colostrum to clear the passage for milk. In the social womb, Thai and Lao mothers might give their newborns to a trusted relative or friend who nurtures well (*liang dii*) to help develop good breastfeeding habits in the newborn. The Thai local regimen adapts Thai infants into Thai society through the nurturing practices of the household they are born into.

This indigenous Thai logic protected mother–infant dyads against the many threats to nurturing practices. While the newborn may lose the advantage of colostrum, the trade-off is the strengthened bond of social reciprocity, drawing the newborn and its mother into the community. Herbal medicines offer another means to dry out the uterus quickly, which might encourage Thai women to feed colostrum to their newborns; but using herbal medicine does not strengthen social relationships.

Across language group, ethnicity, and religion, this pattern of postpartum separation is repeated. After delivery, Lao mothers and infants are expected to rest by the hearth two to three weeks (Breakey and Voulgaropoulos 1968: 51), much as the *juu fai* practices in Thailand. This period of separation and recuperation (usually a month, but less for poor women) is critically important to protect mother and infant when they are vulnerable to spirit loss. Outsider biomedical logic might blame infant vulnerability on women's inadequate nutrition, short birth intervals, and high rates of anemia, contributing to risky births and low birth-weight babies (Ireson-Doolittle and Moreno-Black 2004: 64–66). Regardless of the explanation, the consequences are the same; infant death is familiar and greatly feared.

In Hmong villages, pregnant women and sick people are forbidden to visit the household of a woman who has just given birth, "since they might diminish the new mother's milk supply" (Symonds 2004: 82). Although Hmong mothers value breastmilk, they do not value colostrum, believing it is unhealthy. Another patrilineage mother will breastfeed the newborn for the first few days, establishing the lineage's claim on the infant. The shared substance produces a very powerful medicine, but breastmilk is dangerous if used incorrectly. Lactating women who have recently given birth are not permitted to cook, lest the milk mix with the family food (Symonds 2004: 83). Customs that relieve a new mother of some agricultural work and domestic cooking make space for nurture, strengthening the integrity of the mother–infant dyad through separation in the social womb.

Hmong postpartum practices, as is common in many Southeast Asian communities, reflect the ambiguities of adjusting food restrictions that both help recovery after childbirth and support breastfeeding. Papaya produces "good strong milk," although eating papaya "breaks the humoral rules for avoiding cooling fruits after birth (Symonds 2004: 81). Hmong mothers have to negotiate their consumption of papaya based on what is right for their new infant. Customs have consequences; they are adapted to reflect what works to keep infants alive and growing.

In parts of Java, the newborn child remains with the mother in the social womb for the first forty days after birth; songs and stories are told over the newborn while the mother rests and guests watch over the baby. Uncooked rice and coins are placed on a white cloth with the newborn and placed on the mother's right side. When the cord falls off, the rice that the newborn was placed on is cooked in porridge for a special *hajat* or ritual meal. The placenta is covered with salt and spices, placed in a basket, and wrapped in a white cloth. There are local variations on where the placenta is buried; here too the placenta is considered the sibling of the baby (Wessing 1978: 130). Hair cutting and naming rituals taking place shortly after birth (depending on local custom) are celebrated with communal meals to recognize the fact that the child has become a member of the community. Shared rice meals are critical for creating shared substance.

Pregnancy, birth, and child feeding in Bali are dangerous transitions surrounded with rituals. Mother and baby are both impure at birth and for forty-two days following birth; they are particularly vulnerable to witches for three months. Yet babies are considered divine rather than human until 210 days after birth; these infant deities are free to come and go in the human world until they are bound to the human world by ritual. After the child first touches the ground, has a ritual haircut, and receives a name, he or she is recognized as a human child. Ritual timing and elaboration of these acts depends on the family's social standing, caste membership, and locality (cf. Diener 2000).

Iban and other groups in Borneo make the separation and containment of pregnant women and new mothers explicit. Their ritual throws up a wall of protection around the expectant mother "The Dayak … fence a happy unborn babe whom they cherish" (Andaya 2006: 209). Here the social womb begins during pregnancy.

Whether the idiom is impurity, divinity, weakness, or evil spirits, customs that separate mothers and newborns from regular work routines and provide a period of time for them to relate to each other provide the best chances for infant survival. Throughout Southeast Asia, postpartum rituals were "less a matter of 'purification' than a means of restoring a woman's strength and inner spirit" (Andaya 2006: 214). Once modernity, often through colonialism or missionization, intervened to degrade and ridicule postpartum practices of separation, women lost access to the social womb, this period of recovery after birth. Modernity has no such postpartum customs beyond the six-week check-up, and even discourages the seclusion of new mothers.

Theme 2: Person-Making as Group Work

Following the seclusion of the social womb, infants become social persons and are brought in to the group through being fed, first milk and later, rice. In the Southeast Asian logic of commensality, sharing rice anchors the person in the group. It is the act of eating together that constitutes groups; the group is not prior; in fact, eating together is at the core of identity-making. Eating together restores the whole, restores balance. This form of inclusive commensality contrasts with South Asian logical systems, where groups are prior, and people eat together according to shared group membership (such as caste). In South Asia, exclusive commensality—who you do not eat with—is an important part of identity construction.

According to biomedical lab logic, the early introduction of any food in the form of prelacteal feeds introduce potential contaminants into the vulnerable infant gut and may reduce the consumption of breastmilk, and may thus be dangerous to infants. But the person-making work performed by foods such as rice is important to identity formation. Lao infants are socialized into their commensal circles through sticky rice, the identity-forming food that turns a human infant into a Lao infant. It is so important to draw the newborn into the commensal circle that glutinous rice is introduced to the newborn within a few days of birth.

One popular form given to newborns is a packet of roasted smoked premasticated sticky rice. In the 1960s, 44 percent of mothers gave this pre-chewed rice mixture by two to three days of age (Breakey and Voulgaropoulos 1968: 52). Lao in northeast Thailand and across the Mekong in Lao PDR share many common approaches to child nurture, rooted no doubt in the food shortages experienced in both regions. Mothers in rural northeast Thailand used to masticate rice and bananas and feed it to infants, as is still common in Lao PDR. It was the flavor of the betel juice in the mother's mouth that finally discouraged the practice, rather than nutrition education, according to villagers (Klausner 2000: 85).

By age two, children eat with the family and fend for themselves; because toddlers eat slowly and less efficiently than their older siblings, they are at a disadvantage when they compete with them for the best protein dishes. Toddlers may not be proficient at the motor skills required to form a ball of sticky rice and use it to pinch some vegetables or fish. But they can hold and nibble fistfuls of (dirty) sticky rice. Poor mothers boast how early their infants can "feed themselves," and weaned infants are expected to feed and care for themselves as much as possible (Ireson-Doolittle and Moreno-Black 2004: 66). Sticky rice makes it easy for toddlers to feed themselves, an advantage when their sibling caretakers are as young as six or seven years of age. On the other hand, Lao nurturing practices are learned through sibling caretaking, as children play with real babies rather than dolls.

Southeast Asian ethnographies provide many examples of how children are socialized into sharing food. Children in northeast Thailand are warned that to only eat the best protein dishes (called with-rice dishes), without consuming rice could result in turning them into *phi pawb* spirits, in order to teach children the importance of eating a balance of rice and with-rice dishes (Klausner 2000: 82). If an adult gives a child a choice piece of meat or fish during a meal, that child is rewarded for further portioning the food and giving some to younger siblings. In fact, the child is punished for consuming the food directly, without sharing it. This strengthens the bonds between siblings and establishes the high value placed on restraint around the commensal table; perhaps this makes ascetic practices and fasting especially significant by contrast. A good person shares food; what this sharing accomplishes is more variable.

Theme 3: Vulnerability and Protection

Even with the best of intentions and effective nurturing practices, infants and young children die in large numbers. They are vulnerable beings in need of protection, their souls easily escaping from their container/bodies. Even today, infant mortality rates in some Southeast Asian countries are high—for example, 30.1 per 1,000 live births in Lao PDR, 15 in Cambodia, and 26.4 in Burma according to WHO statistics for 2015.

Protection for infants is particularly well-defined in Bali. To assist the baby in averting supernatural danger, every Balinese child has four sibling-spirits manifested at birth in the blood, waxy vernix coating, amniotic fluid, and placenta/umbilical cord (Diener 2000: 99, 101). After the birth, these products/protectors are buried under the house (and reburied at any new house). The four spirit brothers and sisters of the child continue to reside in the child's body, reminders of the complex balance between inner and outer worlds. As a Balinese healer explained, we often forget our sibling-spirits until near death when they reappear to summon us back to the spirit world (Lansing 1995: 35). Elsewhere in Islamic communities in Indonesia, the introduction of special birth rituals included praying in a newborn's ear to protect them (Andaya 2006: 86).

Buddhist amulets also protect vulnerable infants, although breastfeeding and child feeding is irrelevant to Buddhist textual traditions. Even feeding infants out of *metta-karuna* (loving kindness) is clearly part of the attachment householders have to their offspring, and not the detachment of the Buddhist renouncer. Buddhist institutions reconcile these historical layers of pre-Buddhist customs derived from local fertility cults to support nurture, relying on the nurturing practices of women to feed both monks and children (*liang phra, liang dek*; cf. Van Esterik 1986).

In both mainland and island communities, there is a widespread fear of the spirits of infants and pregnant women who die during childbirth. No doubt, these spirit beliefs are rooted in the devastating experience of actual losses. Women's involvement in curing endured partly because of their fear of the possibility of their own death in childbirth and rebirth as evil spirits (Andaya 2006: 78). In 1818, the high infant mortality rate among Minangkabau mothers in Sumatra prompted mothers to implore the first white woman they had ever seen to touch their children as a preservative from future evil (Andaya 2006: 67). In Southeast Asia, women heal as an extension of nurture; medicinal herbs used in healing are extensions of culinary knowledge (cf. Van Esterik 1988). Postpartum rituals and practices were part of customary knowledge passed on through women, and not necessarily embedded in text-based medical systems such as Ayurvedic and humoral; male healers become the authoritative experts when texts are privileged (cf. Andaya 2006: 129).

In war-torn Laos in the 1960s, only 50 percent of infants survived childhood (Breakey and Voulgaropoulos 1968). Mothers in the 1960s reported they wanted five children; with a 50 percent mortality rate, they would need to conceive ten children to have five survive (Breakey and Voularopoulos 1968: 53). Other surveys confirm the high infant and maternal mortality rates; on average, women give birth to eight children and have five living children; in a more recent small survey in a poor upland area, 17 percent of infants died in the first year and 39 percent died before age eleven (Ireson-Doolittle and Moreno-Black 2004: 64–66). Lao mothers breastfeed their infants until another baby comes along, usually three to four years. After nearly forty years of communist rule, Lao PDR still has a high infant mortality rate. The fact that child survival is so precarious might explain the high birth rate in the country. It certainly explains the popularity of rituals such as *soukhuan* to protect infants.

Like most other Thai and Lao groups, the Shan of Thailand and Burma deal with the vulnerability of babies and young children with protective rituals that keep their soft *khwan* or spirit essence firmly attached to their bodies. Along with ritual bathing of the baby, string bracelets accompanied by blessings from the village elders protect vulnerable infants. Spirit parents watch out for baby (Eberhardt 2006: 78, 79). These *soukhuan* rituals attract wandering souls back in to bodies, or hold the souls in vulnerable people—pregnant women, the sick, infants, travelers. For these events, special ritual foods are displayed and served, rather than everyday foods.

In the past, topknots also offered protection to older children in rural and urban Thailand, part of the pattern of Vedic Brahmanical protective rituals adopted by many Theravada Buddhist countries (Quaritch Wales 1931; Van Esterik 1973). Even Buddhist parents in Thailand had infants who had died or who were about to die christened to keep them safe in Christian cemeteries, although the parents did not convert to Christianity. In Vietnam, Catholic missionaries offered comfort by pledging that baptized women dying in childbirth would find happiness in the afterlife rather than wondering as evil spirits (Andaya 2006: 96, 97).

In the Philippines, "the introduction of wet rice cultivation in Northern Luzon initiated a change in the pantheon" (Kwiatkowski 1998: 146). Ancestor worship was "needed" for ranking descent groups, and ancestors came to interact directly in the lives of the living. But female spirit mediums still performed rituals for infants and children if they were too thin or not eating properly. Ifugao parents had to care for and protect their infants vigilantly, or spirits would take their souls and care for the children properly (Kwiatkowski 1998: 152–54). While spirit worship offered ways of solving the problem of nurture, infant malnutrition was further complicated by the Catholic Church's condemnation of contraception. The more local postpartum protective traditions thrived in rural Southeast Asia, and the more these communities resisted the logic of modernity, the easier it was for women to integrate breastfeeding into their lives, particularly in rice growing communities.

Theme 4: Intergenerational Cycles

In all societies, the intimate relation between the generations, initially between mother and newborn, flows through maternal milk. As we showed in Chapter 3, biological anthropologists are uncovering the staggering amount of information that is communicated from grandmother to mother to child through breastfeeding. But there are other ways to talk about the relation between the generations.

In the mainland, there are hints about the connections between the generations. Among the Shan, Eberhardt notes that newborns do not start life as tabula rasa but exhibit signs that others can read about who they were in a former life (2006: 80). An albino infant born in a Thai village in the 1970s was considered to be a Caucasian foreigner in a past life. In Theravada mainland villages, feeding ancestors rice gives blessings and fertility to those living in the household. Food channels this generalized life force between the generations, represented in Thai as *phujaatajaaj* (maternal and paternal grandparents, meaning the earlier generations and not just one ancestral line).

Island Southeast Asia provides many more ways to link the generations than in the mainland. Bali represents an exception to many of the generalizations made about food and commensality in Southeast Asia. Its unique Hindu-Buddhist history and resistance to Dutch colonialism shapes nurturing practices there. Consider this Balinese example of the relation between infant and adult eating within the life cycle.

Some of the best ethnographic work on children was done by Margaret Mead. Bateson and Mead's photographic analysis of *Balinese Character* (1942) set standards not only in visual anthropology, but also in the analysis of infant and child development. While the culture and personality frame they used is dated, the photographic record illustrates elements of a distinctive infant-feeding style recognizable seventy years later. This is not to say that infant-feeding styles have remained unchanged since the 1940s—only that they provide a unique opportunity to see something about eating and feeding at that time period.

Bateson and Mead are among the rare ethnographers who try to link infant and child feeding to adult eating. Building from the psychological assumptions of their day and using photographs, they separate eating meals and defecation (accompanied by shame) from eating snacks, drinking, and urination (without shame), and suggest that eating pre-chewed food (by infants) is the prototype for eating meals (by adults), while breastfeeding is the prototype for casual snacking and drinking (1942: 107). This hypothesis was developed through observations about the casualness of breastfeeding, often accomplished by turning the nipple upward into the baby's mouth, instead of the downward motion of pushing pre-chewed food into the infant's mouth, replicated in adults by tipping the head back and hunching over food while eating their normal meals. The shame associated with eating is visible in the photographs of sharing food at a funeral where people sit with their right hands closest to the food and their backs toward their neighbors, discouraging interpersonal communication while still eating communally (Bateson and Mead 1942: 112). This is a reminder of the need to keep in mind degrees of commensality, noting not just eating at the same table, but also eating the same food, sharing utensils, socializing (or not) while eating, as well as feeding each other, practiced with lovers and babies.

With breastfeeding, the baby is unconstrained and takes the initiative to breastfeed at will, having free access to the breast. The infant as god is elevated, along with breastmilk. Their photographs also suggest that breastfeeding is associated with fun and pleasure, not the coercion, pressure, or shame of adult meals (Bateson and Mead 1942: 124).

Balinese adults avoid showing emotional responsiveness in interpersonal relations, but enjoy getting babies, who have not yet learned unresponsiveness, to respond. For example, they might ruffle the penis to see the infant respond (Bateson and Mead 1942: 131). Mothers often nurse another woman's child. This act frustrates and angers her child who gradually learns not to show any emotional reaction (Bateson and Mead 1942: 152). Consider, for example, that the same act of shared breastfeeding in Thailand is done to develop good nurturing habits and broaden the child's social network; the same practice in Malaysia functions to create a milk siblingship alliance, not to frustrate the child.

In this Hindu-Buddhist context, babies are reincarnation of known ancestors, and they may also be born with debts owing to beings in the spirit world. These debts must be paid by parents and relatives, reinforcing the life-cycle obligations of one generation to another (cf. Lansing 1995: 31). In the Balinese example, reciprocal relations are not created through shared breastmilk; rather, breastfeeding is casual not sacred. Eating is an obscene or animalistic act done in private (even when eating in a group), with face averted; but bathing and breastfeeding are normal acts performed in public without embarrassment (Lansing 1995: 4). Rice is sacred; rice rituals are sacred; but eating rice is animalistic (Lansing 1995: 26).

These examples of infant-feeding style show how Balinese seek balance between autonomy and connectedness, between the living and the dead through food. Balinese infants develop constitutions that strain to control emotions. They learn the emotional power of eating, that eating is an emotionally charged activity. Breastfeeding helps them learn about ambiguity, frustration, and the balance between good and evil.

The cycles of life so well documented in the islands of Eastern Indonesia link ascending and descending generations. Feeding the dead constructs a commensal relation that aids in the transmission of life force through food shared. Elders in the Austronesian world are closer to the source of life, the world of the ancestors, as are Balinese babies (Janowski 2007: 19). Birth and death are recognized in Southeast Asia as difficult processes requiring skilled nurture. These connections between the nurturing practices at birth and death are made explicit in life-cycle rituals. For example, among the Sasak Muslims of Lombok, mortuary feasts help the dead to become ancestors. The Islamic confession of faith and other sacred verses are recited to ease a person into death and into the ear of a vulnerable newborn to ease it into life (Telle 2007: 128).

In the eastern Indonesian island of Maluku, Muslim mortuary rituals that take place forty days after death mirror the forty days of postpartum seclusion for mothers and newborns, closing the cycle of nurture. After forty days, the deceased becomes part of the collective category of ancestors, just as the infant becomes a recognized part of the community (Kaartinen 2007: 162–66). In Lombok, death, like birth, is a gradual transformation from embodied to disembodied, and birth, from disembodied to embodied social person. The links to rice are made explicit in Lombok, where the spirit leaves the body when the allotted share of rice is done (Telle 2007: 127).

Among the Toraja of Sulawesi, attention focuses on the umbilical cord as the portion of the afterbirth that is symbolically elaborated. The cord is seen as a link between the present and the future. "Ancestors connect people on earth to the upper world; the umbilical cord roots people in the earth and to their houses" (Volkman 1985: 50). The afterbirth is placed in a reed pouch that normally holds the family supply of cooked rice and is buried beside the house. Children are recognized as a form of riches, and siblings as children "cut from the same umbilical cord" (Volkman 1985: 51).

In Western Malaysia on the island of Borneo, frontier groups like the Iban of Sarawak have been described as stressing individualism and personal mobility, combined with mutual dependence that comes from communal longhouse living. Iban means "human and proud of it," much like groups in the mainland where the ethnic labels Khmu and Mien also translate as "human" (cf. Praet 2013: 197). The Iban dry rice cultivators were constantly opening new swidden fields, adapting to new conditions. They were considered egalitarian but conscious of prestige differences. Although rice was a prestige food, success with rice cultivation was unpredictable. Those who faced crop failure might become debt slaves (Sutlive 1978: 26). In their aggressive spread through the hills of Borneo, where they replaced hunting peoples, the Iban harvested the heads of rice and men. Heads were a replacement for the dead and a release for the deceased in a closed cosmology that opposed the world of the living and the "opposite," the world of the dead. This cycle was the first step in the metamorphosis of human into dew to nourish rice for nourishing humans (Sutlive 1978: 28, 29). "Rice nourishes man who dies to give essence to rice, and so the circle of life continues" (Sutlive 1978: 64). Children were highly prized, nursed immediately on demand until three or four years of age and carried in a sarong sling. Weaning was casual (Sutlive 1978: 91–92); the first food an infant tastes after mothers' milk is rice gruel (Sutlive 1978: 64). The Iban refer to household rice bins as the womb of the family, and women have primary access to them (Sutlive 1978: 55). The recognition of interconnections between the generations, visible in the customs in both island and mainland Southeast Asia, is congruent with the newest biomedical breakthroughs about what is passed from generation to generation.

Theme 5: Shared Substance

In the Malay world described by Janet Carsten, commensality begins before birth, when the fetus is nourished by the mother's blood, formed from the food she eats—primarily cooked rice; even in utero, one does not eat alone, but rather the fetus shares the meal with a placental older sibling (1995). Malay siblings become progressively more alike or different depending on whether or not they ate together (Carsten 2004: 74).

The Malays of Rembau, Negeri Sembilan, are descendants of Minangkabau settlers to the Malay mainland who absorbed the local horticulturalists in the 1500s, and introduced wet rice agriculture, Islam, and *adat* (customary) law to the area (Peletz 1988: 18). As among the Minangkabau, rights passed through women, and husbands took up residence in the wife's mother's compound. The youngest daughter then cares for her parents and inherits the parental house. Sisters act as a cooperative unit even after marriage (Peletz 1988: 47). The Malay example demonstrates the importance of siblingship, particularly the bond between sisters. Even before birth, the placenta is treated as an elder sibling who nourished the younger sibling in utero and for forty four days after birth. Villagers consider this to be a complex of great antiquity (Peletz 1988: 50). This customary practice drawing attention to the placenta also provides an adaptive advantage to ensure that the entire placenta is delivered. If the placenta is incompletely delivered, the mother could bleed to death, and any retained placenta would prevent milk production. A girl child's placenta was buried deep under the private section of the mother's house where females sleep; a boy child's placenta is buried in open public areas (Peletz 1988: 50). The midwife (*bidan*) buries the placenta, reciting Koranic verses over a small fire ignited with embers from the kitchen hearth. Some families would rekindle the flame daily while the new mother observed the postpartum dietary taboos for forty four days to dry out the placenta (symbolically) and the uterus (bodily). These practices call to mind the lying by the fire (*juu fai*) practices of Tai groups, where the fire is lit from the cooking hearth.

As a result of these customary practices, children have parallel sex sibling protectors; a girl has an older sister sibling protector and a boy, an older brother, bound together by moral obligations (Peletz 1988: 51). There appears to be less emphasis on the placenta elsewhere on the mainland, although burying the placenta near the house encourages Thai babies to be reborn in the village.

To the Malay, incest, particularly of siblings, is as repugnant as cannibalism and results in the perpetrators' transformation into spirits whose sustenance derives from sucking the blood of postpartum women and newborns (Peletz 1988: 53). Incest within lineage or clan is a grave transgression because the individuals share the same matrilineally transmitted *daging* or meat. Also forbidden is marriage or sexual contact between unrelated persons breastfed by the same woman. These milk siblings also share biological substances—the growth-inducing essences in the breastmilk. Mother's milk nourishes and sustains an infant in the same way that a mother's womb nourished the embryo; consequently, a child contains the *daging* of both the birth mother and the wet nurse (Peletz 1988: 57).

In the mountainous areas of Java, villagers place more stress on household independence after marriage, otherwise the couple are not considered as adults. Only dependents eat in the same kitchen, at the same hearth. Adult children are ashamed of this dependence and make every effort to establish their own households after marriage. If necessary, they set up separate hearths in the same house to show they are independent adults. Although residence is matrilocal, if the new couple eats with her parents, "in the community's eyes, they remain children" (Hefner 1990: 163).

Southeast Asian *adat* law in Malaysia and Indonesia provides negotiating points (not fixed rules) to adapt Islamic sharia law to Hindu-Buddhist communities. Islamic sharia law as practiced in the Middle East recognizes three alternative relationships established through blood, affinity, and milk. In much of the Muslim world, the milk relation is phrased in terms of male proprietorship—milk as paternal substance—rather than milk as conveyor of maternal substance, a refinement of maternal blood. In Southeast Asia, milk siblingship is less about creating alliances outside the kin group and more about shared maternal substance. Here, the maternal bias and the importance of sibling links are stressed.

In Java, as in Malaysia, children of "one breast" (milk siblings) may not marry (*dulur sasusu*). In the past, this restriction might have excluded most of a child's age mates as marriage partners because children were often given the breast by someone other than their mother (Wessing 1978: 140). In larger settlements, marriages may be endogamous, perhaps because there are more children who are not milk siblings.

Wet nurses held positions of power in many courts, including seventeenth-century Aceh (Andaya 2006: 89). In the ancient Siamese capital of Ayuttaya, the Lord mother of a monastery, a former nurse of King Narai, mediated disputes between leading members of the nobility and was invited to sit with royalty (Andaya 2006: 66). Wet nursing was common among the elite families of Makassar of southern Sulawesi in the late eighteenth century. In the eastern Indonesian island of Ternate, the wives of nobles suckled the rulers' children, no doubt to create alliances and incur reciprocal debts (Andaya 2006: 129). Kin, especially siblings, share substance primarily based on milk and rice.

Theme 6: Expanding the Commensal Circle

How does political commensality play out in Southeast Asia? Commensal circles reflect power, privilege, and hierarchy as well as egalitarian sharing. An example from Toraja demonstrates how meat and rice rituals represented different ways of including and excluding people. The Toraja of Sulawesi had two rituals complexes—one based on rice, the other on meat. The one surrounding rice was intrinsically egalitarian, female-centered, and nurturing. It stressed life-holding closure, much like the social womb. The other Torajan complex, meat rituals, surrounds buffalo sacrifice and links to practices of the status-enhancing segments of the commensal circle. This complex is inherently hierarchical, male-centered, and death-managing (Volkman 1985). It is all about establishing ruling centers (sacrifices, shrines, rulers, feasts) and stands quite apart from the container-character and elder-deference of local life. Unlike the closure of rice rituals that contain and protect soul and spirit, meat rituals draw people from far and wide. The uplands of Southeast Asia have expressed this through buffalo sacrifices, feasts of merit, and competitive feasting for status (cf. Kirsch 1973).

Commensality—eating together—entails reciprocity. Reciprocity is not without calculation, in Southeast Asia as in Euro-American communities. As the commensal circle expands and meals are shared more widely, the risks are greater, including the risk of poisoning. In Southeast Asia, food shared beyond the household has broader religious and political meanings.

Sharing food is the most basic means of creating and maintaining social relationships. Refusal to share is a clear sign of distance and enmity (Bloch 1999). Communist Lao PDR is a food insecure country with strong commensal culture even before socialism provided ideological justification for sharing food. Extended families and guests sit around low bamboo tables or mats, select from the same food dishes, eat at the same time, share the same utensils, and interact socially while eating. In rural Lao communities, strangers are easily absorbed into household meals, even in resource poor settings. Food insecurity appears to increase commensality in Lao communities. The Lao meal format is easily adjusted to include extra people (dilute the soup).

Political commensality is very strong in villages and towns, as every effort is made to feed and entertain officials in style, by providing the best food (and access to beautiful daughters). Visitors have noted the unusual degree to which Lao women partake in these rituals of hosting and toasting with local rice wine (*laolao*).

In Lao PDR where hospitality is so important, even food aid may be at risk by customs of hospitality. NGO workers told the story of a Food and Agriculture Organization (FAO) official who was scheduled to visit an impoverished rural area to assess the need for food aid because of rice insufficiency. To prepare for the visitor, the villagers called on all possible obligations from neighboring villages to borrow food in order to put on a feast for the visitor, who promptly determined that the village did not need any food aid. In Lao and other Theravada Buddhist villages, community members feed monks with the best dishes they can afford, and communally share the merit accrued from this act of religious commensality. Following precept day chanting, community members receive extra merit by eating the blessed leftovers that have been provided to the monks.

Throughout much of Indonesia, communal meals referred to as *hajat* among the Sudanese of West Java, and *slametan* elsewhere, involve giving away food with a goal in mind, to bring something or some group into a condition of well-being. *Slametan* meals mark pregnancy rituals at seven months and at several points after the birth. Because birth is such a dangerous time, spirits are invited to protect mother and newborn and are given special foods. Community members eat together because food is a form of power; through prayers and sharing food, the host draws power from the cosmos, rebalancing power between community and cosmos. Women contribute food and labor to the ritual meal that keeps people and spirits in proper balance (cf. Wessing 1978: 65). Participants eat the whole meal in silence (recall Bali). Elsewhere in Java, some of the food is taken home to share with those who could not attend (including children).

Public health officials might want to consider the timing of ritual meals in relation to child feeding. For example, the best, protein-rich foods are made for the monks' alms rounds in the early morning in Theravada Buddhist villages. Leftovers are available for children from the early morning. In the *slametan* feasts, ritual food rich in protein may be more available in the evening after children are asleep.

Other ways of expanding the commensal circle include adoption and fosterage. These means of actively recruiting members into the household are common in Southeast Asia where there is less rigidity around blood lines and lineality. In Southeast Asia, infanticide and abortions are rare; while premarital sex is officially discouraged by the world religions in the region ("eating before being called to dinner," as the Vietnamese say), fertility is prized. In rural rice-growing villages in the mainland, small huts in the rice fields facilitate liaisons; if and when the couples are caught, marriage alliances can be worked out.

Infants born expand the local group and are easily adopted by the mother's family or by someone else in the community (Andaya 2006: 212). This is facilitated by the fact that kinship is not fixed at birth or defined by blood lines, but rather established by eating together and sharing food at the same hearth. This enables fosterage and adoption, common occurrences in Southeast Asia. Feeding a child means that you raised the child. As in central Sulawesi (Schrauwers 1999), kinship and fosterage can be negotiated through feeding. Particularly common is the practice of one sister giving up a newborn child to another, usually childless sibling to raise. There is usually no question about who are the real parents of the baby; they are not the birth parents but the adoptive parents who fed the child in their household. There are, of course, interesting complications, as when the older sister in a northern Thai household "kidnapped" the newborn son of her younger sister who was reluctant to give him away to her childless but wealthy sibling. She eventually agreed to the adoption out of *metta* (loving kindness) for the baby, and the sister returned the baby to the birth mother for breastfeeding, and reclaimed him after weaning. The birth mother becomes the wet nurse, *mae liang* as well as aunt to her son; later in life the child discovers that his aunt is his birth mother and because she breastfed him, the merit from his ordination was transferred to her (Klima 2002: 255).

Among the Iban of Borneo, many women were childless. Sutlive (1978) attributes this to malnutrition, miscarriages because of heavy work, or abortions "lest their husbands lose interest in them and look elsewhere for sexual pleasure." In addition, there was a high infant mortality rate (nearly 50 percent), with possible links to postpartum food taboos that limited maternal diet to rice and salt for one month (Sutlive 1978: 42). Strangers could be adopted through blood brother adoption rituals (Sutlive 1978: 42). Even war captives could become Iban, human.

The Malay in central Sumatra often adopt the children of poor Chinese plantation workers for a substantial payment. They are brought up as Malay, sharing meals, and thus inherit as full members of the family (Kerlogue 2007: 58). In contrast, Malay will seldom allow their children to be adopted out. Transfer of children between households was common in both urban and rural Southeast Asia and Oceania, among both swiddeners and irrigated rice growers. Schrauwers shows how fosterage and adoption in central Sulawesi increased, "eased by a concept of parentage that stresses nurturance and sharing" and was negotiated situationally (Schrauwers 1999: 310–11). He argues that parentage emerges over time and can be exploitative. Austronesian concepts of social identity are not given at birth, and sometimes foster children resist this form of covert slavery, as peasant households tried to substitute free kin labour for wage labour under rapidly changing conditions of labour in a capitalist economy. Fosterage and adoption do not stand alone but are facilitated by an ideology of commensal nurture, even among unilineal descent groups.

Continuity and Change

The ethnographic present used in old ethnographies makes Southeast Asia seem like a region bypassed by modernity—a region lodged in traditional customs of the past. Nothing could be further from the truth. Cities like Jakarta and Bangkok are modern urban centers, end products of complex histories barely hinted at here. Global flows within the region and between regions have not erased nurturing practices; they coexist with cell phones and internet cafes, and other material signs of modernity. But these global flows also made Southeast Asia the fastest growing market for infant formula (Baker, Smith, and Salmon 2016). It is also one region where the economic costs of not breastfeeding have been carefully calculated, along with the economic benefits of breastfeeding associated with potential improvements in cognition through higher IQ and earnings, totaling 1.6 billion US dollars annually. Adequate breastfeeding has the potential to prevent over 12,400 child and maternal deaths per year in the seven Southeast Asian countries studied (Walters et al. 2016).

Commercial baby foods along with appropriate and inappropriate breastmilk substitutes have been available in the region since the 1800s. Chinese traders in coastal towns were the first to have regular access to canned milk from Europe and Australia. Rates of mixed and artificial feeding have been higher among those of Chinese descent for many decades in Bangkok (Stahlie 1962: 183), as in other Southeast Asian cities (cf. Williams 1939). The popularity of using foreign domestic workers as nannies in Singapore relieves mothers of child-care responsibilities.

In the 1950s, UN agencies such as UNICEF distributed dried whole and skim milk powder free of charge to poor pregnant and lactating women, who were not always shown how to reconstitute it. With no dairy industry in the country, cow's milk was imported; when recipients complained they did not like its taste, officials suggested they should mix it with rice (Stahlie 1962: 193). Imagine the appeal of that mixture to a rice-loving lactose intolerant population. By 1955, half the babies surveyed in Thailand were still being breastfed at fifteen months in both rural and urban samples, with Bangkok having the lowest breastfeeding rates. As babies were fed mashed rice and bananas at an early age, clinical beriberi was rare in infants.

A study of breastfeeding in Vientiane province and the capital of Lao PDR in 2007 found that only 19.4 percent of infants were breastfed exclusively at six months while 18.6 were still breastfeeding at two years of age (Phuttakeo et al. 2009: 487). There was more exclusive breastfeeding among rural and minority groups; analysts suggested that marketing and promotion of breastmilk substitutes was less prevalent in less accessible areas. Nevertheless, ads for infant formula from Thailand reached even the most remote areas, and mothers were interested in trying the products they saw advertised on TV (Phuttakeo et al. 2009: 489). The Lao Lum, who made up 80 percent of the sample, gave their infants pre-chewed sticky rice (40 percent), and generally believed that colostrum gave infants diarrhea. At the time of their study, the under-five mortality rate in Lao PDR was 100/1,000 (Phuttakeo et al. 2009: 488). Since the early 2000s, small packets of cheap, inferior Chinese infant formula have been making their way in to rural markets in remote Lao villages. Repackaged in China and marketed across the border, it appeals to the Lao women who have seen the ads on Thai TV although they cannot afford the large cans advertised; no doubt they welcome these small cheap packets with no instructions as an appealing modern substitute.

Modernity brings new food products and disrupts nurture, but it does not reduce its currency. Modern urban Thai women quickly learned that *juu fai* is old-fashioned and that clinic births are safer. If using modern clinics and hospitals come with more cesarean sections and infant formula, at least more children survive, which makes mothers, the national health service, and WHO happy. Fear of dangerous ghosts associated with death in childbirth may have hastened the popularity of birthing in modern clinics. But continuities exist particularly around food sharing and identity.

Breastfeeding's place in Southeast Asian modernity is now shaped more by public health departments and the WHO than hungry ghosts. Long after ghosts have been relegated to premodern superstition, the older reciprocal logic is still reflected in Thai and Lao community-based rituals such as weddings and ordinations. Ritual prayers begin by reference to thanking and paying mothers back for their milk, an explicit reference to the reciprocity entailed in breastfeeding.

Colleagues from the Philippines told the story of a woman who kept the empty tins of infant formula she had used to feed her child. When the child grew up and was about to marry, the mother opened the closet and showed her child exactly how much she had spent on her early feeding. Thai anthropologists responded to this story; one said that her sister had done the same thing. The other commented on the foolishness of the practice because of the cost of the infant formula should be calculated according to the current market price, not on the price the mother paid for the products many years earlier. Weddings and ordinations still begin with reference to paying mothers back for the gift of her breastmilk (Thai, *kha nom*, milk price). The youngest daughter may be breastfed longer to strengthen her obligation to care for her parents in their old age and inherit the parental house.

Nurturing practices survive drastic spatial dislocation, particularly the mobile Hmong who are used to adapting to new locations—another mountain, another country. Both the Hmong and the Vietnamese entered North America as refugees in large numbers in the 1980s. The Hmong value large families. But like the Lao, Hmong mothers expect to lose many infants at birth or shortly after. Hmong population grew more than the American average between 2000 and 2013, probably because families in North America experience fewer infant deaths than in Lao PDR. But Hmong nurturing practices are deeply embedded and seem to have survived the disruption of refugee life and resettlement. Psychometric scales are not the first tool that an anthropologist would turn to when examining nurture and child socialization. But one study of Hmong and white American mothers in urban Minnesota brought to light some surprising differences in nurturing practices. In spite of the poverty and extraordinary cultural adaptation Hmong refugees coming to North America had to make, certain approaches to nurture and child rearing survived intact. Grandmothers and fathers continued to play important roles in child rearing. Hmong toddlers' diet was more balanced than that of the American toddlers. Hmong toddlers had fewer accidents; American babies had three times more burns, trauma, and ingestions of inappropriate substances, with the result that they had more emergency visits and hospitalizations than Hmong babies (Oberg et al. 1986: 404–5). (Hmong families may not trust hospitals.) Hmong mothers scored consistently higher on all mother–child interaction rating scales. Maternal care behavior measured cooperation, acceptance, accessibility, and sensitivity. Hmong mothers were more attentive and responsive to their toddlers. Hmong households supported the mother better than the American households. The conclusion of the psychologists was that in spite of the trauma of refugee experiences, the Hmong child is rich in social interaction, leading to secure attachment and ego resiliency (Oberg et al. 1986: 412).[5]

In an extraordinary story of a Hmong child in California diagnosed with epilepsy, we learn of the American doctors who studied Hmong culture in order to treat their Hmong patients; but those who make use of this cultural knowledge and respect the beliefs and preferences of their Hmong patients, may provide them with suboptimal care (Fadiman 1997: 75). This puts added stress on American doctors caring for Hmong patients: "People in the early years of their medical careers have invested an incredible amount of time and energy and pain in their training, and they have been taught that what they've learned in medical school is the only legitimate way to approach health problems. I think that is why some young doctors go through the roof when Hmong patients reject what we have to offer them" (Fadiman 1997: 76).

Both Hmong and Vietnamese refugees to North America experienced a sharp decline in breastfeeding rates (Romero-Gwynn 1989). In spite of efforts to promote breastfeeding among these populations, mothers relied more on their observations that breastfed babies in Vietnam and Lao PDR were thinner than bottle-fed babies in California, where they received their infant formula free of charge from WIC clinics (Tuttle and Dewey 1994).

A study of Vietnamese refugees resettled in Quebec also confirms the strength of breastfeeding customs even in new socio-geographical spaces. These women found it difficult to breastfeed, not because of a change in beliefs but because of the absence of their own mothers to offer postpartum rituals, including herbal steam baths, and other forms of support. These practices and beliefs are deeply rooted in Vietnamese culture. Better to use commercial formula than risk giving their newborns inadequate milk because of the absence of supportive rituals and appropriate postpartum foods (Groleau, Souliere, and Kirmayer 2006: 524).

In parts of the Philippines, Catholic missions competed with Methodist missions in areas with strong traditions of spirit and ancestor worship. In Ifugao, northern Philippines, women's heavy work load leaves them little time for proper attention to their infant and children's food needs (Kwiatkowski 1998: 202). Public concern about child malnutrition in the 1970s encouraged the aggressive promotion of tonics, vitamins, food supplements, and infant formula, resulting in a decline in the initiation and duration of breastfeeding (Kwiatkowski 1998: 48–49). In rural areas where breastfeeding was highly valued, women were still exposed to food and drug marketing, and many made use of sweetened condensed milk to supplement their breastmilk. The aggressive marketing of these products, and other processed foods set the taste for sweets. In Ifugao, poor children ate only rice and sugar if the family had no meat or vegetables. By providing sugar as a substitute for nutritional food, mothers could fill their children. Even the rice gruel fed to infants to supplement breastmilk was mixed with sugar (Kwiatkowski 1998: 205).

Historicizing Diversity

Considering the incredible diversity of infant-feeding styles and local patterns of nurture emerging from common infant needs and the universal mammalian process of lactation, what can we learn from these ethnographic glimpses into infant-feeding practices in Southeast Asia? What can Southeast Asia teach us about nurture, commensality, identity, and power? Does any of this matter practically or theoretically to anyone outside of Southeast Asia or Southeast Asian studies?

In some parts of the world, breastfeeding is an unproblematic aspect of human existence; in others, it is highly valued and highly charged symbolically, imbued with values beyond nutrition; in others it is a risky process that needs careful management; in still others, it is an act that evokes disgust and an irrational prudery. Customs that protect the mother–infant dyad appear more basic, more fundamental than even religious or medical instructions. The stories suggest that there is wide recognition of infancy as a vulnerable time and breastmilk as a vulnerable product. Thus, social rules in the form of customs exist that protect the integrity of the mother–infant dyad. In Southeast Asia, these involve keeping mothers and infants together around a heat source (*juu fai*) or generally heating up the mother after the coldness of the birth experience, and ideally, relieving her of domestic work for around forty days, the time it takes to fully establish lactation. Outside analysts have identified such practices as old-fashioned, uncivilized, primitive, misogynist, or worse; but we consider them as ways to give women the space to nurture, ways to preserve some of the most basic values of the social group—even when ideological rhetoric stresses the impurity of birth and the birthing woman. The loss of the social womb, encouraged by colonial medical regimes, removed many of postpartum customs from the local repertoire, including women's protected access to special foods and reduction in work loads.

Meals and morality are intimately connected in Southeast Asia. Both are grounded in nurturing practices of great antiquity in the region, and grounded in the activity of growing rice. Here we face a problem. By emphasizing the rural roots of nurturance, and idealizing rural logic, breastfeeding is easily positioned as old-fashioned. It is old-fashioned; it is part of our mammalian heritage, fashioned by generations of tradition-bearing women. Nurture is not modern; it is human.

Why do so many Southeast Asian peoples have similar infant-feeding practices? We see historical continuities that underlie present conditions, suggesting a common origin in the South China Neolithic. This suggests the breastfeeding complex is both ancient and closely connected with wet rice agriculture. After all, farming radically changed the human diet as well as women's roles. Early farmers had to adapt infant feeding to these new conditions (cf. Van Esterik 2011). The breastfeeding complex came to carry a highly refined body of practical knowledge in the form of postpartum customs. That would account for its remarkable stability even as surrounding cultures—the realities we now call Thai, Malay, and many others—have diverged so dramatically. Of course this extraordinary stability amid cultural change further testifies to breastfeeding's importance in maintaining systems of nurture (cf. O'Connor and Van Esterik 2012).

Some of the regional differences seen here may relate to the relation between root crop cultures and wet rice cultures. Successions of communities paid respect to the prior owners of the land, setting precedents, accepting some of the customs and cultural components of prior peoples. The rituals around burying the placenta may be linked to root crop logic: "The supplanting of tubers with rice is a common feature in the myths and rituals of the hill tribes of Southeast Asia" (Sutlive 1978: 63). Divine myths about the replacement of tubers with rice are always linked to females, and refer to mythic times when uncommonly large rice grains grew by themselves (cf. Reynolds and Reynolds 1982). Festivals celebrate ribald women assaulting men with "outlandishly large male organs" (Sutlive 1978: 55), also common in rural villages of the mainland.

The relation between root and rice cultures can best be seen at the margins of Southeast Asia, where Austronesian and Melanesian meet, such as the Indonesian province of Papua. Here, nurturing relations—primarily feeding—can override affinal and blood relations, "diminishing the influence of female blood and of women and wife-givers in general" (Van Oosterhout 2007: 170). In root crop systems of plant regeneration, bodies are reconstructed in a new cycle of life, forging new kinship ties across generations through communal flesh built from sago. Human juices flow, enter new bodies and from bodies, back to the earth and back again through the production of food (Van Oosterhout 2007: 173). Bodies become land that feeds future generations with root crops. Originally bodies could only reproduce through vegetative forms of reproduction, "like shoots from a sago tree," but people longed for sexual reproduction, which meant that humans would die (Van Oosterhout 2007: 175). The decay of a dead body allows the life force to recirculate, saturating the soil with ancestral substance that recirculates as food for the living (Van Oosterhout 2007: 185). In these root crop systems, stress is on male nurture through semen and sago, rather than through maternal milk (Van Oosterhout 2007: 190).

In Papua New Guinea in the 1970s, "Wamirans draw parallels between human beings and taro, and symbolically equate the female realm of human reproduction with the male realm of taro production. Women are said to supply offspring with blood and milk, the main ingredients in the creation and nurturing of life (Kahn 1986: 99). Breastmilk transfers matrilineal substance, and the word for breastfeeding is interchangeable with the word for matrilineal group. In this way, women are believed to control the procreation, nourishment, and growth of human beings (Kahn 1986: 92, 101).

Wet rice cultures have a very different approach to nurturing. A young woman from northeast Thailand working in Bangkok had to leave her breastfeeding baby behind when she traveled to her father's funeral. In traditional Thai logic, derived from the logic of wet rice cultivation and Theravada Buddhism, women are associated with life and attachment, men with death and renunciation; these domains must be kept separate, and so babies do not belong at funerals. Contrast this with Bali, for example, where elements of root crop logic persist in a wet rice context: new life emerges out of the dead decaying body.

Not all postpartum customs in Southeast Asia offer ideal solutions for feeding an infant according to Western biomedical theories. These customs are part of infant-feeding complexes of great antiquity; analysts do not get to choose the pieces they like. Take colostrum for example. Not all mothers throw away colostrum because it is considered intrinsically bad, but rather because it is more important to create strong social relations by having another mother feed a newborn. Often mothers throw away only a few drops, and only once to "clear the passage." The Hmong argue that it only needs to be done for the first child. While the newborn may lose the advantage of colostrum, the trade-off is the strengthened bond of social reciprocity, drawing the newborn and its mother into the community. In these contexts, the social connectivity of breastmilk is valued above its immunological properties.

Southeast Asia has well-developed herbal medical systems. Yet often the galactagogues and herbal medicines such as Javanese *jamu* and Thai *jaa dong* used to increase a women's milk are viewed as old-fashioned traditional customs of little biomedical value. It is healthier to give herbal drinks directly to mothers and indirectly to infants through breastmilk. In contrast, in many Latin American communities, mothers give herbal mixtures directly to an infant in a feeding bottle (cf. Van Esterik 1988: 194).

The Dance of Nurture in Southeast Asia

Dance is always embodied, always about emotion and connectedness. Dance is regional; both folk dances and palace dances link to the places where they were developed. The classical dance tradition of the courts of mainland Southeast Asia harken back to the sacred *devadasi* temple dance traditions of India and require professional classical dance training. In addition, many communities in Southeast Asia practice a participatory circle social dance, known as *ramwong* in Thai and Lao. In the Thai/Lao *ramwong*, women dance a step ahead of the men, conscious of their presence, flirting over their shoulders, and stepping carefully with their own unique style of hands and feet placement. Regardless of skill level, each pair conforms broadly to the group, as they take their place in the circle, dancing to rhythmic music. The Thai version with patriotic lyrics was popularized by Prime Minister Phibun Songkhram in the 1940s as part of the invention of Thai national traditions, but it was based on older, much sexier seasonal folk dance styles, some related to rice production. Some hand motions are reminiscent of classical dance styles, but mostly the gestures reflect local folk dance traditions, easily learned at temple fairs, weddings, and other celebrations.

In Java, *ronggeng* dancer-singers express a pre-Islamic mystical embodiment of the divine, but today they risk arrest under antipornography laws for sexy dancing with male audience members (Foley 2015: 369), as the modern Indonesian state tries to erase the non-Islamic parts of Javanese artistic traditions.

Dance styles, like nurturing practices, build on the historically constituted subsistence practices of their locality (cf. Lomax 1978), including links to *Devi Sri,* the goddess of rice. Both dance styles and nurturing practices are resilient and have adapted to many intrusions, transforming themselves in the process. The next chapter highlights how modernization challenges some of these local customs.

Notes

1. Huber confuses gender difference with gender inequality, a particularly important distinction in Southeast Asia where gender differences are not always used to support gender inequality. Huber argues that continuous cycles of pregnancy and lactation barred women from activities that bring the most prestige and power, at least until the invention of commercial breastmilk substitutes.
2. The term *style* was first used to describe infant-feeding style in urban Kenya, to show how nurturing practices are shaped by local regimens (Elliot and Van Esterik 1986). Others have used the term to refer to frequency and length of breastfeeding as style. Style bears a closer relation to what Kitzinger calls lactational signature (1995). Riordan and Auerbach, in their influential textbook, *Breastfeeding and Human Lactation* (1993: 42–43) referred to the concept of breastfeeding style and used it to address how cultural factors influence infant-feeding practices, including the distinctions between breastfeeding as a process and breastmilk as a product, a distinction emerging out of the concept of style.

3. Although peninsular Malaysia is attached to the mainland, the country also consists of East Malaysia on the island of Borneo, and is most often considered as part of island Southeast Asia.
4. We hope readers will expand this argument by examining similar words in other Southeast Asian languages. Initial conversations suggest that Malay does not have a similar term. The Karen word, *bylaung*, suggests a possible Tibeto Burman variant.
5. The movie about Hmong refugees in California, *Grand Torino*, is a wonderful illustration of family loyalty, nurture and resiliency.

CHAPTER 6

Modernizing Nurture
A Global Shift

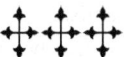

A massive Cartesian makeover that began in the West has now gone global. Sweeping aside earlier ways, it spreads as markets and nation-states remake everyday life. The shift to Cartesian modernity goes in different ways in different places, and yet one commonality is how breastfeeding suffers under conditions of modernity. In Chapter 5 we showed how different local traditions in Southeast Asia handle nurture. In this chapter, we consider how other local regimens of nurture negotiate modernity. We identify some of the forces of modernity that impinge on women's bodies in particular. How does the modern script with its focus on individual autonomy undermine nurture, and particularly breastfeeding, defining it as old-fashioned, premodern, or even "primitive"? Why do people buy into modernity, willingly paying a heavy price to be modern (Latour 1993: 35)?

The Historic Breast-to-Bottle Shift: The Chicago Story

We begin with how this happened in Chicago using Jacqueline Wolf's *Don't Kill Your Baby* (2001). Her story opens in the late nineteenth century when physicians and public health officials discover a plague of dying babies. Thanks to the science of their day, they identify the killer: cow's milk is replacing human milk. Some work to secure safer cow's milk by pasteurization, others develop infant formulas to replace it, and nearly everyone urges mothers to nurse their babies. All these efforts reduce infant mortality, and yet the experts never solve a key mystery: why were so many women failing at breastfeeding? Up until the last quarter of the nineteenth century, everyone had assumed "a mother would and could breastfeed her baby" (Wolf 2001: 74), but suddenly women were bottle feeding, certain their milk was deficient in quality or quantity.

Wolf clarifies what went wrong. One likely cause was the new fashion in scheduled feeding: cutting short breastfeeding episodes by the clock would have reduced mothers' milk production. Doubt did damage too: many people felt that the female body could not meet the unprecedented pressures of modern urban life. Then, too, the ideology of "scientific motherhood" (Apple 1980) not only questioned a woman's intuitions but repudiated the reassuring customs of the past. Is it any wonder that some women lacked enough milk, and many more feared they did? Shifting to cow's milk solved these problems.

Once physicians and public health officials realized the deadly consequences, they instituted breastfeeding campaigns far more confrontational and intrusive than today's mild-mannered "breast is best" advice. Injunctions like "don't kill your baby!" coupled with home visits by nurses exerted a civic and medical authority that is hard to imagine today. Yet even these remarkable efforts failed to reverse the trend. Although the full decline of breastfeeding in North America did not appear until the 1930s and 1940s, Wolf finds "mothers' preference for bottles over breasts ... [was] cemented by the 1910s." To make matters worse, as the medical generation that fought for breastfeeding died off, their successors forgot those public health lessons about the dangers of contaminated milk and the importance of maternal breastfeeding. Many became pro–bottle feeding or at least neutral. Health care professionals would not rediscover breastfeeding's importance until the 1970s.

How could late nineteenth-century American women defy that early medical advice to breastfeed? And how could twentieth-century medicine regress on breastfeeding while progressing elsewhere? Wolf skillfully shows how social currents shaped women's individual decisions:

> Economic pressure and class conflict, as well as changing views of time, efficiency, self-control, health, medicine, sex, marriage, and nature—in short, the social change concomitant with urbanization—prompted women to doubt the efficacy, propriety, and necessity of breastfeeding. (Wolf 2001: 3)

Even as she identifies separate factors, Wolf takes care to show how they interrelate. Take propriety. How could breastfeeding become improper to women whose mothers had breastfed them? Over the course of the nineteenth century, bodily functions became increasingly private, and society became ever more prudish (cf. Brumberg 1988). At the same time, as the birth rate fell in half, marriage became less about having children and more about intimate companionship:

> As the expectation of romance and companionship within marriage altered views of sex, attitudes toward breastfeeding changed. ... A woman's breasts now "belonged" to her husband at least as much as, if not more than, to her infant. (Wolf 2001: 24)

Troubled by how their breasts were at once maternal and sexual, bottle feeding kept the two properly apart.

Throughout her book, Wolf stresses how women made the individual choices that decided what happened overall:

> Women initiated the move from breast to bottle as they embraced complex social, cultural, economic, and intellectual change concomitant with urbanization, change that on the surface had little to do with infant feeding yet affected it profoundly. (Wolf 2001: 5)

In saying mothers chose bottle over breast, Wolf rejects scholarship that depicts women as pawns of men and medicine: "women—all women, for the increasingly common preference for cows' milk crossed class and ethnic lines—and not physicians instigated the move from breast to bottle" (Wolf 2001: 3). Although this is just one society's response to modernity, the story was repeated at other times and in other places.

The Historic Breast-to-Bottle Shift: The Modern Story

Wolf's decades-long story of infant feeding in a single city fits with other progressive North American cities, and the climate of the times. Changes begun in earlier eras and other domains suddenly met in the breast-or-bottle choice. In a few decades, well-functioning traditions died, and today's modern modalities were born. Now deeply rooted, those historic changes quietly yet powerfully impeded breastfeeding. To see how, we first need to retheorize what happened in Chicago.

Conscious Choice or Bodily Betrayal?

Even as we have only praise for Jacqueline Wolf's scholarship, to explain breastfeeding's decline, we need to go beyond attributing the change to women's choices. That individual choice model now dominates public health. In its Cartesian logic, a society's health patterns are the outcome of individual decisions. Here, to make the move to bottles a straightforward consequence of women's choices, the theory must separate the individual (a unique spiritual entity) from society (a generic law-like reality). Yet how separate were they? Humans evolved as social primates; each of us constructs our individuality out of social life; and—like it or not—we embody our social surroundings. In these three regards—phylogeny, ontogeny, and ontology—the Cartesian individual/society distinction does not hold.

To make a strong case that women chose bottle over breast, each option would have to be a viable chosen alternative (rather than bottle feeding by default after failed breastfeeding). For that to happen, a woman would somehow have to separate her sense of self (who she is, what she values, etc.) from the surrounding society that first creates and now influences her. Of course, at one level, every woman can and does consciously choose how to feed her infant. Yet the catch is that her conscious mind is caught up in a body that irresistibly channels its surroundings. Did those who chose the bottle do so freely or were they caught up in mechanistic practices and attitudes that stacked the cards against breastfeeding? And were those who tried to breastfeed but failed betrayed by how their bodies echoed societal patterns?

Take a potentially fateful decision like scheduled feeding. Suppose a woman, in responding to her baby's needs rather than society's imperatives, decided on-demand feeding was right for her child. While she might consciously reject "expert" warnings that such leniency could raise a self-indulgent, lazy alcoholic, could her body still summon the confidence breastfeeding needs? Moreover, if she lived a scheduled life, taking pride in punctuality, treating it as a marker of modern civilized order, could she release her body to adjust to her baby's erratic timing? Not easily. This then is our solution to the Chicago mystery: women who wanted to breastfeed but could not had already developed modern bodies that defied their conscious decisions. And this is our larger explanation for breastfeeding's abrupt decline in the late nineteenth and early twentieth centuries: society had changed and women's bodies had changed with it. The decisive mechanism was embodiment, not choice. In the end, as humans we have a limited capacity to live one way and get our bodies to act another way.

The Societal Crisis

To understand the strength and character of the social currents women were embodying, we need to look outward, beyond infant feeding into the larger society as well as backward in time. Like other progressive North American cities, late nineteenth-century Chicago experienced a distinctively modern crisis. Profound religious (the Reformation), political (the democratic revolution), and economic (laissez faire capitalism) changes—some centuries old, others just beginning—all converged in a single time and place. That social upheaval saw massive immigration, robber baron capitalism, the collapse of the old middle class (tradesmen, yeoman famers), and rise of the new (educated professionals). What Wolf summed up as urbanization might as readily be called secularization or industrialization or bureaucratization or even just modernization. By any name, the radical implications of imagining human life mechanistically—in a methodically soulless and materialist way—had finally come to bear on everyday life and seized ordinary bodies. Suddenly there was "no place of grace" (Lears

1981), no respite from an impersonal market and its amoral outcomes. As the sureties of an earlier day dissolved, an epidemic of neurasthenia, a debilitating depression, swept the middle class. Is it any wonder that some mothers failed at breastfeeding and others did not try? Women were living in a materialist society that lived within them.

The Historic Loss

Even as urban life created conditions that were unfriendly to breastfeeding, it wore away the social capital needed to resist these new ways. As we have shown, success at breastfeeding requires technical knowledge, protective customs, and community support. All of these resources had begun to break apart well before the social upheaval of the late nineteenth century. When the urban crisis came, the support that could have helped women breastfeed under adverse conditions was already in short supply.

The Cultural Solution—A New Body

The societal crisis eventually brought a cultural solution to living with, and within, modern conditions. At this societal turning point, people began working out the coping strategies that have come to characterize a "good person" and a "realistic attitude." This era-shaping shift might be summed up in the sports saying, "When the going gets tough, the tough getting going." So while some people gave up on keeping up, growing cynical or depressed, others took on the pace and intensity of modern life. Embracing the vigorous life, a modern lifestyle stressed exercise, athletics, physical fitness, healthy eating. A hopeful, optimistic, and above all energetic attitude acquired moral force (cf. O'Connor and Van Esterik 2015: Chapter 10).

While corporate monopolies and economic crashes devastated the old middle class and ravaged small towns, a new progressive middle class arose out of urban life to meet the needs of large national organizations. Instead of fighting progress, they embraced the ever-changing modern skills and knowledge it took to keep up. Wanting the same for their children, they organized positive, energetic activities like sports and scouting. Caught in this societal current, women who choose bottle over breast could feel they were doing what was right, or at least inevitable, even if it defied medical advice. And, swept along by these same currents, doctors soon forgot what their predecessors had learned about why babies died.

Modern urban life gave the impression that society was out of control. As distinctions of gender, status, occupation, and ethnicity grew weaker, demands for individual self-control grew stronger. In what Stearns (1999) calls compensatory control, the good person became cleaner, thinner, more self-denying, and more emotionally controlled than ever before. By these standards of bodily discipline, breastfeeding became unseemly. As it inevitably broke all tidy modern lines of cleanliness, control, and autonomy, it was at best an anomaly, at worst an abomination, setting the stage for the disgust reaction to breastfeeding that occasionally resurfaces in Euro-American discourse today.

Defining Modernity

To place the North American story in the broader context of modernization, we need to define modernity, identify some of its characteristics, and focus attention on those features relevant to infant feeding.

What Is Modernity?

For most people, modernity is a stage in human progress. Studies of the grand sweep of history, as we argued at the opening of this book, just ignore matters of care and nurture. Modernity is one of these grand sweeps of history.

Modern is a term that has come to mean improved, rational, scientific, efficient, and current or up to date. *Modernity* describes the state of being modern or contemporary in comparison to what came before—traditional, premodern, ancient, or old-fashioned, and is thus a relative term. When we think the modern era begins depends on what modernity is being contrasted with. The renaissance used the contrast between the ancient and the modern.

Raymond Williams includes modern in his exploration of keywords, noting that the English usage comes from the French term meaning just now, contemporary (1985: 208), clearly a moving definition. The process of modernization, suggests a local alteration or improvement on an old institution, while modern as an adjective suggests a new, modified form. The abstract examination of modernity and modernization is a Western discourse that has been exported throughout the world through the practice of development, often through bilateral and multilateral development institutions established to guide modern social progress after World War II. For example, CIDA, the Canadian International Development Agency, identifies traditional culture as a barrier to development. As societies develop, then, they shed aspects of traditional culture that impede modern progress. These efforts to modernize the developing world are discussed more in Chapter 7.

Colonialism made visible differences that were interpreted as a contrast between traditional and modern. But there are always connections between past and present, hybrid customs and practices, and debts between the generations, as we saw in Southeast Asia. Globalization and capitalism are part of modernity, but in Southeast Asia, for example, globalization has a very long history. For all the problems and anxiety caused by modernity, modern institutions contributed to the reduction of starvation (cf. Goody 1982), maternal and infant mortality, and deaths from polio and smallpox in many parts of the world.

When Is Modernity?

Modernity as a condition in the world associated with late capitalism and industrialization can be studied ethnographically in specific places, particularly in modern institutions like bureaucracies, hospitals, schools, science laboratories, popular culture, and mass media.

Communities around the world adopt features of modernity or define themselves as having passed into modernity at different times and from different histories. In Thailand, royalty is both modern and premodern, whereas in neighboring Lao PDR, royalty is part of the ancient feudal past, while communism is modern. Modernity designates a break in the regular passage of time, dividing ancients from moderns, primitive from enlightened.

The Thai make the comparison between past and present explicit in two phrases, *samai gorn* and *samai mai,* the earlier time period, and the new time period, always shifting what is considered earlier and new. For example, betel chewing is a practice from *samai gorn*; wearing elegant diaper-like sarongs that passed between your legs (*jungkaben*) belongs to an earlier time period, while wearing black nylon stretchy stirrup pants in the 1970s was evidence you were lodged, sweaty, and miserable in *samai mai,* new times.

For the purpose of our discussion, modernity begins in the late nineteenth century when North Americans worked out a response to urbanization, the industrial revolution, and capitalist markets—the time period highlighted in the Chicago story. Utilizing the relativity of the Thai definition, we adopt a distinction that builds on the life-cycle approach: modern is now, contemporary, while traditional refers to practices of our parental and grandparental generation. Thus, we are always modern and nonmodern as we move through the life cycle.

Features of Modernity

Modernity produces new contexts and encourages changes in attitudes. Although there have been attempts to create measurable indices of modernity, here we draw attention to some features of modernity that are elaborated in North America and relevant for infant feeding. What marks us as modern? What is radically new about these changes that brought about modernity? Modernity is about measurable progress. Much like the old General Electric advertisement, "Progress is our most important product," modernity demands constant reform, constant improvement to provide a better life for all.

Modernity values the impersonal, the rational, and the scientific. It requires critiquing false beliefs and liberating ourselves from our prescientific past (Latour

1993: 35), often by attacking custom. The search for scientific progress is endemic to both medicine and science but anathema to custom.

Modern society glorifies individuality and autonomy, and hides the deep dependence we have on one another, including links across the generations. The autonomous individualism of modernity uses the male as the hallmark of adult citizenship, ignoring how maternal embodiment differs from male embodiment (cf. Hausman 2007: 491).

North Americans today value independent, pragmatic people; a good thoroughly modern person is pragmatic, disciplined, reasonable, and able to self-regulate. The work of crafting modern selves to thrive in an empiricist world is a modern project. Modernity requires regulated, clean, autonomous, contained bodies that do not leak. It stresses hygiene that abhors the messiness that cannot be contained without leakages. Moderns have emotional gut responses to bodily fluids like spit, saliva, milk, and blood. In Singapore's march to modernity, even toilets were government regulated, and citizens were fined for spitting or chewing gum (cf. Tarulevicz 2013). Good modern flesh must be fit and tightly managed.

Modernity brings stress; it was widely assumed by Euro-American health professionals that the stress of modern life made breastfeeding impossible (Minchin 2015: 202). Modern urban life brings the stress of constantly making choices, always dealing with strangers (who are lonely); and the stress of loneliness itself, omnipresent under conditions of modernity; loneliness is a modern way of life. Modernity breaks down bridges between biology and custom, past and present, adding yet another source of modern stress, and gives us new pre-scripted paths to follow. As a result, we are forced to choose packages within new consumption frames. Such choices may be forced on people in the absence of accurate information and support, as in the case of breastfeeding.

Secularization and undercutting the authority of religion is another feature of modern life. Although religion can itself be a source of stress and even violence, particularly as it shapes identity politics, the absence of religious authority complicates making choices in the modern world.

Modernity is mobile, deterritorialized. It is modern to move away from home—particularly for adolescents. Immigration separates people and isolates nuclear families, as we saw in the Chicago story. Modern working conditions easily disrupt roots to place and past.

Modernity deconstructs things into bits, breaking up holistic continuities for easier management. Consider the birth continuum, for example. Modernity breaks up the continuity from conception to weaning, supplying new cutoff points along the continuum of care, from pregnancy and birth, to postpartum. These arbitrary points break up the continuity of nurture common in premodern local regimens. Once this continuum is broken into component parts, modern health systems assigned specialties to different stages of reproduction—the gynecologist, the obstetrician, the pediatrician. When midwives were removed from modern hospitals, women lost the one practitioner who could see them through from pregnancy to sevrage. As modern midwives are reintegrated into modern health care systems, they face challenges integrating the premodern and the modern aspects of their work (Davis-Floyd 1996). In the process, we lost local traditions of the postpartum period, often interpreting customs as restrictive and misogynous primitive nonmodern practices. Forty days of ritual impurity, separation, or vulnerability is a small price to pay for having time to rest with a newborn and help with chores. Rituals around the churching of women after childbirth, the lying-in period, and other traces of the social womb lodged in nonmodern practices also mark the period of time it takes for lactation to be firmly established.

Modernity glorifies technology and trusts it to solve, not cause problems. Indeed, rapidly changing technology may be one of the most clearly defined features of modernity. E-mail, electric breast pumps, microwaves, cell phones, fetal monitors, and humanized milk fortifiers all impact on modern infant-feeding practices. Some modern technology has vastly improved lives. And sometimes modern technology coexists with ancient technology. As Latour notes, "I may use an electric drill, but I also use a hammer" (1993: 75). The hammer is hundreds of thousands of years older than the electric drill. Similarly, the miracles of modern surgery are enhanced by having family members attending the patient during recovery, a premodern tradition of continuing value and benefit to modern patients. Technology has allowed us to bypass nurture, to survive, and even to think we thrive without nurture.

Modern technology speeds us up. Modern times are fast times. When humans interact with or are replaced by technology, it is humans who have to speed up, catch up, to match the pace of electronic technology. We are always behind, losing time, wasting time. Breastfeeding is part of the slower pace of life required to nurture a child. Breastfeeding makes women slow down to the infant's pace for a short period of time, as infants and mothers are synchronized to each other. They operate not on clock or linear time but on interaction time and biological time. In the modern world when nurture is not valued, this adjustment in temporal pace is hard to accomplish. Calendar time, like industrial time moves forward like an arrow, obliterating the past behind it. Or as Hannah Arendt explained, life is the time interval between birth and death, and it follows a linear movement that is full of events that tell a story (Arendt 1998: 97).

"Anthropology is here to remind us: the passage of time can be interpreted in several ways—as a cycle or as decadence, as a fall or as instability, as a return or as a continuous presence" (Latour 1993: 68). The future orientation of modernity reminds us to plan for the future rather than enjoy the present. For mothers, this future orientation often includes the early introduction of the feeding bottle in preparation for future separation from their infants. Electric breast pumps are a common but expensive baby shower gift for American mothers without maternity entitlements, modern technology that anticipates future separation.

Breastfeeding and Nurture—Not Modern and Not Not Modern

Breasts and breastfeeding are not modern and not not modern, a paradox that underlies some of the dilemmas of breastfeeding in the modern world. Schechner (1985) used this theater metaphor for dealing with the twice-behaved behavior of performance. We use it to stress the simultaneity of being not modern and not not modern. Breastfeeding tells a human story—a culture-nature, biocultural story—not a modern story. Modern stories are often about individual persons—biographies and autobiographies. Perhaps breastfeeding is the quintessential women's story, one that is not text-based, and often interrupted in the telling: "To understand lived experience, we need narratives, stories of muddled, in-the-midst-of experiences whose only certainties are the beginnings or turning points" (Wikan 2000: 234). While it makes sense to talk about the modernization of hospitals or workplaces, breastfeeding is neither modern, nor capable of being modernized. It fits poorly into the features of modernity described above.

Breastfeeding is personal, not impersonal; it resists being analyzed and pulled apart, it cannot be broken into bits. It is holistic; mothers speak of the moment when breastfeeding starts to feel comfortable and natural. Like the moment when you learn to ride a bike, it is hard to describe in words, but you know the moment when you master any skilled activity.

Over the last two decades, the constituents of breastmilk have been identified, analyzed, and measured by biomedical scientists, and while advocates (and manufacturers) have benefited from that knowledge, breastfeeding is about much more than the nutrients in the product. Product orientation reinforces measurement issues. In a perversion of modernity, human milk has become a measurable commodity, a product with a monetary value that could be compared with other products, as the story below illustrates.

Priceless Milk

The Maternity Protection Coalition (MPC) formed in 1982 from NGOs concerned about the International Labour Organization's maternity protection legislation. There was pressure from other UN agencies to encourage countries to drop maternity entitlements to improve productivity. The MPC lobbied to prevent this and to improve existing legislation. At a meeting I attended in the nineties, I recall tensions with several NGOs who took a very pragmatic approach to women's work, trying to calculate the financial contribution of women's unpaid work, including the work of nurture and care, and assign a monetary value to breastfeeding and breastmilk. Breastfeeding advocates were asked to calculate the price per liter for breastmilk, and many were reluctant to do so. Since some Scandinavian countries include breastmilk in their food consumption tables, we came up with a number based on the current price of banked breastmilk sold to hospitals. But this commodification of human milk made other groups feel as if they were treating mothers like dairy cows being milked. To work with other women's groups, we were forced to reconcile the dangers of commodifying human milk and putting an economic value on something incommensurate and priceless, with the pragmatic need to provide evidence that the work of breastfeeding matters, and that breastfeeding has both costs (including the time, nutrients and opportunity costs for mothers) and huge economic benefits even in industrial resource-rich countries. The net economic value of breastmilk in Australia was estimated around 4 billion Australian dollars/year—minimally (Smith 2013). While putting a price on breastmilk seems offensive, ignoring its value is more offensive. (PVE)

Modern mothers may obsess about measurement to the extent that they may pump and measure their milk in an attempt to know and try to control the amount of milk that their babies consume. But the act of measuring the activity disrupts the activity. The practice of exclusive pumping makes measurement easier, but it is not breastfeeding. Modern North American women looked for total control over infant feeding by measuring their breastmilk output, needing to know the exact amount produced. Normally, output is invisible, except for the odd dribble (and the output at the other end, wet diapers). But it is the breastfed infant who controls the amount of milk consumed and thus, produced, and that amount is difficult to calculate directly.

Breastfeeding refigures the autonomy and rejects the individualism that modernity assumes; breastfeeding is not about autonomy, but interdependence and the creation of social relationships through nurturing practices—the provision of food, care, and emotional support to another person. Breastfeeding exposes the interdependence between people in a way that challenges the modern sensibility.

Modern bodies are neat, disciplined, and controlled. Good modern flesh must be tightly managed. Breasts are particularly difficult to manage; they jiggle, change shape and leak, and are controlled only partially and with difficulty by brassieres (Young 2005). Maternal breastfeeding bodies do not conform to these modern standards. Breastfeeding can even be premodernly messy and inefficient. Premastication, sweaty, leaky breasts and spit ups, even bed sharing and shared breastfeeding, may precipitate a disgust reaction among moderns. The yuck factor inhibits discussion of some of these fears.

Breastfeeding mothers cannot be obsessed with hygiene. Yet the days when nipples were scrubbed with carbolic or boracic acid, alum solutions, or alcohol wipes are not long past (cf. Fildes 1986: 118). Current research suggests that hygiene is not that important for breastfeeding, and that immunity develops best in relation to the impurities in the immediate environment. For example, parents who clean their infants' pacifier by sucking it have infants with reduced risk of allergies (Hesselmar et al. 2013). A breastfeeding mother can never be totally in control of feeding because the activity is coregulated with her infant. That may make breastfeeding particularly difficult for control freaks and perfectionists.

Modern life fears indulgence and sees breastfeeding as indulgent. Older infants are suspected of controlling their mothers and mothers as indulging their children when breastfeeding continues beyond a few months, as if there were a cutoff point when breastfeeding no longer conferred any advantages.

Modern frames of reference emphasize the importance of choice, of a mother's right to choose what suits her best as an individual. With breastfeeding, choices are minimized. A woman's body produces breastmilk by the sixteenth week of her pregnancy; she only has to decide whether or not she will give it to her child. The decision to breastfeed is a profound one for modern mothers and others, but at the moment of decision, it may not be recognized as a choice because the activity takes over her body. If she decides not to breastfeed, there are modern drugs to inhibit lactation. Emphasis on choice distracts from the fact that mothers need to have complete unbiased information, good options to choose from, and structures in place for supporting them when they make their choices.

Expert medical advice may create the illusion of choosing between equal alternatives. The modern "choice" to become a breastfeeding mother, a mixed feeder, an exclusive pumper, a bottle feeder using milk-based or soy-based formulas, or a non-breastfeeder is presented as if it were analogous to the choice among different brands of soap or infant formula.

The modern emphasis on new choices can also inspire antimodern movements, such as "back to the breast" (La Leche League), or back to nature (health foods, cf. Martucci 2015). Modern regimes breed resistance that delights in reversals. Nostalgia for an imagined past is another response to modernity, one not uncommon in Southeast Asia, as we noted in the last chapter.

Breastfeeding is low tech and resistant to the modern time crunch; you cannot speed up a breastfeeding baby, as every mother on her way to a special event knows. Breastmilk is the original slow food. Breastfeeding is not about saving time, but it is about integrating different kinds of time across two distinct bodies through coregulation. Infants operate on biological or physiological time, shaped by the unfolding of their own constitution within the parameters of normal infant development. New mothers operate on their own distinct biological or physiological time, as they recover from childbirth. But they are also fully socialized into industrial, clock, and calendar time, counting the hours or days until they must return to work, until the rains that may damage crops arrive, until dinner needs to be prepared. Breastfeeding is present-oriented in a future-oriented world. In this way, breastfeeding can act much like meditation practice as it requires focused attention on the present moment, particularly in the early weeks after birth.

Modernity inscribes people in time not space, and does not require people to be located where local customs flourish. You can be modern anywhere. In contrast, breastfeeding is always local, always rooted in place, always shaped by local custom. Like blood and soil, breastfeeding lodges people in place; the local taste of the place, the local terroir, establishes taste continuities that pass between the generations. Breastfeeding provides the child's first linkages to place, through taste and the social relationships created through food sharing, as we showed in Chapter 4. The modern assault on local custom damages both commensality and nurture. Breastmilk carries traces of local and even national cuisines; when invoked with nationalism, we see the potential for slippage into the discourse of mastery, as Whitaker (2000) shows with breastfeeding policy in fascist Italy.

Breastfeeding can be difficult for modern mothers; doing it the hard way may include restricting foods and medications, denying North American mothers a relaxing beer or glass of wine, for example. Modernity creates the self-sacrificing mother who has to abstain from what she wants or needs. Eating right or controlling emotions may be important in establishing lactation, but restrictions may become self-limiting and more lax after the postpartum period. Think of how and where mothers in other parts of the world breastfeed. It is WEIRD Euro-American mothers who impose a perfectionism that demands a peaceful environment, a comfortable rocking chair, enriched meals, relaxing music; these are class-based North American standards of what breastfeeding requires.

Technology, Time, and Modern Bodies

Moderns trust technology to solve problems. Of course technology has been solving some problems for people (and primates) since the dawn of humanity (and before). But technology cannot solve the problems of nurture. In fact, technology impinges on infant and women's bodies in unexpected ways. Modernity imposes distinct work patterns, schedules, and time constraints on women and families. Some of the technology invented to adapt to these modern environments such as strollers and cribs distorts infant relations to the maternal body. Just as chairs block the normal capacity of humans to squat, and the boot has blocked the development of the prehensile functions of the foot, bottles, soothers, strollers, cribs, and pumps have blocked the normal hormonal, tactile, and emotional conversations between mothers and infants. "Only with much practice and training can these blockages be overcome" (Ingold 2011: 39).

Because breastfeeding is an embodied practice, how does modernity set up competing embodied practices with the invention of products such as enriched infant formula, humanized milk fortifiers, and breast pumps? Feeding bottles have improved over time, as have the products that are used as breastmilk substitutes. Early containers tried to imitate animals or the human breast. Later items resembled laboratory equipment, part of the complex of scientific feeding, complete with measurements for calibrating the mixture. Glass and plastic bottles provided different advantages and challenges. New forms such as the podee bottle from Australia uses a tube within a feeding bottle to facilitate hands-free self-feeding from any position (cf. Minchin 2015: 215). Some pump manufacturers provide containers that imitate the breast, rather than supplying hard plastic or glass bottles with measurements delineated on the side. The soft silicon breast-shaped container for expressed milk is distinctly different from the glass bottles commonly used for delivering infant formula.

Infant-feeding technology, including bottles, pumps, and nipple shields, along with other gadgets such as pacifiers and plastic-covered breast pads operate "to mediate social anxieties concerning women's proper behavior as mothers" (Hausman 2007: 481). While bottles have been presented as part of the "liberation in a can" strategy by liberal feminists who call for men to share the work of child rearing, they have not freed women from the work of infant feeding, since mothers are often the ones to use the feeding bottles.

In the WEIRD North American world, some women have become breastmilk feeders or exclusive pumpers, rather than breastfeeding mothers. They have come to appreciate the superiority of breastmilk as a product, compared with artificial baby milks, but reject the practice of breastfeeding. We hear of mothers at home with their infants who take twenty minutes with an electric pump to empty their breasts, and then feed their infants with their own breastmilk in bottles, whether they are at home or in public. New gadgets such as the hands-free nursing bra claim to make pumping easier, particularly double pumping. Yet no mothers report the pleasure of pumping, only the discomfort, as we become our own wet nurses.

Sometimes pumping is the only way for an infant to get any breastmilk. When mothers and babies are separated by illness or other unavoidable situations, when mothers have faced abuse or difficult working conditions, then pumping may increase their options and make it easier to provide some breastmilk to their infants. Some mothers use electric pumps until hand expression can be established or they can return to normal breastfeeding. Others use pumps to relieve engorgement or to "pump and dump" their milk to keep up a milk supply when their milk might harm their babies because of medications, for example. It is important to distinguish between mothers who have a choice regarding infant-feeding methods, and those women who do not have a choice. Like wheelchairs and walking, wheelchairs are a great technological innovation for those who cannot walk, but they are not the same as walking. Who would choose to use a wheelchair if they could walk unassisted on their own? Minchin uses an analogy with prostheses; we are grateful for them without thinking they are as good as normal limbs. We use them when needed and constantly try to improve them. "Losing a limb does not alter the normal development of our children or grandchildren. Not being breastfed does" (2015: 461).

Electric breast pumps may be a great technological innovation, but they are no substitute for breastfeeding. Similarly, exclusive pumping instead of breastfeeding your own baby is not the same process as pumping to provide your excess milk to others through milk sharing or banking. The first is a failure to embody nurture, the desire to avoid breastfeeding as a process, the later, an altruistic gift, making a valuable resource available to others as a form of common property.

The growing popularity of pumps in North America raises new research questions. Does exclusive pumping encourage early weaning to infant formula? Is breast pumping harmful to the breast? Does pump use interfere with coregulation by disturbing the regulatory balance between mothers and babies?

Although American women are increasingly encouraged to use electric breast pumps, they also use their babies and their hands to remove milk from their breasts. Mechanical breast pumps are around 100 years old, and the first electric pump was developed in 1991; but the latter practices are as old as our species. Like Latour's example of the hammer and electric drill, some customs survive changes in technology.

The Psalms of the Brothers (*Therakatha*) and Psalms of the Sisters (*Therikatha*) are Buddhist stories of enlightenment in men's and women's lives. Part of the Pali canon of Theravada Buddhism dated from around the first century BC, they are translated and accessible to modern practitioners. But the stories from men's lives are not really accessible, because they refer to premodern tasks and technology such as blacksmithing. The male stories are dated. But the women's stories speak across the generations—stories of being kept awake at night by a fussy baby, of lazy husbands who lose their tempers or who demand sex when their wives are too tired, of burning the dinner, of the rice pot boiling over while they were distracted by children. These stories are as fresh as when they were first told; 2,000 years ago or last week, the messages come through because they are couched in the unchanging vocabulary of nurture.

Although infant-feeding technology can make each generation appear radically different from the one before, breastfeeding makes each generation more dependent on the generation before; lactation does not change, and the customs that support nurture adapt slowly to changed contexts.

Modern Meals

Modernity is predicated on the denial of local traditions and customs. Over the last century, foods that used to be produced, processed, and prepared at home have been produced away from home, by new industrial processes, and made available in both local and distant markets. Industrial technology has produced a number of processed foods that act as substitutes for breastmilk; even poor quality products, inappropriately used, are perceived to solve certain problems for mothers and families. Modern artificial baby foods are much improved over the earliest mixtures developed by Nestlé in the 1860s, composed of malt, milk, sugar, and flour (Minchin 2015: 203). Like olestra and plastic, milk substitutes do not resemble what they were designed to replace.

Although adults may take more risks in trying new foods for themselves, eating foods past the "best before" date, and not obsessing over the quality of their foods (except for those who become literally obsessed with the quality of their foods—orthorexia), are they more vigilant about the foods they provide for their infants and children? Although adults may move readily to adopt "modern" styles of eating, using food to construct and reconstruct their identities, custom still governs infant-feeding practices, particularly when elders participate in feeding infants and young children and when consumption of local foods fashions the infant into an acceptable member of society. Lao families feed infants glutinous rice to make infants "become" Lao; Mexican families use corn to accomplish this.

Is it more common to think of children following "modern" food habits, leaving adults to consume traditional dishes recalled from their own childhoods? Chinese "little emperors" provide evidence for this, requesting faddish new prestige snacks from parents who yield to their children's tastes even knowing the snacks are not healthy (Chee 2000: 53). On the other hand, in Mali, adults do not waste good food on a young child who they say cannot appreciate its taste (Dettwyler 1994). The difference between feeding self and feeding others, and the relation between adult and child meals and their definition as "modern" practice rather than "traditional" custom must be answered ethnographically, a task we began for one region of the world—Southeast Asia—in Chapter 5.

With our modern faith in progress and science, we know more now about vitamins, and micronutrients; but do we eat better food products, developed and improved through the authority of sciences like nutrition? Food as fuel is part of a discourse of modernity developed by nutritional science, the discipline that successfully separated nurture from nutrients.

Modernity and the attrition of customary food practices have given us an excess of choice. Since the 1700s, food choices have steadily increased (Coveney 2000: 8). Choices are forced on people in the absence of information and support, even as modernity breaks down the bridges between biology and custom. With modernity came the range of personal meal choices that can isolate eaters.

Modernity brought us individual portions and dishes, calories, vitamins, health foods, and a lack of trust in the food system. Commensality, as we argued in Chapter 4, requires trust in those who provide and prepare food. Thus, modernity makes commensality more difficult. For eating is a risky business. Throughout recorded history, women have been concerned with the quality of their own breastmilk, and more particularly, with the breastmilk provided by other women through wet nursing. Now women have been made to fear the human milk they purchase online and even the milk in milk banks. Media amplification of these fears followed based on research that found that 75 percent of milk sold online was contaminated with the same kind of bacteria found in human waste (Keim et al. 2013). Although human milk always contains these good bacteria that jumpstart the infant's immune system, the way the information was reported in the popular media would be enough to repulse the reader who knows little about the microbiome of human milk or milk sharing. Although food safety is improving, and regulations mean that there is less adulteration, food scares remain a feature of modern life (Ferrieres 2006; Kjernes, Harvey, and Warde 2007). At the same time, traditional strategies such as wet nursing and postpartum rest declined under the individualized strategies of modern nutrition and biomedicine.

Visceral Knowledge and the Life Cycle

Latour argues that there cannot be an anthropology of the modern world because we were never modern (1993: 7). If we were never modern, then comparison is possible (Latour 1993: 10) because we moderns are much like everyone else. Attention to nurture reinforces how very alike we are by exposing the interdependent links between people, starting with mothers and newborns. And in spite of the great variation in styles of nurture, everywhere, the newborn must be fed or it dies; we must eat—over and over again—from shortly after birth to shortly before we die. This has implications for the life-cycle approach we used in Chapter 4.

Modernity teaches us to be, and to see ourselves as separate autonomous individuals with competing interests, not as links in a larger, more cooperative chain across the generations—the life cycle. Our modern lives suppress the connections between the generations. But nurture requires us to examine what connects us to past and present, linking people together across generations.

Modernity may erode the life-cycle logic where breastfeeding thrives, but it cannot erase the fact that we exist by virtue of the nurture of others. Breastfeeding is a moment that brings interdependence back into focus in an emotionally powerful and potentially threatening way. This is perhaps why in Euro-American societies, some people find breastfeeding offensive, even disgusting and are deeply troubled by doing it, hearing about it, or even seeing it. Princess Michael of Kent made her opinion clear: "My advice to women is don't breastfeed. It's a dreadful practice. I didn't breastfeed. My nanny said it was disgusting" (*Daily Mail,* 10 December 2014).

This erasure of nurture and the life cycle was less visible in the local traditions of Southeast Asia. There, these discourses of nurture and related complexes survive modernity to remain embedded in broader stories of connectedness—to ancestors, to lineages, to food supplies. The cycles of bodies and continuities across generations fits with modern discoveries that the immune system is a complex multigenerational inheritance; "what will become you began in your maternal grandmother's womb" (Minchin 2015: 76, 77).

Breastfeeding assumes—indeed requires—coregulation and can become a model for other kinds of coregulation, other instances of emotional sensitivity to and sympathy for others at other points in the life cycle. The dance of nurture may extend its rhythms into the tense teen years where empathy is often a scarce commodity. Troubled teens who were breastfed on demand can still be calmed by cuddling to reduce stress. Personal stories are supported by the work of Fergusson and Woodward, whose research in New Zealand on the psychosocial outcomes of breastfeeding confirmed that teens who were breastfed as infants for longer durations reported higher levels of parental attachment and maternal bonding, and perceived their mothers as more caring and less overprotective, compared with teens who were bottle-fed as infants (1999: 144).

McKenna's research on cosleeping confirms the responsiveness of breastfed babies who cosleep with their mothers. The cascading effects of bed-sharing include cognitive improvements and psychological adjustment; these babies are generally happier, less fearful and anxious, more emotionally stable, and generally more comfortable in their bodies. These trends continue across the generations as these individuals mimic their own experience when they become parents (McKenna 2000).

This research further suggests that maternal bonding does not contribute to codependence or overprotectiveness. (Of course, one might ask what is wrong with codependence?). If breastfed babies form stronger, longer lasting emotional bonds with their mothers and others, this might also explain why breastfeeding mothers are predisposed to provide more nurturant and caring environments for their children.

Breastfeeding: A Modern Dance?

Is breastfeeding a primitive activity that our modern technologically advanced society has rendered obsolete (Bentley 2014: 66)? Is the dance of nurture a primitive dance that is becoming a modern dance? Modern dance forms developed in the late nineteenth and early twentieth centuries in the United States. Freed from the narrative structures, rigors, and rules of ballet, it stressed free form movement and dancers moving independently of each other rather than in unison. Fit athletic dancers used abstract movements to freely express their emotions.

Partners were not necessary in this new dance form. Modern dance is specific to a particular time and place; although the form has spread to different parts of the world, it is considered an American dance form that consciously rejects the constraints of codified rules and seeks out new, innovative moves.

The modern world is a strange place—a place that creates hybrids around bodies, technologies, and food. Companies have a long history of trying to extract or replicate human milk proteins, fats, and sugars found in breastmilk in order to add them to baby milks. From trying to breed human lactoferrin in Herman, the transgenic bull, to creating genetically engineered components from algae for use in infant formula, modern technology tries to improve on a product perfected through mammalian and human evolution. Some companies tried to produce human milk proteins such as lactoferrin and lysozyme in the seeds of transgenic "breast rice." The developers claim that the food products and dietary supplements that use the proteins from the rice could "help save many of the two million children a year who die from diarrhea and the resulting dehydration and complications" (*Daily Mail*, 8 March 2007). There are currently some 2000 patent applications for human milk components in the US (McClain 2017). Efforts to exploit the components in breastmilk without supporting the producers of the original product, breastfeeding women, draw attention to the modern drive to use technology to solve the problems of child malnutrition without addressing the processes of nurture.

Minchin summarizes some of what we know about the contents of modern infant formula:

> That it is non-sterile, contains fats made by genetically altered marine algae and soil fungi, and may come with industrially produced bacteria as well as foods for those bacteria to grow on; that these substances will affect gut development in ways that cannot be predicted and have not been monitored. (Minchin 2015: 116)

In this chapter, we have focused attention on North American modernity. A logical next step would be to explore how and why Scandinavian modernity differs from North American modernity, and from French, Irish, or Thai modernities. How do their local practices and histories play in to their modern presents? But it is the North American version of modernity that has come to dominate institutions that address global infant-feeding policy. Modernity demands effective and efficient mastery, and it is to these efforts to master nurture that we now turn. The next chapter explores the discourse of mastery that dominates international attempts to improve infant-feeding practices.

PART
IV

Interventions

Part IV examines national and international interventions that promote breastfeeding and optimal young child feeding as part of modernity's march of progress and improvement. In Chapter 7, we draw attention to the institutions that attempt to master nurture as they seek solutions to the universal problem of how to feed a newborn. We show how modern bureaucratic practices themselves can disrupt nurture. In Chapter 8, we return to the biocultural model to remind us that infant feeding is constantly being negotiated between mothers and infants. In the concluding section, we consider advocacy efforts to reposition breastfeeding in the context of broader negotiations around sustaining nurturing practices.

CHAPTER 7

Mastering Nurture
Trying to Get Nurture Right

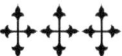

Agata Smeralda entered the magnificent building called the *Spedale di Santa Maria degli Innocenti* (SDI) in Florence on 5 February 1445, shortly after the facility opened on 25 January 1445. She was passed through a rotating shelf in the wall of the Innocenti palace to a woman on the other side. A bell was rung to alert those inside of the new arrival. She was nurtured at SDI with breastmilk purchased from two wet nurses. In spite of receiving breastmilk, Agata died in December of that year. One might expect a foundling orphanage and hospital would be associated with the church or a charitable initiative of a Medici Prince. Not so. It was commissioned by the silk workers guild of Florence. No doubt the guild benefited from having a stream of skilled apprentices, because the Innocenti contracted local artisans to teach trades to boys and girls in the orphanage, especially silk weaving. SDI was built to accommodate the increasing numbers of abandoned (and unbaptized) children in Florence (Grieco 1991: 40).

Like the enlightened self-interest of the silk weavers' guild, contemporary policy makers struggle with how to develop policies to reduce infant deaths. In the 1400s, there were few alternatives to human milk. Some wet nurses came to the Innocenti, some foundlings were farmed out to wet nurses in the region; all were paid for their services, the amounts carefully inscribed and kept in the archives of SDI. Harvesting wheat and raising silkworms, for example, required intensive labor at the hottest season of the year (Grieco 1991: 43). But as paid workers, the wet nurses could return the foundling and end the contract with the Innocenti if their labor was needed elsewhere (Corsini 1991: 68). Just as all mothers must negotiate their time to breastfeed around their work schedules, wet nurses too had to fit breastfeeding in with their other tasks. Perhaps Agata's wet nurses could not fit breastfeeding into their fall harvesting schedules. In fifteenth-century Florence and twenty-first-century Boston or Bangkok, solving problems around infant and child nurture requires examining gender and class inequities, access to resources, women's work schedules, and political will. It is institutions not individuals who take on these tasks.

Despite decades of international and national public health pronouncements about how to feed infants and young children, millions of infants and young children die of malnutrition each year. More than two million of the ten million child deaths each year could be prevented if optimal child feeding were followed, including breastfeeding in the first hour after birth, exclusive breastfeeding for six months, followed by appropriate complementary feeding with continued breastfeeding (Jones et al. 2003). Today, it is not guilds but specialized UN agencies such as WHO and UNICEF who make policy about infant feeding. Their recommendations for optimal infant and young child feeding are based on reviews of current research evidence and clinical practice. In 2016, the *Lancet*'s special issue on breastfeeding estimated that 823,000 annual deaths of children under five and 20,000 annual deaths from breast cancer could be prevented by scaling up breastfeeding (Victora et al. 2016). Guidelines on infant feeding are disseminated to member states through policy documents such as the *Global Strategy for Infant and Young Child Feeding* (World Health Organization 2003). They are implemented by institutions trying to improve infant-feeding practices in different parts of the world—all well-intentioned efforts, but all part of the impossible task of mastering nurture.

From a pragmatic approach to development and change in a world where maternal and infant deaths are all too common, improving infant feeding is promoted as one means to improve economic development: "Inappropriate feeding practices and their consequences are major obstacles to sustainable economic development and poverty reduction" (Moran and Dykes 2009: 198). It is thus prudent policy to try and improve infant-feeding practices.

Globally, it has been estimated that 85 percent of mothers do not conform to current infant-feeding recommendations; less than 35 percent of infants are exclusively breastfed for even the first four months of life (World Health Organization 2003). It seems that neither mothers in the Global North nor Global South do what they are told. Sellen asks why normative practices differ so dramatically from recommended ones, arguing that there are "advantages to developing policy directives broadly concordant with evolved, species-typical patterns and the collective folk wisdom of human societies" (2001: 2707). Recognizing the importance of these passed down biocultural practices such as the social womb and the commensal circle might be a useful first step for international public health policy. Interventions that ignore biocultural nurturing practices are bound to fail, and fail they have. Sellen identifies this crisis of theory as a tension between focus on "individuals as actors in a social vacuum and an epidemiological focus on population groups as homogeneous units" (Sellen 2002b: 224).

This chapter examines how interventions to improve infant feeding relate to nurturing practices. This requires examining the practices of institutions—particularly the UN specialized agencies, such as WHO and UNICEF, the key institutions that control information and policy implementation related to infant feeding. These institutions rely on evidence-based biomedical science to provide the master metanarrative guiding program interventions, and they are seldom informed by anthropological evidence, beyond the use of local ethnography to improve program compliance or to adapt the KAP (knowledge, attitudes, practices) sections of survey instruments to local conditions (cf. Van Esterik 2012b). In itself, the information generated from KAP surveys is incomplete without placing the information in the context of historically passed down biocultural practices.

UN agencies are modern, rational, scientific, and pragmatic institutions, committed to measurable progress, expressed through indicators such as the Millennium Development Goals (MDG), or more recently, Sustainable Development Goals (SDG). Like all modern bureaucracies, they are organized in ways that break the immensity of tasks into manageable bits for improved efficiency and accountability. This "cutting into bits" allows agencies to codify, quantify, and control interventions around infant and young child feeding, to master nurture. This is mastery as total control over people and institutions

We look at the mismatch between global recommendations and local practice, not by examining ethnographic literature as Sellen (2001) has done for the period from 1873 to 1998, but by trying to take up what Sellen calls the "crisis of theory"—the "absence of a coherent theory of human social action" (Sellen 2002b: 224). This book is part of the developmentment of such a theory, beginning from the possibility that errors in thinking about child nurture have drawn us to ask the wrong questions (Chapter 2), and continuing in Chapter 3 to review lessons from human phylogeny and ontogeny.

Mastering nurture works on the assumption that there is one correct way to feed an infant, without negotiation or adjustment for individual differences. The title of Nathoo and Ostry's 2009 book, *The One Best Way: Breastfeeding History, Politics and Policy in Canada* says it all.

A phrase like "the one best way to feed an infant" epitomizes the logic of many past public health approaches to infant feeding. Advertising for baby food products often co-opted the idea that there is one best way to feed an infant, and it includes their products. Subtle and not so subtle suggestions that if you cannot be certain about your diet, the safety of your environment (free from toxins), or your schedule, or if you are uncomfortable about breastfeeding in church, in a doctor's office or anywhere in public, then use our product and do not breastfeed. If you have concerns about the quantity or quality of your milk, then do not breastfeed.

Ironically, the more modern health professionals identify the ideal conditions for breastfeeding, the more they encourage the belief that breastfeeding success is unattainable and thus more infants have to be fed artificially: "health care professionals in the US have been found to reinforce the view that breastfeeding is difficult, inconvenient, time-consuming and even painful, and to actively discourage certain categories of mothers from breastfeeding" (Sellen 2002a: 23). This has been a particular problem for African American mothers in the United States, who are assumed to be uninterested in breastfeeding, a racist attitude that is being challenged by groups supporting black breastfeeding mothers, such as Black Mothers Breastfeeding Association, Black Women do Breastfeed, and ROSE (Reaching Our Sisters Everywhere). Of course, lecturing others about what to eat and particularly about how to feed and care for children has never been effective because these are not the independent pragmatic acts of individuals but rather nurturing practices embedded in local customs that often include iconic rituals and moral gestures.

In the real world, breastfeeding and infant care in general invite uncertainty. Mastery implies certainty; measurable indicators provide the illusion of certainty in an uncertain world. Few mothers of newborns feel certain of anything except the love they feel for their child and their desire for restful recovery after childbirth. The mastery demanded by policy interventions from day one ignores the individual constitutions of mothers and infants and contingencies of life, as well as the trial-and-error knowledge that mothers acquire about feeding infants and solving breastfeeding problems themselves.

Interventions to improve infant feeding are usually lodged in public health models whose lab logic and clinical logic rarely fit everyday breastfeeding. After many failures, policy makers and researchers have learned that they need to fill in the culture box (cf. Van Esterik 2012b).

The Culture Box

In 1980, I joined Michael Latham and a team of researchers working on infant-feeding practices of the urban poor in Bangkok, Thailand; Semarang, Central Java; Bogota, Colombia; and Nairobi, Kenya. It was Latham who taught me how to negotiate the boundaries between research and advocacy discourse. Working with an interdisciplinary team was also instructive, as we all examined breastfeeding from disparate disciplinary perspectives. Instead of trying to construct a transdisciplinary framework, as a junior member of the consortium, I absorbed the dominant public health and epidemiological stance on the research, and adopted the role of anthropologist as naysayer, arguing at every opportunity for the team to consider cultural factors and the local meaning of breastfeeding. At a very early meeting, the team showed me a small box labeled "culture" among a large number of variables such as ever breastfed, maternal employment, and health status on a large conceptual framework drawn on a whiteboard; that culture box was to be my responsibility. In frustration at the narrowness of the domain—consisting of beliefs and attitudes, I took what I thought was an erasable marker and drew a box around the entire framework, claiming that it was all culture. Unfortunately, it was a permanent marker, and I had a faint pink reminder on the board of what was taken to be my empire building for the remainder of the study. One day, one of the public health professionals leading the study shouted at me in frustration: "Will you stop telling me what anthropology can do for nutrition and public health and just show me?" This was probably the most useful professional advice I ever received, and I continue to pass it on to my students. (PVE)

Rather than trying to stuff culture into linear reductionist models, we need to develop models of relational practices that are better suited to analyzing processes like nurture and care. Relational models also make the best use of ethnographic, cultural, and biological evidence collected by anthropologists. Moran and Dykes recognize breastfeeding as relationally oriented but suggest that this is more obvious in less industrialized cultures (2009: 198). We argue that nurture and care activities are always and everywhere relational activities.

Policy Making and Cultural Coherence

As we argued in the last chapter, modernity takes problems out of the hands of God and cuts tasks to fit human skills, with the result that perhaps for the first time in history, humans are "alone to take care of things human" (Bauman 1997: 170). Infant feeding is particularly frightening for moderns. This is the terrifying challenge facing every new mother who delivers a baby and then must decide how to keep it alive. The landscape of new motherhood becomes filled with objects that might harm a newborn, including vaccinations (cf. Bliss 2014). The life of a new human rests on her judgment, skill, and choices made under the pressure of the transforming peak experience of birth. Into this dramatic moment come new feeding options created by modernity claiming to offer solutions to the problem of nurture.

In the past, premodern solutions to problems like hunger were considered to be in the hands of God. Agatha was baptized by SDI. At her death, she joined the angels. Modern policy making must deal with the manageable bits that are the responsibility of humans. This gives policy makers almost God-like power; is it any wonder that embedded in this culture of empowerment they may get delusions of omnipotence?

Policy is a set of flexible principles or protocols to guide decisions to achieve a rational outcome; it is a statement of intent implemented as procedures, often preceded by comparing alternatives and setting priorities. Policy matters, but not too much. Bad policy does damage; does good policy do good or just avoid damage? We should not underestimate how small bureaucratic policy decisions like changing budget lines, merging projects, or altering insurance rules can result in unanticipated consequences. Consider, for example, what the impact of raising the fees for dumping garbage has had on recycling or giving tax breaks for employers who support their breastfeeding employees. Regulations by state or multilateral agencies are clearly a form of mastery, an exertion of power over others. How effective have regulations about infant feeding been? Regulating the baby food industry works, albeit slowly and only if someone is monitoring. Changes have come about in marketing practices, as the most blatant activities to promote infant formula are less common in some parts of the world. On the other hand, the baby food business is booming far beyond the needs that adoptive parents or chemotherapy patients have for commercial baby milks.

We need infant-feeding policy. Society has a large stake in maternal nurture, and throughout the world, communities have to deal with infants who were not nurtured or inadequately nurtured. In such cases, social interventions such as orphanages or fosterage may be needed—inadequate, resented but needed. But policy that attempts to micromanage breastfeeding directly does not work. Policies that regulate the promotion of competing products help, when they are enforced. For example, keeping the promotional activities of infant formula companies out of government health clinics in Ghana, or fining employers who prevent women from breastfeeding in Indonesia may be locally appropriate steps; but drafting a law requiring women to breastfeed for two years, as the UAE did in January 2014, was criticized for being too rigid and for criminalizing women when they were most vulnerable.

UN agencies like UNICEF and WHO work with universal policy—all or nothing solutions, black or white, one size fits all, because they cannot negotiate the gray of local traditions. The "uncontaminated purity" (Code 2006: 43) of the discourse of mastery is unsuited to the chaotic and contextual complexities of nurture. Nor can infant-feeding policy deal with the individuality, intersubjectivity, and cultural embeddedness of the everyday lives of mothers and infants, and that is what understanding breastfeeding requires. Nurture is a relationship not a thing, and relationships cannot be reduced to their parts.

Policy work breaks apart wholes like nurture, reducing them to their parts, and suggesting interventions on the parts we have some control over, including new programs, new standards, new definitions, new categories, and new regulations. But once divided into parts, policy cannot solve the problem of infant and child malnutrition holistically because it cannot address the underlying process of nurture.

NGOs face the same challenge. For example, individuals contribute a mosaic of activities to social movements, each hooking up a piece of the puzzle without ever having seen the complete picture on the cover of the box. But policy only works on the assumption that we know a priori how all the pieces fit back together—what the finished picture looks like. In fact, with our current explanatory frameworks, we cannot fully explain infant-feeding choices in North America, let alone those in the rest of the world. The coherence of infant feeding once came from biocultural practices such as the social womb and the commensal circle, pieces that tied the whole together. Rather than build on these biocultural practices, institutions misconstrued infant and child feeding as technological problems amenable to business logic.

As we argued in the last chapter, the logic of modernity erases nurture while providing a totalizing metanarrative of progress. Other logics dominate in other parts of the world. Societies such as those in Southeast Asia we described in Chapter 5 often work from holistic views of the world that provide answers to "the big questions." While the modern world assumes progress, it generally avoids the big questions, while trying to master details. Do the subordinate discourses of holism still exist under conditions of modernity? Perhaps they are brought out in the stress of birth and the awesome responsibility of infant nurture. This is why the social womb with its local and familial customs is so important.

National and global health policy takes breastfeeding and infant feeding to a higher level of abstraction and further from the local regimens where policies are implemented, denying policy makers the opportunity to observe how nurture works locally. Policy assumes linear cause and effect instead of something like conditional sequencing happening over time, each action conditioning the next, so that events come to take on lives of their own. For example, once a woman begins to bottle-feed a newborn, certain other things happen, other steps become easier or harder; once a woman begins to breastfeed, certain other things happen, other steps become easier or harder. There is a cascading effect to this seemingly simple decision about how to feed an infant that is not reflected in policy-making work, either in documents, programs, or practices.

Although anthropologists understand contingencies well, immersed as they are in the local, policy makers have no way to deal with these ever-changing realities. Anthropologists can advise on the conditioned synchronicity of the local to policy makers who must develop and implement standardized universal guidelines. The new ethnology builds on human commonalities rather than single ethnographic cases, and so might be more useful for policy makers.

UN bureaucracies are mandated to intervene, to improve, to solve problems, but as Bateson explained about his reluctance to take on political appointments: "political life seemed to demand action based on insufficient data and precise language before any conceptual clarity had been achieved" (Harries-Jones 1995: 31). Agencies do not like to see universal policy altered in any way, as Nichter describes in his analysis of a top-down tuberculosis control program (2008: 109).

If we wait until all evidence is in, interventions are too late, and policy making becomes irrelevant. For example, WHO policies addressing the transmission of HIV through breastmilk changed several times from 2003 to 2010. Policy directives regarding breastfeeding and HIV improved over time, as more research became available or was taken more seriously (cf. Mathews 2015). But there is always lag time for the word to get out; health workers trained on earlier policies are not always aware of or believe the new policy changes. And what happens when policy gets it wrong? How do you forget a bad policy based on wrong information or outdated research when so many actions have been taken on the basis of that policy? And what happens when policy-worthy issues become unfashionable?

In the 1990s, infant and child malnutrition threatened to become a global embarrassment. But it evidently did not embarrass governments enough to extend programs on breastfeeding that could improve the situation. Instead, "breastfeeding seems to have disappeared from the development and child rights agendas. Is this a result of the HIV and infant feeding controversy, or of pressure from the infant-feeding industry? Or is breastfeeding merely no longer fashionable? The European blueprint also noted the European governments' general lack of commitment to allocate sufficient funding to breastfeeding initiatives (EU Project 2004: 12). The amount of talk generated about breastfeeding vastly exceeds increased budgets or improvements in infant-feeding practices. There is too much talk, too many documents produced, and too many media messages generated, and this makes people think the problem is solved.

In a world where politicians and political culture celebrate motherhood and family values, why do so many governments and societies fail to support women by ensuring they have what they need to nurture their families? This is particularly surprising when support for breastfeeding is among the least expensive of all health interventions (cf. Horton et al. 1996; Black et al. 2013).

Finding the Right Box

In order to master infant feeding, policy interventions require organized categories with easily measured and managed indicators. Indicators help consolidate power in the hands of those with expert knowledge by influencing the allocation of resources and the nature of political decisions (Merry 2011). Neither biomedical evidence, nor ethnographic evidence suggests any self-evident categorical schemes that would capture and simplify the diversity of nurturing practices in the world. But interventions based on policy guidelines require some categorical answers, some benchmarks such as the importance of beginning breastfeeding in the first hour after birth or delaying the introduction of complementary foods until six months; this allows practitioners to behave "as if" exclusive breastfeeding for six months was the only possible option for every newborn, for example, or acting "as if" every parent wants their infant to survive.

Breastfeeding as a subject has many homes, but is a priority in none (Labbok 2012: 41). To master breastfeeding, practitioners must understand the consequences of choosing one home over another. We list some of the real and potential homes below, noting also where breastfeeding is absent.

Food Security

Breastfeeding is seldom lodged in efforts to improve household food security or food sovereignty; although breastfeeding is food security for infants, human milk is anomalous, as it is neither grown agriculturally nor produced industrially. It is the only food product produced by humans within their bodies. The bodies producing this food are female bodies; this is a fact of the human condition. All food products, including human milk, take their place in local commensal circles. Like these other products, human milk can be banked, shared, given a cash value, and sold. It is the only food for newborns that provides them with the "highest possible attainment of health," linking breastfeeding to the Convention on the Rights of the Child. But women cannot be coerced into giving this product to their children. Thus society has had to provide alternatives—always inferior, often fatal. Breastfeeding costs women in time, nutrients, and opportunities. Using alternatives to breastmilk also costs mothers, households, and communities, both the direct costs of the product, and the indirect costs of medical care and child death. But it is society that should bear these costs, not mothers. While human milk fits in the food security box, breastfeeding is much more than food security.

Public Health

Although public health is the most likely home for breastfeeding programs, it cannot always address the breastfeeding situation of individual mothers, but rather must consider the best outcome for the majority (Labbok 2012: 47). Public health programs such as maternal and child health (MCH) and sexual and reproductive health (SRH) shape how breastfeeding is integrated into intervention programs.

MCH. MCH is a box where mothers and children belong together because of the nature of maternal reproductive work; the health and nutritional status of mothers and infants are intimately linked, particularly through the social womb (cf. World Health Organization 2003: 5). MCH encourages a temporal focus on the first 1,000 days, conception to two years—the period when the connections between the generations are most obvious, where the overlap between generations of women—grandmothers, new mothers, and newborns are most beneficial to the next generation. Hrdy (2009: 290) has provided ample evidence to show the importance of maternal grandmothers in increasing child survival, concluding that nurture is an art form passed on through the generations through the experience of nurturing and being nurtured.

MCH provides a category in an institutional bureaucracy and a budget line for projects. Some would argue that this pairing of mother and child is too narrow, a zero-sum game that pits mothers against their children or subsumes mothers' needs as relevant only as they relate to the needs of their children. Patriarchal and protective approaches to women and children based on English common law can be patronizing. Keeping women in late pregnancy out of dangerous mines may be patronizing, but it is a small price to pay for increased maternal and infant survival. We argue that the mother–child link is a foundational relationship not a category, and that placing breastfeeding in the category of MCH makes sense on that basis, and that the association of women with children does not weaken women's rights.

SRH. SRH is another box where breastfeeding might reside. Breasts are sexual; breastfeeding is a crucial part of the reproductive process. But breastfeeding is invisible in the reproductive rights movement; or as phrased by a reproductive rights conference organizer faced with a breastfeeding poster presentation, "We only do below the waist." Instead, interest centers on contraception and abortion. In the past, religious and secular authorities advised on and regulated wet nursing, but did little to support breastfeeding mothers.

Reproductive health is no doubt a useful category, as it emphasizes the important role of childbearing to women's health. At the International Conference on Population and Development held in Cairo 1994 reproductive health was explicitly linked to reproductive rights, including the right to a satisfying and safe sex life. These rights were expanded during the Beijing conference (1995), and women's rights to sexual pleasure as well as reproductive health care were specified. Many groups challenged this progressive stance (including the Vatican and many Islamic countries), since SRH also addresses highly contested issues, including violence against women and abortion. All global documents related to SRH reflect carefully negotiated language. For example, Merry reports that representatives to a UN conference from Pakistan would accept language that acknowledged widows as vulnerable women in return for removing reference to sexual orientation (2006: 60).

In addition, since Cairo and Beijing, women's sexual rights and gay men's sexual rights have moved along separate but parallel tracks. For both groups, breastfeeding rights are not even on the horizon. Yet bodily integrity and stigma are equally important to gay men denied their sexual rights and HIV-positive women denied their right to breastfeed.

What are the policy and praxis implications of the categorization that places breastfeeding in MCH rather than SRH? Both MCH and SRH require addressing the elephant in the room—the fear that support for breastfeeding will become another means of defining women by their biological functions, reducing women to their breasts. SRH activists would reject the conservative maternal feminism potential of some mother-to-mother breastfeeding support groups for example. MCH appears inherently conservative because of the complete dependence of all human newborns on nurturing care through provision of maternal milk or substitutes, and the need for protection of the mother–infant dyad during this postpartum period.

Strengthening the linkages between SRH and breastfeeding requires acknowledging and resolving the tensions between movements. Just as assisted reproductive technology (ART) could be incorporated into prolife perspectives as easily as into reproductive choice agendas, so too can breastfeeding. The tension around feminist support for infertility treatments (cf. Thompson 2005: 56) parallels the tension around feminist support for breastfeeding. Petchesky (2005) discusses the formulation of the right of bodily integrity, a new terrain for human rights activism, and how these need to be recast in the age of HIV/AIDS. Although some question the privileging of women's bodies as bearers of sexual rights, a more useful question might be how sexual rights, reproductive rights, and maternal rights are integrated in the bodies of breastfeeding women.

Keeping Out of the Dissenter Box: HIV and Infant Feeding

Some boxes present more challenges than others. Breastfeeding has found a home in the AIDS box, but it is not a good fit with breastfeeding support or the general understanding of HIV/AIDS treatment and care; instead it lives in the very narrow specialized box of PMTCT (prevention of mother-to-child transmission). Infant-feeding choices are always negotiated, always a tradeoff between what is best for mothers and infants, and what is feasible in the context of people's everyday lives. Never have these choices been more devastatingly difficult for women and society than in the last few decades when AIDS emerged as a global pandemic. Unlike breastfeeding policy, HIV/AIDS policy faces the problem of constantly having to integrate new information concerning the basic biology of the disease. The exact mechanisms of transmission are still unclear, and it is difficult to distinguish between intrauterine, perinatal, and postnatal transmission through breastfeeding. In addition to these scientific uncertainties, stigma, disinformation, gender inequalities, and the manufacture of doubt complicate the situation. Breastfeeding advocacy groups were also faced with the need to revise their messages around HIV/AIDS and breastfeeding or risk getting put in the "dissenter box."

International AIDS conferences are shaped by nonbinding documents produced at earlier conferences and at UN agencies. Meanwhile, breastfeeding activists were trying to amplify the evidence that exclusive breastfeeding is an effective intervention to prevent infant death. The risk of transmission of HIV through breastmilk creates an impossible dilemma for many mothers who are HIV-positive. Although epidemiological and biomedical research on the transmission of HIV through breastmilk and PMTCT projects seek to find ways to reduce the rates of transmission, this route of transmission is a relatively minor concern for most AIDS researchers who must consider the need for more effective prevention and better access to treatment worldwide. But it is of central importance to child-feeding advocates who have seen programs to support breastfeeding decimated over the past few decades. The reduction in facilities to support maternal and child health generally was a direct result of American policies to remove support for services that could be construed as linked in any way to women's reproductive rights. The "ABC" (abstinence, be faithful, use condoms) criteria for some American AIDS funding was considered at best inadequate, at worst, insulting, ineffectual, and unrealistic for women, offering them nothing relevant for solving their infant-feeding dilemmas (cf. Van Esterik 2012a: 156). As a result, PMTCT programs to prevent transmission of HIV to newborns often undermined other child-feeding programs, particularly in the Global South.

Breastfeeding advocacy groups in particular faced the anger of AIDS activists for drawing attention to pregnant mothers and newborns, rather than to women per se. AIDS activists directed attention to sex workers, ignoring the fact that sex workers are also mothers. Treatment was often directed to women only to prevent transmission to their infants. "Risk categories" in the early 1980s included the 4Hs—"homosexuals, hemophiliacs, heroin addicts, and Haitians," with the implication that breastfed newborns do not "deserve" to get AIDS. In the Global North, HIV-positive pregnant women usually receive antiretroviral therapy in late pregnancy, and are required to replacement feed from birth. No breastfeeding is permitted, and women who breastfeed a child knowing they are HIV-positive could be prosecuted for child abuse or have their children removed (cf. Hausman 2011).

In the Global South, replacement feeds were not always available when needed, nor free of charge. Because of difficulties surrounding both exclusive breastfeeding and exclusive replacement feeding, infants often received mixed feeds, the option most likely to kill young babies in areas where replacement feeding was not AFASS (affordable, feasible, acceptable, sustainable, and safe). When replacement feeds were given, there was seldom follow-up on the survival of infants of HIV-positive mothers who were given them. These substitutes still require a clean reliable water source, adequate conditions for sterilization or hygienic preparation, and cash for purchase. Problems such as fecal content in feeding bottles and over dilution did not disappear in the context of HIV/AIDS. These problems were painfully exposed in Botswana, a country praised for its good PMTCT program using replacement feeds. From November 2005 to February 2006, following heavy rains and flooding, more than 500 infants died from diarrhea after replacement feeding. Risk factors for death included not being breastfed. But the discourse had changed. The old rhetoric of the breast-bottle controversy becomes a tragic, ironic double bind, advocacy inside out, where companies supplying the replacement feeds of infant formula were heralded as "the good guys," and the breastfeeding advocates, "the bad guys" with their heads in the sand, ignoring the "fact" that "breastmilk causes AIDS." The AIDS box brings out the bifurcation between the Global North and Global South, contrasting the dilemmas of modernization in the North and the dilemmas of underdevelopment, poverty, and traditional customs in the South (cf. Peake and Rieker 2013). These epistemological arguments around categories and rights are important in some academic discourses and not in others. For activists concerned with infant malnutrition, the arguments are not central to accomplishing their work, although they may affect their budgets.

Bureaucratic Process and Document Production

UN agencies make policy to guide nation-states; they have different constituencies, including NGOs and private industry, and work on behalf of over 190 nations. Documents have important roles to play in coordinating these constituencies, and regulating ways of engaging with others. Texts help create the illusion of uniform conditions, necessary for interventions. Dorothy Smith refers to the texts and discourses produced by bureaucracies that regulate beyond their local settings as relations of ruling. Discursive events—past and present, spoken and written statements—are shaped by and create distinctive forms of power (cf. Smith 2005). To fully explore the relations of ruling of regulatory agencies would require an institutional ethnography of UN agencies like WHO and UNICEF,[1] a task beyond the scope of this book. Nevertheless, the documents produced out of these agencies provide important evidence about how the work of mastering nurture proceeds.

Documents are key actors in the coordination of actions, things, and people in the service of a policy goal, and child feeding is no exception. Consider the Innocenti Declaration and related documents. In 1990, a global initiative sponsored by a number of bilateral and multilateral agencies resulted in the adoption by thirty governments of the Innocenti Declaration on the Protection, Support, and Promotion of breastfeeding. For optimal breastfeeding:

> All women should be enabled to practice exclusive breastfeeding and all infants should be fed exclusively on breastmilk from birth to four to six months of age. Thereafter, children should continue to be breastfed, while receiving appropriate and adequate complementary foods, for up to two years of age or beyond.

In order to bring this about,

> Efforts should be made to increase women's confidence in their ability to breastfeed. Such empowerment involves the removal of constraints and influences that manipulate perceptions and behavior towards breastfeeding, often by subtle and indirect means. This requires sensitivity, continued vigilance, and a responsive and comprehensive communications strategy involving all media and addressed to all levels of society. Furthermore, obstacles to breastfeeding within the health system, the workplace and the community must be eliminated. (WHO/UNICEF 1990)

This carefully worded statement on breastfeeding offers a challenge to change many priorities of the modern world. The language stresses the empowerment of women to breastfeed, rather than their duty to breastfeed, a change that should appeal to women's health advocates and enable them to be more supportive of breastfeeding programs.

To celebrate the fifteenth anniversary of the declaration in 2005 and publicize fifteen years of progress since the original Innocenti Declaration, UNICEF proposed a publication to be launched at a special event. The committee planning the publication and the celebration chose to contract for a single document that integrated multiple voices, rather than a compendium of separate statements. The publication would review policy and program initiatives by UN agencies and NGOs around breastfeeding and child feeding, and would be launched at an event in Florence, Italy, to celebrate fifteen years of progress based on the Innocenti Declaration.[2]

The Innocenti +15 document was constructed from pieces of texts, all lodged in very different discourses, with different histories and different agendas. NGOs contributed stories of activities with groups of mothers or local case studies outlining their accomplishments. UN agencies and national governments submitted official reports and position papers about infant feeding, in addition to statistical tables that could show changes in breastfeeding rates and child survival as a result of interventions. One challenge in preparing the long document was reconciling and working with the distinct discourses of each contributor; each group had different priorities and agendas that affected how they spoke about the past, present, and future of breastfeeding advocacy.

NGOs who enter into policy debates at international meetings know how to use language as UN insiders would, or at least to use agreed upon words and phrases from earlier UN documents. They are encouraged to have policy papers written in UN style. Even single words can make a difference. For example, the United States, Australia, and Brazil rejected reference to an international policy "agenda" in favor of the less committal "dialogue" during preparation of another policy document (Dimitrov 2005: 9). NGOs and academics do not always speak the same language, even academics who claim to have a foot in both camps.

Who Let the Academic In?

> UN meetings were also occasions for less formal advocacy work with local grassroots women's organizations who used the occasions of these meetings for lobbying and advocacy activities. I recall one poster-making meeting when I tried to correct the translation of a poster to read breastfeeding "cultures" instead of breastfeeding "culture." After a hastily translated lecture on the meaning of culture, the group leader asked, "Who let the academic in?" and I was banished to coloring posters on the floor. Years later I remember that story and wonder who was "right." Should we talk about breastfeeding cultures? Yes, in that the plural term suggests some of the variation in customs associated with breastfeeding in different localities; no, when it downplays the uniqueness of every mother–infant pair on the one hand, and the universality of the human pattern of nurture on the other. At least I learned to color between the lines. (PVE)

The circulation of key policy documents, many known only by their initials, is part of the aesthetics of bureaucratic practice. Phrases and initials such as BFHI (Baby Friendly Hospital Initiative), the Code, Ten Steps, and EBF (exclusive breastfeeding) are well known from past breastfeeding documents. The Innocenti +15 publication was part of a chain of events, documents and practices stretching forward from the original Innocenti Declaration (1990) to the *Global Strategy for Infant and Young Child Feeding* (2003), and backward to the International Code of Marketing of Breastmilk Substitutes (1981). These documents address the problem of infant and young child feeding from different viewpoints and perspectives, but they are all elements of a set, links in a chain, and their words and practices are embedded in each other.

> As "language" is quoted and repeated from one conference document to the next and as states begin to conform their practices, or at least their discourse, to the norms expressed therein, some of what is agreed upon at global conferences gradually will become rules of "customary international law." (Riles 2001: 8)

While the Innocenti +15 document proceeds from past, to present and future, from the Innocenti Declaration to the *Global Strategy for Infant and Young Child Feeding,* with the International Code of Marketing of Breastmilk Substitutes embedded in both, in fact, this is an arbitrary separation of what are deeply interconnected documents and processes. This layering of documents is more mechanical and literal than is implied by a term such as Foucaultian genealogy. It is more like a palimpsest. Earlier documents set agreed upon language that does not need to be reexamined or debated (cf. Riles 2001; Merry 2006). Yet words and phrases are themselves products of compromises. Each new document in the hands of new writers is treated as a closed system with no history, with the newest policy document simply replacing earlier documents referred to as settled text. Language from the Innocenti Declaration on the empowerment of women has been slower to appear in the breastfeeding advocacy and child nutrition literature. Empowerment of women does not qualify as settled language, except among NGOs.

Fighting over words—past and present—has become the reality for international institutions. But words matter to NGOs too. As one experienced NGO leader explained, "Bad language can be used against us." NGOs also need to master legal language if they make links to human rights, using phrases like maternal rights, reproductive rights, and child rights appropriately. NGOs have lost UN funding for projects that refer to breastfeeding as the right of the child. Under the convention on the Rights of the Child, rights and obligations are carefully spelled out so that a woman who does not breastfeed is not liable if she fails to deliver something that she owes her infant.

NGOs remind their network members for whom English may be their second or third language to avoid terms like prolonged breastfeeding, in favor of a more neutral term such as continued breastfeeding, or to consider when using the term, human milk, is more effective than using breastmilk; after all, we talk about cow's milk not udder milk. Such distinctions may be irrelevant in some languages or have very different connotations in others. Some might ask why so much energy is spent fighting over words in policy documents; the answer is that the words matter and have a very long life span.

Measureable goals and targets are part of the work of mastering nurture, and numbers are not apolitical. Martin and Lynch refer to the disputes about counts, estimates, and measurement as the numero-politics of counting, or counting as contextual performance (2009: 243, 246). Indicators are important parts of the politics of accountability in both UN agencies and NGOs to show progress toward benchmarks such as the MDGs, for example. In fact, governments that do not want to take action often drop demands for "quantifiable global targets" and support "voluntary commitments" (cf. Dimitrov 2005: 11). Most agencies and NGOs need numbers for budgets and setting priorities. NGOs often record numbers of people participating in community-based health promotion events rather than health outcomes. Thus, numbers—accurate or not—act as sign and symbol of shared objectives and intentions. But numbers do not always guide policy decisions. For example, while around three million children under five die from malnutrition every year, around 190,000 die from AIDS. Yet more funding goes to HIV than breastfeeding support.

To make a long story, short, the long document that was produced was unacceptable to both UNICEF and WHO. Within a very few days, UNICEF had redrafted and condensed 150 pages into 60 pages, the Innocenti +15 short document. The paragraphs cut from the long document provide clues about how documents are produced as truth, and what is considered unsuitable or challenging to that truth. Most of the paragraphs that disappeared contained analyses of power, poverty, globalization, and gender—subjects that could not be adequately supported by biomedical citations. There was no place in the document to explore or even acknowledge the power differentials and dynamics between underfunded NGOs, international bureaucracies with complex accountability structures, and the agendas of national governments. Any sign of mothers—past or present—giving birth and nurturing infants under difficult conditions disappeared.

Gender

UN infant-feeding policy is constrained by "governance feminism" with its global regulatory infrastructure of targets, outcomes, and accountability (Peake and Rieker 2013: 10). Gender inequities, sexism, and violence against women were unpopular subjects with Innocenti +15 document reviewers. For example, the poverty of women-headed households was dropped because there was no agreement among agencies about measurement of indicators. Numbers produce a world without particulars of context and history, creating certainty and lack of ambiguity (Merry 2011).

All phrasing regarding gender inequalities in the document had to be watered down, sanitized, and supported with citations from UNIFEM, or other UN sources. Because UN women's programs at the time generally ignored breastfeeding as a feminist issue, trying to make the links with infant and child malnutrition was difficult. But, as Stephen Lewis argues, women were never a top priority in UN country programming (2005: 125). More recent efforts at gender mainstreaming in the UN meant that gender and women were everyone's business and nobody's business, all accountable and no one accountable. "There is no greater emblem of international hypocrisy than the promise of women's rights," wrote Lewis in his call for a UN agency devoted to women's equality (2005: 129).

Partnerships

Discussions of the effectiveness of NGOs and breastfeeding support groups like La Leche League and International Lactation Consultants Association (ILCA) were muted. Paragraphs questioning why so much critical breastfeeding support work is done by volunteers rather than budgeted through the health care system were also cut. The idealized image of cooperation between UN agencies and NGOs expressed in the long document was cut in the short document, because by the time the document was ready to be reviewed, the gaping disparities between NGOs and UN discourses became painfully visible. The underlying concern of the UN agencies was to identify the obstacles to consensus among groups committed to support breastfeeding rather than to figure out the obstacles to breastfeeding in local contexts and why interventions did not work, which is precisely the knowledge that local NGOs brought to the table.

Globalization

Other serious disagreements concerned globalization, poverty, and corporate influence on health policy, topics that did not fit well into the ever-narrowing discussions of the causes of infant and child malnutrition and the growing UN interest in public-private partnerships (PPP).

In early drafts of the long document, the effects of globalization were perhaps too negatively defined, rather than considering that globalization has both negative and positive aspects. As Marion Nestle explains, "globalization has improved the social, dietary, and material resources of many populations, but it has also heightened economic and health inequities" (2003: 271). However, by focusing attention on corporate-led globalization, the long document made a strong case against globalization in relation to infant-feeding policy, including, first

> The potential loss of national identity and autonomy to multinational corporations bent on maximizing profits. The second is the possibility that international regulatory bodies established to deal with globalization issues might make decisions that favor corporate interests at the expense of public welfare and social justice, especially in the areas of health, environmental protection and food safety. From a business perspective, globalization is about open markets, low wages, and minimal regulations. (Nestle 2003: 236)

In the final document, references to the marketing of breastmilk substitutes were gradually reduced and restricted to sections on the implementation of the International Code of Marketing of Breastmilk Substitutes, and not permitted to spill out into discussions of globalization, health care, corporate power, poverty, or the position and condition of women. These issues were not considered part of WHO or UNICEF's mandate, in spite of the fact that they determined how women fed their children.

UN conferences are what Stephen Lewis calls a marathon talkfest with a declaration at the end, thousands of power-point presentations and "throbbing intellectual rumination" (2005: 73, 87). The Innocenti +15 was no exception. As Dimitrov notes about UN documents: "We produce texts only to prove we have been here" (2005: 11, 18). In the case of the Innocenti +15, it became clear after the fact that writing the document (which was translated into Italian for the event) was a precondition for holding the event. The UN needed a document to launch, in spite of the fact that groups could not agree on its content. The text was the pretext for the meeting. The short document was finally published in April 2007 in time for the celebration in Florence, Italy. The paper was neither a UN policy document for a UN agency nor an independent statement of the author's position, nor a compilation of other approved documents. It was neither fish nor fowl; words in these spaces between are hard to pin down textually and often hard to find materially.

The 1990 Innocenti Declaration on the protection, promotion, and support of breastfeeding was unique in its recognition that support for breastfeeding was a universal good, not a policy that only applied to some countries. It was the first UN policy document related to infant feeding that did not target industrial and developing countries separately. All were expected to meet the same targets, respect the same principles, just as policy and regulations around environmental issues and climate change must apply globally.

This policy initiative had the potential to add new and powerful unifying language. But child nutrition policy can carry unstated underlying assumptions—that all women in the Global North can replacement feed safely, and do not value breastfeeding; that all women in the Global South value breastfeeding and cannot replacement feed safely, and that breastmilk and milk- or soy-based replacement feeds are equivalent. Barston argues that infant formula does not kill in the developed West; thus discussions about the developing world (including global policy documents like the Innocenti Declaration) are irrelevant to Americans (2012: 157). False assumptions such as these are retained in texts that continue to shape discourses and direct action related to infant feeding.

In the process of creating the Innocenti +15 document, UN agencies effectively depoliticized child feeding, silenced the NGOs working in this area, and reconstituted the relations of power between the UN and the baby food industry, as UN agencies were already anticipating the shift to PPP.

What resists representation in the institutions that master nurture is the life situation of mothers and their children. In UN documents, they belong in the photograph section not the policy section. Instead of prefacing the document with a personal story of a particular infant, Agata, the infant whose story opened this chapter, the writers of the short document substituted "Children can't wait. Their day is today"; the generic child replaced a specific child.

Corporations and the Neoliberal Mastery of Nurture

The rigidity of mastery and the certainty associated with measurement also suits the corporate agenda of baby food corporations where standardization is the route to maximize profit. Baby food corporations cannot master nurture, but corporations themselves can be mastered—with difficulty, political will, much effort, and only partially. It is becoming increasingly difficult for politicians to regulate corporations; instead they ask consumers to buy more expensive, less toxic soap, for example (Klein 2014: 200), or choose a baby food with fewer preservatives. Klein calls this the "open for business" approach, compatible with the idea that infant feeding, like climate change, is a narrow technical problem with profitable solutions (2014: 205, 210). But the discourse of mastery is a language corporations understand.

Legal work on maternity protection, human rights, and code monitoring is probably the only advocacy initiative that effectively employs mastery. But national efforts to legislate the code to limit the promotion of infant formula are filled with loopholes that only lawyers can negotiate. Even when national legislation is in place, few countries effectively implement and monitor it (de Schutter 2011: 10).

How do food companies contribute to the mastery of nurture and support the work of institutions that master nurture? For a start, UN agencies prefer to address the problem of child malnutrition by partnering with coalitions of food corporations, not with small local NGOs. The donor environment has changed with the growth of deregulation and the increasing influence of corporations on multilateral agencies. The UN agencies and the food corporations now speak the same language—the language of international business; they share a neoliberal attitude where business flourishes, and it has quickly transformed UN culture, facilitating the use of language and concepts supportive of their common goals. These goals include sidetracking regulatory tools in favor of voluntary codes and self-regulation. Governments also understand and listen to Davos culture; it makes sense to them, and so they force it on other elements of civil society, including NGOs who are forced to use logical frameworks to monitor the efficiency of programs. Strathern (2000) refers to this logic as audit culture.

Corporate crime flourishes under these neoliberal conditions:

> These are the glory days of global capitalism. The mix of technology and economic integration transforming the world has created unparalleled prosperity ... having joined the global labor force, hundreds of millions of people in developing countries have won the chance to escape squalor and poverty. ("Globalization: The Rise of Inequality" 2007: 15)

This optimistic assessment preceded the economic collapse of 2008 that damaged households and NGOs that help mothers in the Global North and Global South. NGOs that support breastfeeding have had increasing difficulties raising funds over the past decade. But food corporations weathered the financial crisis and even managed to profit from the problems faced by bilateral and multilateral agencies. The Euromonitor (2001) estimated the annual world market for commercial baby milks and foods at nearly 17 billion US dollars, and forecasted its increase to nearly 20 billion US dollars by 2005 (Euromonitor International 2001). In fact, by 2006, the market was well over 25 billion US dollars, and by 2011, it had grown to over 42 billion US dollars (Euromonitor International 2011). The market for baby milk is projected to reach 70.6 billion US dollars by 2019 (Rollins et al. 2016). Between 1997 and 2004, the market in commercial baby food had grown by 90 percent (Kimura 2013: 117), and the most rapid growth has been in Southeast Asia (Baker et al. 2016). Not breastfeeding is associated with economic losses of about 302 billion US dollars annually (Rollins et al. 2016). Ours is not a world of exclusively breastfed babies. In comparison, "The value of all arms transfer *agreements* with developing nations by the United States and foreign countries was over 71.5 billion USD. This was a substantial increase from 32.7 billion USD in 2010. In 2011, the value of all arms *deliveries* to developing nations was 28 billion USD, the highest total in these deliveries values since 2004" (Grimmet and Kerr 2012).[3]

The increasing numbers of market-driven approaches to addressing the problem of infant and child malnutrition are facilitated by PPP, also known as multi-stakeholder initiatives (MSI). These alliances with food corporations have drawn funding away from local infant and young child-feeding support programs, and encouraged medicalized, technical solutions to the problem of malnutrition, while discouraging humanitarian interventions that address the underlying root causes of poverty and hunger. This shift to technical interventions has resulted in the neglect of other community-based social interventions (Sengupta 2011: 251). These alliances thrive as governments reduce spending on social programs and remove safety nets.

The Global Alliance for Improved Nutrition (GAIN), a PPP alliance of over 600 (mostly) food companies, promotes processed, fortified, and ready-to-eat foods for the poor in developing countries. It includes global companies such as Ajinomoto, Cargill, Coca-Cola, Danone, Kraft, Pepsico, and many others. The alliance began by focusing on micronutrient deficiencies, but soon offered a wider range of "business solutions" and "enabling environments" for companies interested in nutrition for the poor. UNICEF has been particularly supportive, lauding their "cost-effective food fortification initiatives that promise to improve the health and productivity of the poorest nations" (Sengupta 2011: 256). By fortifying low-cost processed foods like cookies and instant noodles for low-income markets, these food corporations reinforce the habit of eating cookies and other cheap processed foods rather than the value of the micronutrient (Kimura 2013: 167). In addition to creating a market for their expensive products, fortification solves the compliance problem and eliminates the need for nutrition education for mothers (Kimura 2013: 50).

Until May 2009, Danone, the second largest baby food manufacturer, sat on the Board of Directors of GAIN. Advocacy groups objected to this obvious conflict of interest—having such a significant manufacturer of baby foods and one that violated the Code on the Board of an alliance to "improve" child nutrition. Danone is still a member of GAIN, although it is identified as a known violator of the code (Lhotska, Bellows, and Scherbaum 2012: 33). Danone began marketing their fortified yogurt in countries like Bangladesh in 2006 in competition with local, richer buffalo curd yogurt.

Other large coalitions between UN agencies, governments, donors, private industry, and academia such as Scaling Up Nutrition (SUN) offer even more technical solutions to the problem of malnutrition. The project, costing around 10 billion US dollars per year, is promoted through the World Bank, as well as other bilateral and multilateral agencies. Of the thirteen nutrition interventions in the package that national governments are encouraged to support, ten involve commercial products such as vitamin and micronutrient supplements, and fortified foods (Horton et al. 2010).

Conflicts of interest affect more than just infants; Ajinomoto, another GAIN member, recommends MSG to stimulate the appetite of seniors through nutrition education materials on healthy eating put out by the Academy of Nutrition and Dietetics, the professional association of 74,000 registered dietitians. When the academy also endorsed Kraft's processed cheese slices with their "Kids Eat Right" logo after receiving payment from Kraft, some members of the academy complained that the group was selling out to industry (Blackmore 2015). But the problem of conflict of interest is much clearer in the case of infant and young child feeding because of the ethical complexity of research and the fact that caregivers must make the feeding decision on behalf of infants and children.

The UN encourages these business alliances through the Global Contract, a 1999 business initiative that provides principles that have been used to thwart efforts to regulate harmful business practices (Lhotska et al. 2012: 31). The same business logic also underlies corporate social responsibility initiatives promoted by the UN Global compact (Merry 2011: 2).

GAIN and SUN are not accountable the way that a single corporation like Nestlé was; we cannot boycott them. These large well-funded business coalitions build new markets for quick-fix solutions such as micronutrient supplements and fortified foods; they draw attention away from strengthening indigenous food cultures, and the nurturing practices associated with them. Although the nutritionism that views food as a vehicle for delivering nutrients is the basis for these business enterprises, both food and nurture disappear from consideration, along with hunger and poverty. These partnerships open the door to new and more complex conflicts of interest in the regulatory environment. Some of the food companies in GAIN and SUN have a significant influence on the Codex Alimentarius, a review committee of the UN's FAO that sets food safety standards. At a meeting in November 2011, 40 percent of meeting delegates were food industry, many representing BINGOs (business interest NGOs), and were part of (or heading) government delegations. For example, the Mexican delegation, which made many industry-friendly interventions, was 100 percent industry. GAIN lobbied the Codex Alimentarius to permit promotional health claims on infant food products. To curb well-documented abuses, advocates wanted more safeguards for baby foods, such as regulations that would prevent defatted cotton-seed flour or irradiated ingredients from being used in their manufacture; however, the industry-dominated meeting did not take up these suggestions (Baby Milk Action 2009). They were more interested in creating new markets for processed foods and allowing advertising for products directed to infants over six months of age than improving products already on the market (International Baby Food Action Network 2012).

In addition to UN regulatory bodies like Codex Alimentarius, every national government has agencies to advise on the risks associated with the national food supply. Although we would like to think that these food safety regulations are based on objective science, there is growing evidence of the influence of the food industry on these regulatory bodies. The International Life Sciences Institute (ILSI), an industry lobbying group for the food, chemical, and pharmaceutical industry has a substantial presence on the European Food Safety Authority (EFSA), where ILSI members have encouraged industry-friendly policies concerning pesticides residues, genetically modified crops, the sweetener aspartame (made by Ajinomoto), and the use of a known endocrine disruptor, BPA (bisphenol A), in food containers (Holland, Robinson, and Harbinson 2012).

Pesticides, chemical additives, and persistent organic pollutants (POPs) occur in both the general food supply and baby foods. As everyone carries chemical residues in their bodies, they also exist in breastmilk. This continues to be a concern to breastfeeding advocates, but with more collaborative work on message integration with environmental activists who understand the complexity of the issue, there are fewer sensationalist headlines about breastfeeding mothers downloading toxins into their infants. Curiously, there are few comparable stories about the toxins in sperm, a substance more vulnerable to toxins than women's eggs (Daniels 2006: 118).

Commercial marketing strategies for infant formula develop and sustain the cultural perception that artificial infant feeding carries no risks. Messages that claim that infant formula is risk-free have been more effective than campaigns that say there are no risks to eating beef or unpasteurized cheese, for example. Media amplification of risk scares many consumers away from consuming their favorite cheeses after they are alerted about the risks. Why are the risks from unpasteurized cheese more believable than risks associated with infant formula? Perhaps the risks in infant formula are just too great to contemplate, compared with risks to products that you can easily do without, such as unpasteurized cheeses. This is all the more difficult to understand when mothers are so sensitive to the quality of their own milk; long standing fears have made women so skeptical of their own diet and body that they may "think" their way into insufficient milk. But at the same time, mothers may be so accepting of the quality of what they use to substitute for their breastmilk that they react to media scares about an industrial accident in a baby food factory by choosing another brand of infant formula, confident that the regulatory system will protect them from obvious defects like melamine in milk-based infant formula or arsenic levels in organic formula (or more recently a lizard in a sealed can in Singapore).

Enterobacter sakazakii, renamed Cronobacter sakazakii in 2008, is a pathogenic food-borne microorganism found in unopened tins of powdered infant formula. Recent outbreaks of infections have confirmed that the problem is not always in the mode of preparing and filling bottles, but may be intrinsic to the industrial processing of powdered infant formula itself. These infections can be fatal for newborns and young infants, and include meningitis, necrotizing enterocolitis, and sepsis. The bacteria increase rapidly in the warm milk, and could enter the milk by three routes: first, from the raw materials used in the production of the infant formula; second, from contamination following pasteurization; and third, during reconstitution. To date, the number of deaths worldwide is unknown, because of the difficulty of testing for specific strains and because not all incidents are reported or attributed to Cronobacter sakazakii. Although newborns are most at risk, follow-up formulas for older infants are often given to infants less than six months of age; these products may be manufactured in less hygienic facilities (Food and Agriculture Organization/World Health Organization 2008). For example, 16.9 percent of the milk-based baby foods tested in Shaanxi, China in 2010 and 2012 tested positive for Cronobracter sakazakii, many of them antibiotic resistant; the authors conclude that this presents a potential health risk for consumers (Zhen 2016).

Testing the safety of infant formula is an ongoing process. Strategies to address this problem include mandatory labels warning that powdered infant formula is not a sterile product; explaining how to prepare infant formula more safely by raising the temperature of the water mixed with powdered infant formula to no less than 70 degrees C.; and making the dangers more widely known. Manufacturers object to this as it draws attention to the intrinsic risk in the powdered infant formula, and in the process, inactivates the (unnecessary) heat-sensitive probiotics added to infant formula. But activists question the safety of the probiotics and the industry-funded research that claims any benefits to the added probiotics in the first place. Critics of breastfeeding advocates argue that they exaggerate the risks of using infant formula; damage caused by Cronobacter sakazakii and related bacteria provide evidence that this criticism is unwarranted; there is no way to ensure safe formula feeding, only safer formula feeding.

Many NGOs are becoming concerned about the increasing complexity of conflicts of interest obvious when pharmaceutical companies and food companies sit on regulatory bodies and participate in policy and research discussions. GAIN participates in UNICEF's policy making, although they have a clear conflict of interest in program implementation (Sengupta 2011: 256). The UN has no comprehensive framework or agreed-upon definition to deal with individual and institutional conflicts of interests (Lhotska et al. 2012: 32). However, there is growing public support for addressing issues like conflict of interest and stopping harmful trade deals (Klein 2014: 153).

Close cooperation between baby food industries and policy makers and researchers produces potential for conflict of interest. "In North America and Europe, it's virtually impossible to do public interest work of any scale—in academia or journalism or activism—without taking money of questionable origin" (Klein 2014: 198). Industry-funded articles, reviews of literature, and ghost writing also have a strong impact on research and policy development. Activists insist that industry-funded research should not be considered reliable. But if industry does not sponsor research, should public money pay for research that the corporate partner wants done, when the benefits from the resulting knowledge and products then revert to become the private property of the commercial partner? Should public money fund research studies that identify constituents in human milk that companies will then try to copy and insert into their products to create the impression of improving the product to make it appear to be closer to human milk? Such adjustments improve profits not products. To be fair, the distinctions between public and private funding sources are not always clear. A more nuanced critique around conflict of interest would also examine the negative results from clinical trials, and the results that were never published.

Although consumer preferences for foods (not just baby foods) have always been shaped by commercial interests, breastfeeding advocates are concerned about the degree to which commercial interests are driving the marketing of new food products for infants and for processed foods in general. Why does the UN allow a food corporation to take on the role of a nutrition educator for children (Lhotska et al. 2012: 34)? Of course, fortification projects eliminate the need for nutrition education, saving the government even more money.

In addition to UN agencies, universities also encourage researchers to partner with industry. Most academics prefer having no direct commercial partner who might try to influence research topics, outcomes, or the way results are reported. Many NGOs warned of the dangers of conflicts of interest in these business partnerships. But the market-driven approach to child feeding is not universally condemned. At a meeting of North American breastfeeding activists, a consultant took WABA to task for writing a letter to WHO and UNICEF urging them to reconsider their partnership with GAIN because of these conflicts of interest. She was concerned that the letter might have angered GAIN to such an extent that they would not want to work with NGOs because they were too "antibusiness."

PPP are eagerly funded by the new superheroes, the super-rich philanthrocapitalists (cf. Bishop and Green 2009). The Gates Foundation, a primary funder of GAIN, has an endowment of 60 billion US dollars; its stock portfolio includes McDonald's, Coca-Cola, Monsanto, Proctor and Gamble, Kraft, Nestlé, Johnson and Johnson, Glaxo-Smith-Kline, Walmart, and Costco, almost a quarter of that of the entire UN system (Baby Milk Action 2009). Gates argues in print and social media that business practices of accountability and measurable outcomes are the answer to improving interventions to end child malnutrition, arguing that market incentives drive change, and that profits can be made by doing good. Child malnutrition has become a profitable business. Corporate social responsibility is good for business (Merry 2011), but critics point out that it is unaccountable power (McGoey 2015). Philanthrocapitalism has the potential for positive good but only if accountable to the public and fully engaged in public debates. Otherwise it can be read as an example of how the rich can save the poor and keep getting wealthier, or as profit-making disguised as corporate social responsibility.

Manufacturing Doubt

Ignorance as a deliberate and strategic ploy plays a critical but unanalyzed part in the mastery of nurture. The role of ignorance has been carefully examined in the tobacco industry, and the parallels with the baby food industry are helpful. Tobacco companies tried to obfuscate the link between smoking and lung cancer, an example of strategically imposed ignorance created when opponents of regulation try to manufacture uncertainty by calling into question the validity of the science (Smithson 2008: 215). Ignorance is maintained by mechanisms such as deliberate neglect, secrecy and suppression, document destruction, appeal to tradition, and selectivity. "Doubt is our product," the words of a tobacco company memo, are equally applicable to infant formula manufacturers who downplay the risks of infant formula in general and their brands, in particular. They exploit the doubt some women feel about their own milk and manufacture doubt about contemporary research on human milk, with potentially serious consequences.

To further their ends, they produce their own industry research, often without acknowledging the obvious conflicts of interest. False health claims such as advertising that using a particular brand of infant formula boosts the immune system, or that a particular additive increases visual acuity in infants can be fought, but the cases are difficult to prosecute, particularly in countries that have not legislated the International Code of Marketing of Breastmilk Substitutes. As with the tobacco companies, baby food manufacturers claim the right to keep trade secrets for business advantage (Proctor 2008: 9). But as the advantages of human milk began to be more widely publicized, baby food companies responded much as the tobacco companies did about the health effects of smoking, arguing that the research was flawed or that "the evidence is not all in."

What food companies do not tell us (keeping us in ignorance not because they do not know but because they do not want us to know) is that infant formula is not a sterile product and that powdered infant formula may contain dangerous bacterial pathogens such as Cronobacter sakazakii, or that ready-to-feed bottles of infant formula may contain printers ink; or that feeding bottles may contain BPA, a known carcinogen classified in Canada as a toxic substance. Newborns have difficulty eliminating BPA, as their livers are not yet fully developed.

When breastfeeding advocates turned their attention to publicizing the dangers of infant formula rather than repeating that "breast is best," food companies turned to manufacturing reasonable doubt about the research on the risks of infant formula, arguing that the hazards are not yet proven, and casting doubts about the advantages of human milk. When cornered on a single outcome, such as breast and ovarian cancer rates, they call for more research to slow down the already slow passage toward regulations that might limit their profitability. As with any health argument that invokes cancer, responses include that there is "always room for disagreement," and cancer has "complicated causes" (Proctor 2008: 12). Baby food companies might also call for red herring research to avoid examining the genuine hazards of commercial baby foods. They may appear to alter practices so they can claim to be self-regulating, thus undercutting the need for regulation.

Ignorance is more than a void but an active choice, a deliberate strategic ploy often employing disinformation to create doubt and uncertainty that could reach a state of paranoia. As with the tobacco lobby, publications and reports lauding breastmilk substitutes and casting doubt on research that showed the advantages of human milk were sent to doctors in an attempt to ally them more closely with industry.[4] Scientific journals make much of their profit by selling reprints to authors. Academics not aligned with industry can seldom afford these reprints, let alone mailing costs.

Where the tobacco lobby hired historians to rewrite the history of smoking and the tobacco industry, saying that "history is messy," the infant formula companies preferred using anthropologists to argue that culture is complex and that culture, not marketing, shapes infant-feeding decisions (cf. Raphael 1976; Gussler 1980; Maher 1992). It is challenging for anthropologists to explore the cultural complexity of infant feeding and the customs that support new mothers without having their ethnographies cited as evidence that marketing practices of baby food companies or health care practices are not the problem. "Culture" is the problem.

Another common strategy is to attack industry critics and whistleblowers, particularly advocacy groups. A manager of Nestlé Brazil referred to them as Marxists marching under the banner of Christ, out to undermine the free enterprise system (Senate Hearing, 1978: 135). In Canada, NGOs that threaten corporate power may find themselves losing their charitable status or facing tax audits. In other parts of the world, threats may be more physical. A 2014 documentary film, *The Tigers,* tells the story of the threats against a whistleblower from Pakistan, a former salesman for Nestlé products whose job was to convince Pakistani doctors to promote Nestlé infant formula.[5]

Industry spokespersons raise the standards of proof so high that nothing could satisfy them except "more research" (Proctor 2008: 18). Research is also controlled by funding and defunding certain areas of inquiry. Current efforts include research to identify newborns that "have to be fed" infant formula, or who exhibit allergic reactions to their mother's milk, both extremely rare occurrences. Most research protocols could never meet industry standards of proof because they are limited by ethical standards.

Randomized double-blind studies of breastfed and artificially fed infants are unethical, because one method of feeding is known to be superior to the other. In fact, all mass uncontrolled trials on infant-feeding methods are unethical, as infants should never be experimental subjects. Universities bar many kinds of research that might entail risks to human subjects, have strings attached, use animals, or are done for the military or solely for profit. Experiments may be banned when the cost of gaining knowledge is judged to be too high (Proctor 2008: 21–22). But industry research often slips between the cracks of review committees. When industry participates in and funds academic research, there is a danger that ethics committees may rubber-stamp ethics approvals and survey protocols that require more scrutiny. For example, a study in Indonesia referred to as the Daffodil study was approved by the ethics board in an Indonesian university, even though infants cannot ethically be used to test for ingredient safety. In the Daffodil study, ingredients designed to affect respiratory and digestive systems of infants zero to four months were to be added to infant formula. Economic incentives to poor families who agree to have their infants be experimented upon are not ethical. Clinical trials cannot prove the safety of infant formulas or commercial baby foods, when vulnerable infants most likely to be damaged by unsafe products are excluded from trials—as they should be. The trials were halted after a media campaign by local activists in 2013 (Faizal 2013).

Although efforts to improve breastmilk substitutes are necessary, along with precautions to ensure their relative safety, the resulting experimental products should be compared with each other, not with breastmilk. If a constituent is found to be safe and useful, then its inclusion in all infant formulas should be mandatory in order to reduce the risks of artificial feeding.

We already know enough about human milk to act to promote and protect it, while acknowledging the extent of our ignorance, our desire to reduce the ignorance deficit and replace it with knowledge (cf. Proctor 2008: 25, 4). As we saw in Chapter 3, ongoing research is providing new information about human milk at a rapid rate. Efforts to reduce the ignorance deficit about human milk are a far cry from manufacturing ignorance by the suppression or distortion of knowledge.

International Baby Food Action Network's (IBFAN) Legal Update exposed industry tactics to discourage legislators from enacting a strong code. In Fiji, Nestlé pulled product from the shelves to create an artificial shortage of infant formula, to spread the idea that limiting the promotion and marketing for infant formula through legislation would result in product shortages (International Baby Food Action Network 2013a: 3). The Philippines has been a leader in advocacy for infant and young child feeding. In 2005, they planned revisions to update their 1986 Milk Code regulations to implement new World Health Assembly (WHA) resolutions and strengthen standards on the marketing of baby foods. Philippine regulations include a ban on advertising and promotion of breastmilk substitutes for children up to two years of age, with an absolute ban on false health and nutrition claims. The largest American and European baby food companies appealed to the Supreme Court, arguing the regulation constituted a constraint on freedom of trade. At the same time, the US Chamber of Commerce in the Philippines exerted pressure on the Philippines government to intervene in the case, warning President Arroyo of "the risk to the reputation of the Philippines as a stable and viable destination for investment" if she did not "reexamine this regulatory decision." Four days later, 15 August 2006, the courts reversed their earlier decision and suspended the regulations to limit inappropriate promotional practices targeting new mothers and health professionals.

International Policy and NGOs

In *Human Rights and Gender Violence* (2006), Sally Merry uses the international human rights movement against violence to women as a site for understanding how new categories of meaning emerge from transnational practices. Her book explores how global law is translated into the vernacular by NGO activists who mediate these different meanings. Her examination of the interface between local and global activism revealed three forms of cultural flows between global and local spaces—transnational consensus building, transnational program transplants, and the localization of transnational knowledge (Merry 2006: 20). We can apply this framework to international public health efforts to improve infant and young child feeding.

Efforts at transnational consensus building to improve child nutrition span the Protein Advisory Group (PAG) meetings of the 1960s to the *Global Strategy for Infant and Young Child Feeding*. Earlier in this chapter, we assessed the importance of official UN documents and resolutions, as they struggled to collect clinical evidence for the best way to feed infants and young children and put it into practice in hospitals, households, and communities around the world. We have seen the emphasis on wording, rather than evidence, because evidence is assumed to be agreed upon by earlier documents and on procedures for negotiating consensus. These negotiations include finding vague phrases acceptable to all to blur differences in assumptions between global and local partners, as in the negotiations for the Innocenti +15 document. Once documents are officially approved and vetted through legal departments, they are translated into UN languages and move from the global to the local level.

At the end of the process, there may be minimal evidence for arguments behind particular positions taken, because wordings are compromises, resulting from negotiations and the bracketing of contentious issues (cf. Riles 2001). For example, the International Code of Marketing of Breastmilk Substitutes is a compromise document, weakened by industry and attempts to keep the United States in negotiations. Huge literature reviews are contracted to justify positions taken, resulting in not lack of evidence but surplus of evidence, often without addressing the contradictions and ambiguities embedded in documents and practices, and even in the research itself. In the case of violence against women, Merry writes: "The notion that cultural diversity should be respected is awkwardly juxtaposed to the assumption that religion and culture are barriers to women's equality" (2006: 47). Nowhere is there room for local nurturing practices that support new mothers.

Other cultural flows between global and local include program transplants such as the BFHI, PMTCT, and infant-feeding counseling guidelines. For nations and communities that adopt these programs, global documents and resolutions matter a great deal. When programs end, budgets end; salaries end. But often program vocabulary persists through training manuals, for example. BFHI has entered the vernacular, often in ways that frustrate local practitioners who argue that hospitals should be mother-friendly not baby-friendly.

Local NGOs and health clinics have to reframe WHO/UNICEF documents and guidelines to fit local circumstances. Relations between mastering nurture and negotiating nurture occur at the local level, as UN documents are translated into practices recognizable in local regimens, ideally to become embedded in social practice, local habitus. UN documents and guidelines are also used by policy makers to guide national policy, but it is national policy makers who negotiate the challenge of translation, not the UN.

A phrase like AFASS has not entered the vernacular but remains a specialist term for HIV workers. Its use provides a shorthand way to avoid talking more directly about corporate involvement in replacement feeding and poverty conditions. Similarly, PMTCT has almost entered the vernacular as it is cited regularly at international AIDS conferences to avoid direct discussions of breastfeeding practices and the transmission of HIV through breastmilk. Phrases like BFHI, AFASS, and PMTCT may well remain long after projects end, or policies have been changed. (Who remembers the UNICEF initiative called GOBI, promoting Growth monitoring, Oral rehydration, Breastfeeding, and Immunization?) If documents, policies, and guidelines are found to be flawed or ineffective, how are they withdrawn after the language and logic has been adopted and translated into the vernacular? The interface between local and global activism is best exemplified through the work of international NGOs to localize global or transnational knowledge. UN documents and programs are not enough; agencies depend on NGOs to disseminate information and to generate public support and sometimes government discomfort (Merry 2006: 71). NGOs that know the agreed upon UN language do better at lobbying at UN meetings (cf. Merry 2006: 55).

NGOs lobby for phrasing, explain issues in local terms, develop and research new issues, make interventions when invited, and are particularly effective in social mobilization and publicizing violations of UN resolutions, including code violations. Transnational knowledge localization for improving infant and young child feeding is accomplished through social mobilization strategies such as World Breastfeeding Week (WBW) and code monitoring activities carried out primarily by international NGOs like IBFAN's Code Documentation Center in Penang. Other larger NGOs like CARE or Save the Children may have more formal contractual roles in implementing UN strategies. Local actors in large and small NGOs who participate in international networks, participate in national and international meetings and take information home to be translated literally and figuratively into local campaigns.

NGOs mobilize outrage (cf. Merry 2006: 70), and according to Stephen Lewis, they should continue to do so. In his keynote address opening a WABA-UNICEF conference on HIV and infant feeding, he reminded the NGO members present that they were meant

> to harass and irritate and goad and enrage all the comfortable, conventional, institutional arrangements in the field of breastfeeding. … It's terribly important, I think, that WABA, in a respectful but determined way, launches criticism, even of its friends. (WABA-UNICEF 2002: 16)

However, when core and program funding may come from these same institutions, power differentials can have immediate and devastating consequences for NGOs, while even blatantly bad policy decisions are unlikely to seriously affect UN personnel or projects.

The UN and its specialized agencies are not the only institutions engaged in mastering nurture. The *Global Strategy* makes reference to "collaboration between governments, international organizations and other concerned parties" (#9), including in this definition of concerned parties, commercial enterprises (Richter 2005: 2). UN agencies could not master nurture without help from NGOs, governments, and corporations. The *Global Strategy* takes a more holistic view of infant feeding than the Innocenti Declaration by including complementary feeding.

Mastering Breastfeeding?

What are the consequences of providing universal standards, global recommendations, and guidelines for exclusive breastfeeding, knowing that in many parts of the world, these standards may never be met? Do UN agencies marginalize themselves in the struggle to promote child survival by developing universal standards that most women in the world do not know about, or cannot meet? And yet experts say exclusive breastfeeding is ideal based on the best evidence to date, thus justifying one standard for all. But what if the identification of the one best solution (exclusive breastfeeding), results in poor practices? Will mothers become so upset when they fail to breastfeed exclusively that they will never try again, thinking, why bother, reasoning if they cannot breastfeed exclusively, then there is no point in bothering to breastfeed at all? Efforts to create the highest standard for all can become the worst experience for many. Exclusive breastfeeding, if promoted rigidly or intolerantly, sets experts up as missionaries for breastfeeding, creating potential for all or nothing, black or white alternatives, the best and the rest opposition, much like breast or bottle feeding. More significantly, universal policy cannot negotiate with local traditions and may encourage premature closure for things we do not know about and cannot even imagine. This is what makes ethnography so critically important for infant-feeding research.

Attempts to master nurture fail because they ignore or cannot address nurturing practices—all the varied maternal, parental, and social efforts to keep infants and children alive and thriving. In this chapter, we have explored how breastfeeding and breastfeeding policy become institutionalized. We suggest that breastfeeding rules work against, and even repudiate, relationships like nurture. Much like food programs that deny commensality by defining food sharing as program leakage, breastfeeding programs that deny nurture give participants the feeling of being watched, both locally and globally. Trying to "master breastfeeding" reinforces the masculine metaphors emerging out of public health, including targets, goals, and bullets, setting us on paths too narrow to fit the reality at the end. Mastery can occur at all levels—global policy, implementing institutions, or a husband who insists his wife use infant formula.

The struggle over the Innocenti publication, and the complexity of policy making around HIV/AIDS reflects one reality—the UN reality; the experiences of mothers who must nurture newborns (and often fail due to lack of resources) provide an array of other realities. When document production and distribution increases the distance between the realities of poverty households, and the UN, for example, document production becomes another route to mastery. The UN reality is the dominant view represented in documents. Mothers' realities are better understood through mother-to-mother support groups, both lay and professional (which is why mother support groups were annoyed that peer support was cut from the Innocenti messages), and through ethnographic research.

If UNICEF and WHO are missionaries for universal statements like the *Global Strategy*, driven by its search for adequate funding levels, preceded by gaining approvals for agreed upon language, anthropologists are missionaries for the local, for understanding the diversified traditions and everyday compromises of women nurturing newborns, and the human commonalities we have identified, including the social womb and the commensal circle. The particulars of locality are needed because public health models are ill-equipped to address the underlying causes that make it difficult for women to breastfeed and nurture their children—gender inequities, poverty, and corporate-led globalization. Feeding—even breastfeeding—does not solve all problems of infant survival.

The March toward Mastery

Mastery as a noun refers to expert skill or outstanding ability; this mastery is what the mother–infant dyad develops over time. There is a place for a master dancer or a dance master to help develop these skills when necessary. But no audience would mistake the repetitive exercises of a Cecchetti ballet exam for a performance. Rigid training helps students acquire mastery of dance techniques according to a master teacher like Cecchetti. But such mastery is not a dance performance; it is mastery of a skill set.

This chapter has been more concerned with mastery as total control over people and situations. UN policy, NGOs, and hospitals may try to dance to this tune; it is also what corporations strive for, to master or control a market. Theirs is not a dance of nurture, but a march—rigid steps to music that draw people into lockstep with other people, yet not necessarily responsive to each other. Marches encourage synchronism but not intimacy. Often this is a march to music that only bureaucrats can hear, no doubt good moral people with good intentions, bent on creating *The Future We Want* (the title of the UN report from the Rio summit on Sustainable Development 2009) based on individualism and accountability (Peake and Rieker 2013: 10). The last chapter shifts attention from mastery to negotiation.

Notes

1. The ethnography of institutions like the UN differs from the institutional ethnography that Smith develops; in her work, institutional ethnographies examine how people produce institutions "in the course of their everyday doings" (2005: 13).
2. I was contracted by UNICEF to prepare the long document. I met the conditions of the contract but could not address the critiques of WHO and UNICEF in the few hours remaining in the contract. In addition, I had no experience with the politics of font size, logos, and track changes, important techniques in the discourse of mastery. As a first-time "pen for hire," it was difficult to accept that UN agencies owned my words and could do with them what they liked. (PVE)
3. Fidel Castro made a related comparison at the meeting of the World Health Assembly in 1998. He noted that it would take 3% of the amount of money spent on military worldwide (800 billion USD) to provide basic health care to the whole world
4. I was caught in this process. Reprints of a paper on insufficient milk authored by an anthropologist working for Ross Labs (Gussler 1980) were widely circulated by the company to North American pediatricians. The critique and response to Gussler's paper that I coauthored was less widely circulated because we did not have access to the funds to purchase multiple copies of reprints or the address lists of pediatricians available to Ross Labs. (PVE)
5. After his family was threatened, he eventually arrived in Canada as a refugee where he now drives a taxi near Toronto.

CHAPTER 8

Negotiating Nurture
Yesterday's Lessons, Tomorrow's Hope

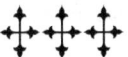

> Ecological knowings are enacted and ecological principles derived within a transformative, interrogating, and renewing imaginary—a loosely integrated system of images, metaphors, tacit assumptions, ways of thinking—a guiding metaphorics that departs radically from the imaginary through and within which epistemologies of mastery are derived and enacted.
>
> —(Code 2006: 29)

Chapter 8 takes us back to the larger pattern, to ask the big questions about why infant feeding matters and why nurture cannot be mastered bureaucratically. Naturally occurring systems like care and nurture are never perfect, always changing as they adapt to new circumstances. How then can we restore a viable realistic approach to infant feeding and negotiate nurture? Consider an ecology of infant feeding building on local biologies rather than the mastery of an activity. Lock refers to the way that "the biological and the social are co-produced and dialectically reproduced, and the primary site where this engagement takes place is the subjectively experienced, socialized body. ... The material and the social are *both* contingent—both local" (2001: 484). Local biologies are not context-free knowledges. But until we historicize our traditions of nurture, we cannot understand (nor negotiate with, in the case of UN agencies) the diversity of infant-feeding patterns in the world today. We began this task for one region of the world, Southeast Asia, in Chapter 5.

Every system of infant feeding has known, unknown, and unknowable tradeoffs. Every mother–infant pair must negotiate these trade-offs within different cultural settings. Substitutes to maternal breastfeeding have always been a part of infant-feeding complexes. For mothers everywhere, past and present, infant feeding is always a case of negotiating options, acknowledging the many complex tradeoffs, and optimizing the mother–child unit (rather than maximizing milk production or the duration of breastfeeding). People who promote breastfeeding do not always remember this, as we argued in Chapter 7. Negotiation is relational work, full of compromises, nudging the system to make strategic adjustments so as not to generate knee-jerk opposition and backlash that generates the "breast Nazi" language that permeates public culture and incites the mommy wars.

How do we nudge nurturing practices to fit today's postindustrial reality without generating a backlash? Newborn babies epitomize nudge theory (cf. Thaler and Sunstein 2008) as they push gently to gain their mothers' attention and signal their wish to breastfeed by licking and massaging their mothers' breasts even before they are hungry; many mothers resist the nudge. Should breastfeeding advocates follow the babies' approach and take nudge theory more seriously, nudging mothers to initiate or continue breastfeeding without sounding like they are forcing them or taking away their right to choose? By nudging more subtly, we may encounter less backlash against breastfeeding and breastfeeding advocacy in the Global North.

Nurturing practices are very different from business practices or even health practices; they are, however, easy to identify even in contemporary modern Western society. These thoughtful empathetic practices that occur spontaneously (even among other primates) are not restricted to feeding. Letter writing, urban gardening, cuddling frightened toddlers or reading to children, and mentoring students are nurturing practices. In modern Euro-American life, nurturing practices emerge in the face of tragedies like the shooting at the Boston marathon, April 2013. Both empathetic selfless practices and communal action followed the shock of the attack. Street picnics when the power goes out in urban neighborhoods are also common occurrences. Solidarity in the face of disaster is well understood. Newspapers lauded the Chinese firefighter who breastfed a newborn rescued from the earthquake in 2014, an incident that contrasts with the reports of Chinese parents who pay a monthly fee to have their children's teacher provide hugs to their children (Bethune 2014).

Less well understood is the rapidly eroding empathetic sociability in everyday life, when good neighbors are defined as people who keep their distance, leave you alone, not bother you, and respect your privacy (cf. Bethune 2014). To counter this erosion, nurturing opportunities have appeared in cyberspace in the form of internet support groups. *Meal Train* helps organize meals for someone who is sick or in need of help (mealtrain.com); mealbaby.com provides the same service for women who have just had a baby. *Patients Like Me* began as a non-profit site for people to share their experiences with medical treatments; the data sharing site is now for profit (patientslikeme.com). Many hospitals have websites that allow friends and relations who cannot be there in person to receive information about hospitalized patients and leave messages of encouragement and sympathy. Senior support networks (such as stayingput.com and housingcare.com) help seniors age in place. Many online self-help groups exchange information on specific diseases such as breast cancer. The rise in informal community breastmilk sharing networks such as *Eats on Feets* (eatsonfeets.org) and *Human Milk for Human Babies* (hm4hb.net) is part of this trend. Women who donate their expressed milk informally to their peers or through milk banks do so overwhelmingly to help others (over 70 percent, Gribble 2014). In 2013, UNICEF India launched a health phone app in over sixty languages to provide health information, including breastfeeding and complementary feeding advice for mothers. The Australian Breastfeeding Association is collaborating with Google Glass in a trial to help breastfeeding mothers, particularly in remote locations. The live stream will allow breastfeeding counselors to see what mothers see while they are breastfeeding and offer assistance, to adjust a latch, for example.

These technological innovations are helpful substitutes for face-to-face support in the modern urban world. Perhaps these methods also let people who could be there face-to-face "off the hook." But digital networking cannot replace the face-to-face and physical contact required for strengthening nurturing practices, nor develop the skills of negotiating across difference. Nor do they solve the problem of passing practices to the next generation; transmission is more easily accomplished in small-scale societies where children in different age groups play together and learn their nurturing practices directly from caring for younger children. In North America, these skills are learned from caring for eggs or dolls. Programs such as the Roots of Empathy in Canada bring babies and mothers in to classrooms to teach empathy; in other schools, students have to care for raw eggs for a week to learn how to treat and care for infants (cf. Gordon 2005). But egg handling does not necessarily lead to social sensibility; bullying may be one result of lack of empathy and social sensitivity.

The dance of nurture is a far cry from the financial negotiations that ask women to mentally calculate how much more money could be made by devoting time to affluent careers rather than to time-consuming nurturing practices like breastfeeding or making baby food. Globally, not all women have the option of affluent careers. Books like *Lean In* by Sheryl Sandberg (2013) present an ethnocentric Euro-American perspective on nurture that is deeply rooted in affluence and choice, and destructive to collective action. Although Sandberg is sympathetic to breastfeeding, having breastfed her own children, her books stress the need for breast pumps rather than maternity entitlements or social support:

> Breastfeeding makes mother the logical and biological choice for caretaking but the advent of the modern day breast pump has changed the equation. At Google, I would lock my office door and pump during conference calls. (Sandberg 2013: 124)

It is up to the enterprising woman to fit nurture in where she can.

Books like those by Wolf (2010), Barston (2012), and Jung (2015) fuel the fires of the mommy wars by denying the evidence ("voodoo science") for the superiority of breastfeeding, or citing it as evidence to further a cult of total motherhood. The media picks up on any story that can simplify an otherwise complex situation; their argument is simple: science got it wrong, breastmilk is not best. Citations from these books are recirculated as evidence that "lactivists" try to force women to breastfeed against their will.

An Outstretched Hand

A colleague once referred to writing a book as an outstretched hand extended to others who can then take the next steps. Thus far, we have opened up new conversations about breastfeeding and nurture, and suggested some steps that anthropologists and others might take. We began with the doom and gloom metanarratives about the human condition. This modern story we have been telling ourselves reflects our human need for a consistent narrative to make sense of the senseless worlds we inhabit; stories about the rise and fall of civilizations, of power and progress, ignore nurture. While we deal with crises, we have not been paying enough attention to those highly evolved mediating structures that protect people from exploitative forces, while characterizing customs as traditions of the past, not current compromises. Anthropology has been complicit in these absences, as its subfields drift farther apart, making it difficult to address biocultural hybrids like breastfeeding.

The challenges of the modern world are frightening, and they offer no solutions about how to nurture in the modern world. What ideologies and structures make it easy to ignore nurture? Why do we let nurture go so easily without a fight? Placing nurture as a biocultural hybrid in its broadest possible context, including identifying the sets of customs around the social womb and commensal circles, is a place to start.

Chapter 2 explored in more theoretical depth why past approaches to breastfeeding based on Cartesian dualisms have not solved problems, answered questions, or improved the quality of life for breastfeeding women. The oppositions between nurturing women and aggressive men, working mothers and stay-at-home mothers, breastfeeding mothers and bottle-feeding mothers have not helped either analysis or advocacy. Such oppositions obscure how cultural complexes provide context, and how immediate material conditions can trump cultural complexes. Taking knowledge out of these true-or-false oppositions opens up opportunities to consider other bodies of knowledge created through other practices of knowing; for example, we contrasted lab logic and clinic logic with the field logic of the ethnographer and proposed a new synthesis; the New Ethnology brings these other bodies of knowledge into play to examine mother–infant interaction as a social universal, a biosocial hybrid, that can flourish only with support and protection.

Chapter 3 showed how breastfeeding is embedded in biocultural life. It tells the human story; recovering nurture requires reclaiming our biocultural heritage. Nurture makes tradeoffs, negotiates, and compromises to sustain the dance. Nurture is not wired-in. There is particular danger in treating nurture as a part of the natural capacity of women; it is equally dangerous to develop cultural theories that ignore biology and the physiological basis of lactation. The fear of biological essentialism has discouraged the development of biocultural frames for analyzing breastfeeding as a biocultural hybrid. We argued that human phylogeny makes our bodily functioning dependent on our social surroundings, necessitating the development of the social womb in human communities, where new mothers can be supported. Without these sympathetic surroundings, women may have difficulty breastfeeding.

Like other breastfeeding advocates, we assume that breastfeeding is normal, not best, and expect that further research will uncover new properties of human milk and reveal new truths about the role of breastfeeding in building human constitutions. Current and future scientific evidence about the effects of breastfeeding on human development and the constituents in human milk will remain true whether or not critics believe the evidence.

In Chapter 4, we saw how the new infant is gradually integrated into the commensal circle. The chapter provides a temporal/developmental frame for putting breastfeeding and infant feeding into the context of the broader food system and the life cycle. Without inclusion of infant and young child feeding into discussions of food systems, we lose the opportunity for insights into food socialization and the long-term impact of infant feeding on the health and eating habits of adults. By reintegrating infant-feeding experiences into food studies, we have the potential for further developing a life-cycle approach to the intergenerational transmission of taste preferences, food habits, and the potential sociality of meals. In addition, the pattern of infant feeding in the first few days influences subsequent feeding practices (Southall and Schwartz 2000; Minchin 2015). Initial experiences with food and eating can set activity patterns for life, and these patterns, as well as the mother and grandmother's diet during pregnancy, may have a profound influence on adult health (Kuzawa and Quinn 2009). We argue for the importance of life-cycle approaches including looking at pregnancy and breastfeeding across the generations, and linking adult eating patterns back to infant-feeding patterns.

Chapter 5 demonstrated how breastfeeding developed in one region of the world. The ethnographic snapshots of infant feeding in Southeast Asia provides glimpses into how local nurturing practices are expressed, reminding us that there are a plurality of ways to nurture. Regional approaches are comparative and require knowledge of the historical precedents underlying current nurturing practices. In Southeast Asia, nurture is political, highly valued, variable, and manipulated through kinship but not limited to kin relations. Often rice meals provide the idiom for connectedness through shared substance. Other parts of the world might frame infant feeding around different idioms such as fertility, or different core foods such as corn or wheat.

Postpartum practices in Southeast Asia remain important for strengthening the social relations that anchor ethnic and feminine identity, even after hospital births and contraception reduced the need for spirit intervention to prevent maternal and infant deaths. But occasional infant deaths continue to signify the failure of the community to nurture its present and future members.

Chapter 6 told the modern story of breastfeeding, beginning with a case study of Chicago where modernity began to rule our bodily lives. We argued that breastfeeding is outside the model of improvement, progress, and perfectibility characteristic of mainstream middle-class North American modernity. Breastfeeding as a way to nurture newborns is part of our primate heritage and is as good as it gets—full stop.

People live and act in a world of received forms; even modernity is a product of received forms. Some features of modernity have an impact on breastfeeding, including the stress of choice and the measurement of time. In many contexts, modernity ignores or disrupts nurture, making it irrelevant to modern life. Take, for example, modernity's hostility toward local postpartum customs, many of which supported nurturing practices. The pressures of modern life diminish our sense of community, undermine social connectedness, and discourage paternal nurture (Hrdy 2009: 286, 288). The controlled, modern disciplined body as machine may be efficient, but it is not necessarily good at nurturing.

When nurturing practices are coded as custom and passed from generation to generation, customary knowledge about infant feeding is retained if it works and if there are no serious disruptions to its transmission. New religions, government regimes, or conditions of work may mean that customs that used to be effective no longer fit, and are thus adjusted or replaced. But nurturing practices are resilient and have adapted to many modern intrusions, transforming themselves in the process.

In Chapter 7 we looked at institutional efforts to address some of the problems caused by modernity, and why attempts to master nurture bureaucratically fail. This is the modern story told in a bureaucratic voice. Health care workers nagged women to breastfeed and then blamed them for their failures. It is thus not surprising that well-intentioned people have not solved infant-feeding problems. We cannot go back in time to restore enabling customs that were trashed by modernity. Nor should we romanticize the past; traditional postpartum customs were not perfect because they were always compromises.

Part of the arrogance of modernity is thinking it can fix all mistakes with technology. Once UN agencies align themselves with free-market forces, they become even more intolerant of local solutions to problems and more attracted to the silver bullets offered by neoliberal business solutions, conveniently forgetting that business practices are organized to maximize profit not health. In this concluding section, we consider how breastfeeding advocates might address some of these challenges and why anthropology is positioned to help.

Rethinking Advocacy

Advocacy has a necessary role in protecting breastfeeding and nurturing practices. There is a division of labor among breastfeeding advocacy groups, along with many shared values. Peer support groups such as La Leche League help women where they are, avoiding politics wherever possible. Recently, the organization has worked more closely with activist groups such as WABA and IBFAN, acknowledging that someone has to do the political work around maternity entitlements and corporate monitoring in order to make the structural changes that will allow peer support groups to do their work with individual mothers more effectively. Breastfeeding advocacy in the 1970s and 1980s focused on boycotts and code development. The Nestlé boycott, begun in 1976, remains the longest and most successful food boycott in North American history. The campaigns to limit the unethical promotion of infant formula spread from industrial to developing countries through the creation of loose networks of consumer activist and women's health groups. "Suck-ins" and boycotting stores where breastfeeding mothers were not welcome were ad hoc responses to corporate rule breaking, after the fact. In the 1970s and 1980s, Nestlé was vulnerable to the threat to its brand image; it was relatively easy to demonize the unethical profit-driven promotional practices of the baby food industry. In the era of PPP and corporate social responsibility, the picture is more complex.

Groups such as IBFAN were part of the process of lobbying and drafting a code to regulate the promotion of breastmilk substitutes. The WHA passed the International Code of Marketing of Breastmilk Substitutes in 1981 (with only one negative vote from the United States). In 2013, only 19 percent of countries had passed laws incorporating all code recommendations, 17 percent had passed the code into national law, but few had fully implemented the code (IBFAN-ASIA 2013: 26). This is not surprising:

> Challenges include a lack of political will to legislate and enforce the Code, continued interference from manufacturers and distributors in governments' efforts to initiate or strengthen Code monitoring and enforcement measures, lack of sufficient data and expertise on Code-related matters, absence of coordination among responsible stakeholders, and limited national and international resources for legislation, monitoring and enforcement. (World Health Organization, UNICEF, and International Baby Food Action Network 2016)

Anticorporate watchdogs at the Code Documentation Centre in Penang, as well as other IBFAN and WABA groups around the world, look at the broader connections between food and pharmaceutical corporations and policy making, including the problem of conflict of interest. These activists may be militant, relentless, media savvy, and easily misunderstood, but they are very few in number. They may occasionally get it wrong or overstate a case, but there is no doubt about their values or their impact. This was publicly recognized when IBFAN was named the recipient of the alternative Nobel Prize in 1998. Governments make promises to support UN conventions and regulations that they never intend to keep; they need to know that someone is watching.

Breastfeeding advocacy groups that monitor the baby food corporations have a long, successful history of engaging with these industries. The boycott story is particularly relevant because it brought NGO players to UN policy meetings (FAO, WHO, UNICEF) and made industry participation in policy making more visible. Public interest NGOs (PINGOs) successfully fought to restrict the participation of BINGOs (business interest NGOs) in health and nutrition policy making. The groups moved beyond public awareness to actually change policies with regard to the role of the food industry in policy making.

Lactivism is a term applied to activists who support and promote breastfeeding. It is not a term used by activists to refer to themselves. It includes mothers who enjoy breastfeeding, peers who help other mothers solve breastfeeding problems, and academic researchers who admit their "biases" toward breastfeeding, as well as NGOs who work on the assumption that breastfeeding is normal. Militant lactivism is a term that could be applied to those who are willing to confront, in person and in writing, the forces aligned against breastfeeding; their militancy is never directed against mothers who do not breastfeed, but against the promotional practices of formula companies. In fact, in an effort not to offend, many advocates, including researchers, delayed documenting and publicizing the risks of infant formula in order to avoid making mothers who use infant formula feel guilty for their decision. For example, *Environmental Health Perspectives* published a report showing that both powdered infant formula and well water may be a source of arsenic and that breastfed babies have lower arsenic exposure (Carignan et al. 2015). Reporting on the study: "Parents who need to use formula to feed their infants shouldn't feel badly about the new findings, said Katherine Cottingham, one of the study's lead authors" (Seaman 2015).

Faircloth's book, *Militant Lactivism* (2013) is a useful ethnography of extended breastfeeding among middle-class families in England and France, but it is not an ethnography of militant lactivism. Not all breastfeeding mothers practice attachment parenting, and few have the means and energy to monitor or lobby baby food companies, at least until their children are older. Of course, authors may not always have control over their book titles. Lactivists also host internet sites and blogs such as *Alpha Parent* and *The Badass Breastfeeder,* exchange information, and generally try to keep breastfeeding on the public agenda. Of course, militant lactivists can also be guilty of trying to master nurture if they become too aggressive or fail to respect the integrity of the mother–infant dyad.

Media may sensationalize research and advocacy in ways that do a disservice to the public. Headlines such as: "Breastfeeding: Protect Us from the Breastapo: Stop Attacking Mothers Who Feed Their Children on Formula, says Anna Maxted" (*The Telegraph,* 11 May 2011), creating straw (wo)men to grab media attention. Although critics accuse militant lactivists of trying to force women to breastfeed against their will, this has never been their intention or practice. One cannot (and should not try to) force a woman to breastfeed against her will; her body (and her baby) will rebel.

There is radical and restorative potential in breastfeeding activism because supporting the mother–infant relation requires altering priorities in the modern world, such as shifting gender hierarchies and reducing social inequities, in order to remove economic and social barriers to breastfeeding. Changes to marketing practices of baby foods require overturning entrenched capitalist corporate strategies that undermine breastfeeding and nurturing practices. Denying parents the time to nurture their children, and then offering them commodities such as ready-to-feed infant formula or convenience fast foods that replace time-intensive caring practices like child feeding to "save time" undercuts nurturing practices.

A Vague Utopia

In 1995, I was part of a small delegation invited to the Pontifical Academy of Sciences at the Vatican by the Jesuit group on faith and science. Doctors and nutritionists presented papers on current clinical research on breastfeeding. As the lone anthropologist in the delegation, I spoke about the cultural context of breastfeeding; my presentation included Playboy slides of bare-breasted women selling everything from vacuum cleaners to cars, to raise questions about the sexual representations of the breast in Western societies. Needless to say, the images were unlike the tables of nutrients and milk volume in the other presentations, but they were well received. Several priests told stories about breasts and breastfeeding; one French priest was disturbed to recall a topless woman being forced to leave a topless beach in the south of France when she began breastfeeding her infant.

We were told very suddenly that Pope John Paul II would receive us. I had false expectations about the visit, fearing that if he agreed that breastfeeding was important to infants' and women's health, he might make some kind of papal order for Catholic women to breastfeed. Unlike his predecessor Pope Pius XII who urged Catholic mothers, if at all possible, to nourish their children themselves, Pope John Paul II

> recognized the context in which such decisions are made, including the marketing strategies of infant formula companies, poor public health policies, and the need to harmonize work schedules with family time. He did not play on the dream of the angelic mother and child evoking the peace and nurture we yearn for, reflected in the paintings of the maternal lactating virgin we passed on the way out of the Vatican. But he recognized that breastfeeding "can create a bond of love and security between mother and child and enable the child to assert its presence as a person through interacting with the mother" (Solemn Papal Audience 1996: 289). He left us with the question that has stayed with me over the years: "Is this a vague utopia, or is it the obligatory path to the genuine well-being of society?" (Solemn Papal Audience 1996: 290). In January 2015, Pope Francis further normalized breastfeeding by inviting mothers attending a baptism service in the Sistine Chapel to breastfeed their children whenever they were hungry. (PVE)

It is utopian to think we can eliminate corporate power or end gender hierarchies, but activists can hold corporations accountable for the quality of their products, their promotional practices, and even their support for initiatives such as maternity entitlements. Civil society can challenge corporate efforts to discredit science and scientists who disagree with industry-funded research.

It is also utopian to think that advocates or public health professionals can resolve the contradictions of breastfeeding; the vulnerabilities and tensions are built in to the work of nurturing the next generation. Although breastfeeding rates change over the years, this does not mean that we should view breastfeeding as a lifestyle choice that moves in and out of fashion like hem lengths; it is a part of our human heritage that may well be at risk without extra vigilance and support.

Disability studies may provide some useful directions for transforming advocacy work. All social movements share the problem of refusing to acknowledge the common humanity shared by the oppressor and the oppressed (Morris 2001: 6). Using biomedical criteria of best practices, the "good" and "bad" practices are always intertwined with each other and with other aspects of society. Building on the assumption that humans, like other social primates, take care of one another, breastfeeding advocacy requires a feminist ethics of care—interdependence, relationships, and responsibility not autonomy, independence, and individual rights (Morris 2001: 13). Following disability advocacy, how do we shift breastfeeding advocacy into the social model (society needs fixing) rather than the medical model (the defective individual needs fixing)?

Interpreting infant feeding becomes a much more complex problem when we move beyond lab logic to bring in other kinds of evidence. While labs and clinics are at the forefront of trying to measure the health consequences of exclusive breastfeeding or bottle feeding, much more is at stake than can be documented by fragmenting wholes such as the mother–infant relation, the life cycle, and the social obligations of nurture. Breaking these practices apart will always produce ambiguities, a fact that antiscience arguments can always exploit. The evidence is never all in and never will be.

Advocacy is made more difficult when there are disagreements about results among lab scientists and clinicians. As with the case of climate change, advocates are faced with offering clumsy solutions to wicked problems—problems with unclear alternatives that offer threats to entrenched interests (Raynor 2006). Activists, like ethnographers, are more attuned to real life, but more likely than ethnographers to select evidence, cherry-pick what furthers the cause. Over the last decade, breastfeeding activists have attempted to be even more accountable to lab and clinic evidence by providing detailed footnotes to back their written reports and press releases. Although their advocacy work takes them far beyond the science to address the political and ethical issues surrounding promotional practices of baby food companies, the accountability to science is there in the small print. This is particularly evident in the work on pre- and probiotics in baby foods, and the chemical residues in human milk.

The more we learn about how breastfeeding works biologically, the more baby food companies try to reproduce the constituents found naturally in human milk to boost the appeal of the products they sell. They do little but boost the cost of the products, and thus company profits. And sometimes the additions can do damage. Infant formula companies add variable amounts of iron to their products, suggesting that the lack of iron in breastfed infants is a problem. But this added iron promotes the growth of pathogenic bacteria that feed on iron, disrupting the balance of bacteria in the infant gut. The addition of iron to these products undermines a delicate adaptive mechanism and increases the risk of infant illness (Quinn 2014: 10).

Advocates need to know how to access, interpret, and make sense of the complex science underlying every development in the biochemical analysis of human milk before they can communicate widely to the general public in multiple languages. They reach their publics by distilling, simplifying, and reducing arguments to sound bites, such as the themes and action folders for WBW or the Ten Steps to Successful Breastfeeding. This is a complex task for voluntary workers to undertake. These volunteers should be congratulated for making the science available to a broad audience, and not dismissed as "lactoloonies."

Repositioning Breastfeeding in Social Movements

Breastfeeding, like environmental issues, neither trumps nor distracts from other causes like poverty, hunger, or human rights; it supercharges them. Klein argues that climate change is not a separate movement but an opportunity to unite different issues and movements (2014: 157). Breastfeeding, too, is part of the effort to change the world; however, it is seldom viewed as a progressive movement. Single issue causes like climate change may see breastfeeding as a distraction from their priority goals rather than recognize how breastfeeding fits into an overarching narrative about nurturing future generations and the planet. However, by carefully integrating tactics and goals, all become part of the grand project of building a nontoxic shockproof economy (Klein 2014: 153, 154). Ingold explores these options through the concept of meshworld, interwoven threads entangling lines of life, growth, and movement (2011: 63). Nurture is the glue holding that meshworld together.

The work of creating allies in the breastfeeding movement and developing new constituencies is ongoing. The movement cannot just preach to the converted and hope that other advocacy groups will use their scarce resources to support breastfeeding. Even if groups choose not to get involved, it is important to be aware of common issues so that messages are not at cross-purposes, as for example, when breast cancer activists refer to breasts as toxic waste dumps, fat-loving toxic sponges soaking up the poisons in the world around them, or environmentalists refer to breastmilk as the world's most polluted food. To create allies, we need to find the commonalities in different single issue campaigns, all based on very different premises. How can we nudge feminist groups, human rights groups, environmental health groups, and antiglobalization campaigns into a more explicit relationship with nurture? How can we shift the frames so that breastfeeding and nurture play a role in improving our understanding of ecological processes, women's empowerment, food sovereignty, and even heritage preservation?

Global Health and Environmental Movements

Environmental health groups are natural allies for breastfeeding, particularly groups focusing on water and toxic chemical contaminants. Could one imagine a stronger motivation for cleaning up industrial waste than the thought of our children's children drinking our waste products? Recently, IBFAN has published evidence showing how infant formula production and use damages the environment. Their publication, *Formula for Disaster,* documents the significant carbon footprint of industrial production and household preparation of infant formula. But it can be a hard sell.

"You Do Your Issue, I'll Do Mine"

In 1999, WABA sent me as an NGO delegate to the intergovernmental negotiations on persistent organic pollutants (POPs), which ultimately resulted in the Stockholm Treaty to ban the production of some of the world's most toxic POPs. I had just written *Risks, Rights and Regulation: Communicating About Risks and Infant Feeding* (2002), about the contaminants and chemical residues in breastmilk, and needed to learn more about how best to develop a joint communication strategy to allow environmental groups and breastfeeding groups to work together. We stood shoulder to shoulder with environmental activists, all of us wearing paper-mache pregnant bellies and breasts, trying to shame the delegates into developing strong legislation to end the use of POPs. As breastfeeding advocates, we kept a low profile, while Greenpeace campaigned around the theme of protecting breastmilk, "the world's most polluted food." When we tried to suggest how dangerous it was to talk about contaminants in breastmilk this way, without talking about the toxins in water, cow's milk, and other replacement feeds, we were told (by a very aggressive male), "You do your issue, I'll do mine." Later messages from breastfeeding groups tried to stress the fact that human milk was simply a noninvasive source of samples for testing levels of contamination, and not a reflection of the amount of contamination in human milk. This separation of single-issue advocacy causes was painfully obvious in this case, as it was in the case of breastfeeding and HIV/AIDS. (PVE)

Nichter's work on global health does not discuss breastfeeding per se, focusing instead on the importance of monitoring industries that promote pharmaceuticals, tobacco, and infant formula in a less than ethical manner, and the international agreements that attempt to regulate such practices (2008: 170). But his analysis of syndemic problems can usefully be applied to bottle feeding or early weaning; syndemic problems are synergistic, intertwined with other mutually reinforcing health, environmental, social, and economic problems facing a population (Nichter 2008: 157).

Building on his concept of syndemic relationships, consider artificial infant-feeding practices in the context of poor quality water or an uncertain water supply. Contaminated water used to mix powdered baby milks or given directly to infants (on the false assumption that breastfed babies need water when they are thirsty) both increase the risk of diarrhea. An unreliable water supply results in people storing water in containers. Containers become breeding grounds for vectors of malaria and dengue fever. But advocacy programs on water seldom consider infant and young child feeding, in spite of the increasing evidence of persistent toxic metals like arsenic from pesticides and herbicides found in groundwater. Drinking water standards are established with adults in mind, not infants and young children. More disturbing are the attempts by companies like Nestlé to privatize and control public water and turn it in to a profitable commodity.

Breastfeeding in these same environmental contexts would provide synergetic advantages. Exclusively breastfed infants need no water, reducing the need to store water in the household. Also, breastfeeding conveys some protection against malaria. Families become less dependent on breastmilk substitutes and drugs to suppress diarrhea, freeing up cash in households and in health centers, for needed drugs like antibiotics.

Poor funding for the health system increases the appeal of pharmaceutical "gifts," including treatments for diarrhea and provision of new baby food products to "solve digestive problems." Companies whose products cause problems and who can also provide drugs to solve the problem they caused are doubly blessed. This synergy between industry and health systems is well documented but easily ignored.

Breastfeeding also supports efforts to address overpopulation by increasing child spacing through lactation amenorrhea, and encouraging women to have fewer but healthier children. Just as population problems exist in the context of other interconnected problems of the environment, economics and education, for example, solving the problem of nurture could simultaneously contribute to reducing population pressure.

Women's Movement

The issue of breastfeeding is almost invisible in the women's movement, either because it is taken for granted in some parts of the world, or totally out of women's consciousness in other parts of the world. The preparatory meetings for the Beijing Conference for Women, September 1995, were not receptive to the inclusion of breastfeeding promotion in their action plans. Instead, women who raised the issue were dismissed as "pro-Vatican."

Feminism Light

The Conference on Women held in Beijing in 1995 provided another opportunity to consider breastfeeding from a global perspective. Unfortunately, at the preparatory conference in New York, all references to breastfeeding were deleted from document sections on women's health, human rights, and employment. One reference under structural adjustment was bracketed and not discussed until the Beijing meeting. The Beijing conference devoted most effort to addressing questions around diverse feminisms, human rights, and violence against women. One American delegate called breastfeeding issues "feminism light" suggesting that breastfeeding was not a serious feminist issue compared with subjects like domestic violence, for example. I remember feeling vaguely disappointed with myself, as I sat in our pink booth full of breastfeeding posters, providing information linking breastfeeding to women's empowerment and rights. WABA provided a rocking chair, snacks, and drinks for breastfeeding mothers—a valuable service, much appreciated by delegates who were also new mothers. I recall more vividly the antagonistic questions from workshop participants about women's right to choose whether to breast or bottle feed, and comments about the need for modern women to seek profitable work away from their infants. Some participants nodded in agreement; others tried to counter her arguments. Later we found that the questions came from young women who were "Nestlé interns," paid to attend workshops related to infant feeding, raise questions about "women's right to choose," and report back to Nestlé. The use of student interns was another effective marketing strategy for the companies.

I felt I had nothing to contribute to the NGOs concerned with violence against women who dominated the Beijing conference. I have since worked to remedy this feeling of discomfort by addressing the infant-feeding challenges of women survivors of childhood sexual abuse (CSA) with a colleague in Saskatoon who worked with these mothers, including many First Nations women (cf. Wood and Van Esterik 2010). (PVE)

Breastfeeding can be a divisive issue in national or regional women's organizations in developed and developing countries. For example, national women's organizations were not immediately supportive of Brazil's breastfeeding initiatives because they saw it as a means of isolating women in their homes. Similarly, women's groups in India protested against the government's legislation to control the marketing of infant formula in the country, calling the bill "draconian," fearing it would do "untold damage to women's careers and force them back to the kitchen."

In the 1990s, Norway had the highest incidence and duration of breastfeeding in Europe and indeed among all developed countries (98 percent leaving hospital, 75 percent at six months). But those figures represent an increase of about 30 percent since the 1970s (Helsing 1990: 73), following sustained policy changes to support breastfeeding mothers. The links between feminism and reproductive choice provided the conditions for the success of breastfeeding policy in Norway. The crucial choice for Scandinavian women is whether or not to have children; women who chose to have children expect that society must provide parents with support. Breastfeeding becomes the natural choice because structural conditions that support mothers are already in place: humanized hospital routines, protection of workers' rights including generous maternity entitlements (both paid leaves and lactation breaks), strong mother-to-mother support groups, including support for women who cannot or choose not to breastfeed, well-regulated breastmilk banks, and a careful monitoring of the promotion of breastmilk substitutes (Heiberg Endresen and Helsing 1995). In Scandinavian countries, efforts to support breastfeeding have been more strongly supported by the women's movement:

> The new feminist movement in Norway has encouraged women's self-confidence and pride—both prerequisites for breastfeeding. Unlike similar movements, the Norwegian feminist movement has never seen a contradiction between women's liberation and breastfeeding. (Baumslag 1989: xvi)

Maternal mortality rate is a good measure of the status of women in a society, and Norway has one of the lowest maternal mortality rates in the world (5 per 100,000 live births in 2015). Although women with higher education breastfeed more, mothers employed outside the home have a higher prevalence and duration of breastfeeding than those working at home, regardless of educational level (Helsing 1990). In Scandinavia, feminist movements have been positive toward breastfeeding, and breastfeeding issues have been easily integrated with other concerns of women, including increasing the number of women in political life. In these countries, maternity entitlements and breastfeeding support have complemented other policy objectives.

There has been a long but unexamined history of women who do not want to breastfeed but are told they must (usually by males), as well as a long history of women who want to breastfeed and are told by persons or circumstances that they cannot. (Believe it or not, redheads are still told to expect problems with breastfeeding.) It is critically important that we try and understand the decisions made regarding infant feeding of both the former and the latter mothers, or breastfeeding advocates will continue to be the focus of feminist ire that attacks breastfeeding advocacy as a plot to promote "total motherhood" and to make women breastfeed against their will. Joan Wolf (2010) gives us this in spades.

Even more complex is the problem of understanding women who say they want to breastfeed but really do not want to, or are disgusted by the practice. It is not politically correct to admit disgust at the process, but some people have no hesitation at expressing such views, as we saw in the comments of Princess Michael of Kent, widely circulated in the *Daily Mail*. She reiterates an opinion expressed by Queen Victoria who called breastfeeding "a horror."

The breastfeeding movement will soon face a paradox. The more successful breastfeeding becomes as an accepted, normal part of women's reproductive lives, the more devastating it will be for women not to be able to breastfeed—for whatever reason. As breastfeeding cultures become more established, they will need to develop ways to support mothers who feel they have had unsuccessful breastfeeding experiences so that they will not feel guilty, ashamed, or resentful of breastfeeding mothers, and too discouraged to try again.

It is often a challenge to avoid sending messages that make breastfeeding just another burden on women, another attempt to promote women's domesticity, particularly if public health messages are Western in origin. The dangers of backlash with regard to breastfeeding promotion are substantial in Euro-American settings, fueled by the media's love of conflict. Magazine articles and blog entries document personal stories of women who found breastfeeding an unpleasant sacrifice are common. The agony of breastfeeding, the dark side of breastfeeding, the bad experiences of individual women, cannot be ignored when they have such a prominent place in popular culture in North America. Social media has made these stories more prominent. Among the many oldest culturally specific "gotchas" is the phrase echoed by both industry and women who bottle feed: "Better to bottle feed with love than breastfeed with reluctance."

Many feminist groups are more conscious of not making women who do not breastfeed feel guilty than they are in fighting for the supports new mothers need to breastfeed. Breastfeeding advocates must be prepared to deal with these critical discourses effectively or lose support from women's organizations.

The antagonism to breastfeeding that exists in many parts of the North American women's movement results in difficulties in establishing breastfeeding as a priority in international women's meetings. This antagonism or apathy will be particularly destructive for efforts to implement infant-feeding policy if it is not countered by efforts to revalue women's power to breastfeed and nurture and reintegrate nurturant power into feminist theory. If this involves reinventing maternal feminism, then let it be a new maternal discourse that does not support the ideological hegemony of pro-natalism, the cult of total motherhood nor a romanticized motherhood.

Women did not create this bottle-feeding culture alone; men created the substitutes for human milk and the technology that "freed" women from breastfeeding. Men invented the pumps that further freed women from close contact with their infants. The misogyny of modernity, which pulled apart the human body into its constituent parts, encouraged the ideology that valued breasts for sexuality and advertising, not for nurture. There are already many public meanings of women's bodies in circulation. It may therefore be difficult to build new self-representation around bodies, for how do we de-eroticize, and de-colonize the female breast (Miles 1991: 181), or as Giles (2012) asks, how do we re-eroticize breastfeeding?

Women's issues and feminist issues are intertwined, each moving along their own trajectories. Some focus on advancing women's claims to equality and respect, others on attacking male privilege and power; but the issues remain intertwined. Nurturing has to bridge differences. Most nurturing practices are not gendered, with the exception of those around birth and breastfeeding.

Although breastfeeding can be usefully considered a feminist issue, and a woman's issue, it is first and foremost a human issue, relevant to men and to all members of society, because society benefits from women's reproductive work. As Haraway notes, "All women's practice is not feminist, and men's practice can be feminist" (1989: 287). Men would not survive to adulthood if they had not been nurtured; they too must nurture the next generation.

Human Rights

If breastfeeding is a human issue and not simply a women's issue, would human rights groups be valuable allies in the breastfeeding movement? While it sets universal standards, it does not prescribe a specific course of action; that is a matter for states to determine; thus, human rights activists target states (Claeyes and Lambek 2014: 3). Breastfeeding advocates debate how and when to use human rights frameworks and tools; like many anthropologists, some breastfeeding advocates feel the human rights discourse is too narrow and legalistic to encompass the complexities of breastfeeding. Human rights discourse recognizes the obligation of the state to respect, protect, promote, and fulfill rights. Rights discourse is very much about legal power; rights are made visible by their violation. Some anthropologists have successfully integrated their work with human rights (Merry 2001, 2006; Marchione and Messer 2010) usually paying particular attention to local efforts to vernacularize rights and acknowledging how the meaning of both rights and culture changes over time (Merry 2001, 2006).

The right to food is considered a second-generation right, with some arguing that malnutrition needs to be seen as a violation of human rights, a failure of the state to fulfill the right to food. The public generally accepts the right of the state to regulate food safety and food advertising, but not to tell citizens what they can and cannot eat. Thus, efforts to limit sugar or the size of soft drinks sold at fast-food restaurants in New York City, for example, was met with protests.

The movement for food sovereignty began with La Via Campesina and other farmers' collectives in a move to go beyond the right of individuals to be food secure. Food sovereignty refers to the right of communities, peoples, and states to democratically determine their own food and agricultural policies. Food sovereignty makes explicit the need to dismantle the corporate food regime and return control over the food system to local producers and consumers. It builds on a rights-based system but goes beyond, stressing the importance of repoliticizing food politics (Claeyes and Lambek 2014: 25). States need to regulate the actions of corporations to ensure they do not violate the right to food, as well as to regulate in support of the right to food. Breastfeeding protection fits well with negative rights—the right not to have states or corporations interfere with the way people acquire food (Lambek 2014: 101). Like food security, breastfeeding protection should be considered a global public good that requires cooperation among countries (cf. de Schutter 2011).

The right to food has been a more effective discourse for food activists than for breastfeeding activists. It has been used to promote food sovereignty and security, but that promotion seldom includes infant feeding, in spite of the fact that breastfeeding provides food security for infants.

Allies and Silos

> In 1996, I prepared a WABA Activity Sheet on breastfeeding as food security for the World Food Summit. I carried the brochures to Rome but could find no place to put them—once again, no place for breastfeeding. I settled into a small space beside a booth explaining local sustainable food systems in Peru. The NGO, Via Campesina, wanted their space back and suggested I go and squeeze in beside a pro-life group promoting natural child spacing. I wanted to stay. I told them I would move if they could identify a better example of a local sustainable food system that did not rely on global inputs than breastfeeding; they could not; I stayed, and we exchanged materials, integrated our messages, and became allies. (PVE)

The former UN reporter on the right to food, Olivier de Schutter (2011), argued that the right to food requires direct intervention by states because self-regulation of the agri-food industry is ineffective, arguing that regulatory human rights–based frameworks are more effective than nonbinding voluntary codes such as the International Code of Marketing of Breastmilk Substitutes.

The most effective use of human rights has been the efforts to regulate and control business activities in order to prevent the violation of child rights (Lhotska et al. 2012: 32). Breastfeeding advocacy groups have explored how legally binding human rights instruments could be used to expose and eliminate harmful business practices of the baby food industries. Initially, as breastfeeding advocates first began using human rights language, some programs tried to promote the child's right to breastmilk without adequate consideration of maternity entitlements and other supports for mothers. Some states such as the UAE have tried to compel mothers to breastfeed. Such approaches would be damaging to women in the long run. Other advocacy materials developed the argument that mothers have a right to breastfeed, while other groups argued that the state has an obligation to ensure that mothers are informed of the risks of infant formula use, or the risks of not breastfeeding. No one benefits when infants' and mothers' rights are pitted against one another; they are joint right holders. If the state is the duty bearer, the state may be pressured to provide proper supports for breastfeeding mothers, using the UN human rights processes. But in the current financial climate, states are less inclined to regulate the food and pharmaceutical corporations promoting baby food.

How does the rights discourse work with or within systems of nurture? Human rights arose out of the Western notion of law as a reformist ideology, and out of Western theory and practice. Human rights follows the fragmenting logic of modernity, breaking apart wholes such as nurture into individualized constituent parts; it is about individual legal rights and presumes the existence of an autonomous individual whose rights are either respected or denied. Breastfeeding reveals the ambiguous position of rights in the rhetoric of choice (cf. Bartlett 2005: 167) where breastfeeding has been positioned as a human right, a woman's right, a child's right, and a reproductive right; all these rights involve the right to choose, variously defined. More recently, Western women also claim the right not to breastfeed as an act of resistance to what they perceive as pressure to breastfeed their infants against their will.

Our model stresses that there are no individuals apart from society; infant feeding is never accomplished outside of household and community contexts. Breastfeeding is about a relationship between two people and never about the right of an autonomous individual (cf. Van Esterik 1999). Framing breastfeeding around rights too easily slips into an oppositional discourse opposing a mother's right to choose, and the infant's right to mother's milk. The rights discourse has largely replaced this relationship discourse as a way of framing breastfeeding. Rights separate people, while relationships bind people together.

In spite of the complexities surrounding breastfeeding and human rights, the movement could find potential allies among groups that advocate for group or collective rights (such as women's rights, indigenous rights, or children's rights). Intuitively, collective rights seem inappropriate, as breastfeeding is such an intimate personal activity. But if breastfeeding is understood as a relationship between two people, it also partakes of collective material bodies and accumulated customary knowledge of all women in a community and of all past generations. While parents judge what is in the best interests of the child, groups also share an interest in a child's well-being. Breastfeeding advocates seek more synergy between these discourses, strategizing when to use rights discourse and work within the human rights frame and when to develop a relational discourse more compatible with breastfeeding.

Heritage Foods

Imagine if breastfeeding support were conceived of as part of the extra-jurisdictional obligations owed to all people, part of our collective human heritage? Instead of rights, consider heritage: the UN system itself might provide an alternative framing. In 2012, Washoku, the "traditional" dietary culture of Japan consisting of soup and three side dishes was identified as a "living human treasure of humanity" by UNESCO's intangible cultural heritage (ICH) program. Washoku, derived from a courtly ascetic accompaniment to the tea ceremony, is not exactly food of the people, nor is it threatened. When the award was made in 2013, the Japanese recognized its importance for stimulating tourism and Japanese food exports.[1]

The UNESCO award is supposed to honor things of universal but intangible value, perhaps to get away from the Niagara Falls/Taj Mahal wonders of the world model of heritage. According to the UNESCO website:

> Intangible Cultural Heritage means the practices, representations, expressions, knowledge, skills—as well as the instruments, objects, artifacts and cultural spaces associated therewith—that communities, groups and, in some cases, individuals recognize as part of their cultural heritage. This intangible cultural heritage, transmitted from generation to generation, is constantly re-created by communities and groups in response to their environment, their interaction with nature and their history, and provides them with a sense of identity and continuity, thus promoting respect for cultural diversity and human creativity. For the purposes of this Convention, consideration will be given solely to such intangible cultural heritage as is compatible with existing international human rights instruments, as well as with the requirements of mutual respect among communities, groups and individuals, and of sustainable development.

UNESCO disburses funds to support the maintenance of recognized ICH items. Some recent examples include horse-riding games of Azerbaijan, Mongolian calligraphy, big shoulder-borne processional structures, making and sharing kimchi, Mediterranean diet, knotted woven bags of Papua, falconry, Ecuadorian straw hats, training puppeteers, tight rope walking in Korea, Mariachi bands of Mexico, Chinese acupuncture, French lace making, Indonesian batik, classical ballet of Cambodia, Indonesian puppet theater, Turkish coffee culture, and in 2010, the gastronomic meal of France.

What if we argued that human milk and the postpartum customs that support breastfeeding are part of our human heritage? A campaign for recognizing the importance of breastfeeding customs would stress the cultural context of support passed from generation to generation—and the nurturing practices that help new mothers as living human treasures provide this treasured food to the next generation. Just as we can argue that human milk is the original slow food, could we elevate and fund our work by putting UNESCO to the work of identifying a food that has more universal human value than human milk? With careful review of the research base, we might even be able to claim breastmilk as an endangered product, as the modern world throws up more and more obstacles to breastfeeding mothers in the form of toxins, chemical residues, hormone-disrupting chemicals, poverty, and isolation. If human milk were given the protection and safeguarding awarded to kimchi, for example, UNESCO would be obligated to "help garner international co-operation and assistance so interested parties can take adequate safeguarding measures"; UNESCO would then share the best safeguarding practices and pressure states "to promote and safeguard these treasures" (www.UNESCO.org/culture/ich).

Nurturing Optimism

The UNESCO campaign could provide an opportunity to identify postpartum practices that need to be better supported, including recognizing the nurturing potential of males, fathers, and grandmothers (cf. Hrdy 2009), and reevaluating those customs that were destroyed unintentionally through the well-meaning interventions of modernity. In some cases, interventions might act to preserve customs, but simply acknowledging the importance of birth customs and local postpartum supports would be valuable. Nurturing practices might also include the availability of objects such as baby slings or clothing styles that facilitate breastfeeding.

Consider the following as nudges toward negotiating nurture:

- Acknowledge that both the physiology and the social dynamics of breastfeeding can go wrong. In such cases, timely skilled assistance and support needs to be available.
- Provide enabling structures such as skilled assistance, rest periods for new mothers, maternity and paternity leaves, workplace creches, and flexible but consistent work shifts for new parents.
- Respect the local (particularly rituals and practices associated with the postpartum period), if it has no negative impact even if it defies the reductive logic of the lab.
- Recognize the uniqueness of infant foods, and exempt them from the usual promotional marketing practices of food and drug companies; find other products to promote.
- Add constituents to all formula and not just one brand if they have been independently tested and found to be useful. Efforts to improve infant formula are commendable harm reduction strategies, valuable as long as they are evidence-based, not accompanied by health claims and across the board. We cannot make infant formula safe, but we can make it safer.
- Include detailed contents of baby milks, including full disclosure of individual constituents.
- Insure that men, women, and non-breastfeeding mothers benefit from arguments and policies to support breastfeeding mothers, by emphasizing women's rights to control their own bodies including the right not to have children.

- Ensure that medical histories ask detailed questions about how patients were fed as infants.
- Include details regarding mode of feeding in models and research protocols on a wide range of health issues such as autism, obesity and allergies.
- Provide and publicize cost-benefit analyses for programs that support maternal and child health, including the costs of not breastfeeding (cf. Walters et al. 2016).

Love alone is not enough. We need enabling structures.

Reclaiming Anthropology's Place: The New Ethnology

Why should policy makers turn to anthropology to solve the mystery around the rise and fall of breastfeeding and other nurturing practices? What do economists and psychologists offer that anthropologists cannot? While they are better able to control variables, they slight cultural and historical context. Anthropologists appear to be less effective at influencing policy and even capturing the imagination of the public. Are we too open-ended, too accepting of diversity to be useful to policy makers? Our focus on the particular puts us in a good position to observe how institutions change over time, but who is interested in what anthropologists have to say about how systems change?

In the end, anthropology does have answers. The answers are just not silver bullets. Both ethnographers and biological anthropologists know a great deal about how to go about the work of understanding differences. There is no generic human; anthropology knows this to its very bones. Ruth Benedict said it best: the purpose of anthropology is to make the world safe for human differences.[2] Anthropology has a deep understanding and acceptance of diversity, and has given up on the search for unanimity and consensus (unlike the UN bureaucracy with its inability to accept and work with diversity, where well-intentioned arrogance keeps different agencies fighting for control and power).

The New Ethnology draws ethnography back to human commonalities by providing a middle ground between explanations claiming universal validity and those that only apply to "my village." It draws the subfields back into a new biocultural conversation—one that includes history, comparison, the life cycle, and holism, and operates across all bodies of evidence. It lets us think about the general in the particular, or as both embedded in one another. The ethnological point of view (Wittgenstein 1984) is not new; it means comparing two or more contexts, describing their differences from a standpoint outside to see things more objectively (Martin 2013: 157). The particular and global, universal and relativist, then, become false oppositions, "since all analysis straddles both" (Parkin 2007: 19). Or put more simply, both/and, not either/or. In the specifics of every mother–infant pair, we have the potential to see general patterns that may take us closer to understanding nurture through understanding breastfeeding in its totality.

Biocultural processes like breastfeeding require collaboration between biological and cultural anthropologists, a difficult task considering the increasing separation and specialization of the subfields. Medical anthropology reintegrated them somewhat, offering a new synthesis based on concepts such as local biologies (Lock 2001). Lab logic and clinic logic can strengthen ethnographic field observations about breastfeeding. Interest in life cycles and the links between generations has been muted in contemporary cultural anthropology. Here the New Ethnology can take a lead from the biological anthropologists who are going beyond genetics with their interest in epigenetics and life history models. Our approach to the life cycle is less competitive than life history models and more like a dance.

The New Ethnology has a place for life-cycle approaches that link overlapping generations, reabsorbing the insights from old culture and personality approaches and affect theory. Recollections of one's own childhood experiences, including memories and dreams of being breastfed, can be sources of evidence. They raise questions about whether nurture is encoded deep in human brains below the level of conscious intentionality as affect theory proposes, or is it developed through custom, heritage, and social experience? Or both?

The New Ethnology does not assume that all culture-crossing regularities are biology, pure, and timeless. Just the opposite: it supposes that all humans and their groups are highly historical creatures whose piecemeal, local solutions to universal problems like nurturing a newborn are passed down and borrowed widely. Adaptive complexes like the social womb and commensal circles require approaches such as the New Ethnology to explain how human constitutions are shaped over lifetimes.

Anthropologists are missionaries for the local, for avoiding closure and foregrounding statements and observations in "the real world," the field, wherever that might be. A century ago, ethnology tried to make sense of the vast diversity in the world by seeking underlying biological and cultural universals. Current practitioners are seldom comparative and no longer attempt to create massive all-encompassing frameworks for comparing civilizations, although many anthropologists remain drawn to holism, perhaps regretting the loss of interest in linking the specific, the local to "the big picture." For example, Philippe Descola (2013) returns to the grand intellectual synthesis in his comparative ethnology of ontological regimes.

The New Ethnology embraces comparison; but comparative work requires that we come to grips with the issue of commensurablity. This is particularly complex when policy and advocacy both operate across the Global North and Global South. Infant-feeding research and advocacy is full of examples of WEIRD passing as universal. Comparison and commensurability does not assume uniformity—far from it. The new holism is clearly not about totalizing integration, wholes, or reductionism, but rather, in the words of Ingold, about currents of discourse that flow into one another: "anything, caught at a particular moment, enfolds within its own constitution the history of relations that brought it there" (2007: 209). It is through historical processes that we can see how biology and ecology are integrated into cultural systems. We provided a glimpse into these patterns in one region of the world, Southeast Asia.

The New Ethnology leaves a place for advocacy and engagement as a key part of the discipline. It grounds advocacy by respecting difference and addressing practical solutions to real problems. Neither biological nor cultural universals motivate activism. Instead, grounded observations about human activities contribute to making generalizations based on patterns and regularities, rather than ideologies. Case-based knowledge empowers activism and allows activists to move forward. Currently, individual anthropologists who take on "the big problems" do so as citizens in the spirit of speculative journalism rather than from their disciplinary base (cf. Ortner 1998). The New Ethnology could provide evidence about enabling structures that support breastfeeding without forcing Cartesian choices. Activism has a particularly important role when the evidence is not all in. Evidence will never be all in; but using the precautionary principle, action can be taken now. Activists still need to be accountable to lab logic in their documents and presentations; their traces are visible in the citations in small print and footnotes.

Anthropology says delay categorical answers until you know just a bit more about local conditions. Understand the situation first before you suggest how to change it, always delaying coming to a definitive conclusion—which makes us undesirable consultants. Anthropologists know the realities of compromise and negotiation; even applied anthropology—a subfield that once aimed to "solve problems"—does not have the quick answers that neoliberal business models expect. The need for quick answers made the move to business solutions both appealing and understandable to policy makers. Within this logic, public private partnerships made perfect sense. The promise of quick answers endeared economists and accountants to large bureaucracies such as the UN agencies that implement global strategies on subjects like infant and young child feeding. Authoritative scientific knowledge based on lab logic and clinical logic inspired masterful interventions such as fortifying baby foods, all the while ignoring nurture. Good science does not always lead to good policy, and the politics of policy making does not always respect good science. To make sense of processes of nurture such as breastfeeding, we require historical and cultural specificity.

Moving Forward

Theoretical work on breastfeeding has been polarized between essentialist and determinist explanations, contrasting the regulated/cultural/mind with the free expression/natural/body. This is resolved in our work through the activity focus, treating breastfeeding as having its own integrity. We have created a road through a theoretical jungle; the motivation and intentions of people who use the road is irrelevant to the argument. That is, it is unimportant whether women breastfeed for reasons of compassion, convenience, attachment parenting, traditional custom, duty, a desire to space their children or to obtain trace elements and micronutrients for their children. For many women, breastfeeding is the only way to keep their newborns alive. Whatever the motivation, breastfeeding is first and foremost, normal for humans. What is often overlooked is that the activity can take over a person's life, much like monasticism, elite athletics, or anorexia (cf. O'Connor and Van Esterik 2015).

Although motivations for breastfeeding can be divergent for cultural as well as personal reasons, women may still accept or express the same premise: that not breastfeeding a child would be like rejecting the child, not giving it the best possible start in life. Imagine a Scandinavian woman and a Bangladeshi woman expressing that view. Most Scandinavian women would be speaking from the context of choice, while the Bangladeshi women may speak of doing their duty, in the context of an oppressive patriarchy. In neither case is breastfeeding itself empowering. In the Scandinavian case, power has already been won through political transformation, and the enabling structures that support breastfeeding are already in place as a result of women's past political and economic empowerment; in the Bangladeshi case, breastfeeding has nothing to do with empowerment in the political and economic arena, and efforts to politicize breastfeeding would be seen as neither helpful for breastfeeding women nor supportive of political change, making global campaigns around the message, *breastfeeding empowers women,* risky.[3]

Knowing women's motivations for breastfeeding are primarily relevant for experts trying to change behavior from the outside and better target breastfeeding promotional messages. In interdisciplinary projects, anthropologists are expected to explain the meaning of breastfeeding as part of an exotic belief system that could then be tapped as part of KAP surveys to improve health messages. But looking at breastfeeding as an activity minimizes the importance of cultural meaning. The wide range of motivations, experiences, and breastfeeding strategies of women means that efforts to find the one best way end up promoting politically correct breastfeeding. While exclusive breastfeeding may be the one best way according to the lab logic of health authorities, there is neither one best way to breastfeed nor one best way to nurture children. Even among our closest animal relatives, "There is no one, universal pattern of infant care among primates" (Hrdy 2009: 83).

Mothers often ask "experts" the right way to feed an infant, or the right way to breastfeed. If breastfeeding is always a negotiation between mother and infant, then mother and infant pairs are the experts; there is no one way to do it right—whatever works for a mother and her infant is right.

Breastfeeding is both a health practice that women perform to provide nutrients and more to their children, and a person-making practice—a way to relate to a new human. It is also an expression of the mother's inner person, part of her individual identity, who she is in society. Infant formula companies understood this latter fact perhaps better than breastfeeding advocates, and exploited it very effectively to promote formula use in developing countries in the past few decades. Recall the Nairobi advertising billboards that contrasted "modern African women" bottle feeding (and smiling) and "traditional African women" breastfeeding (and frowning).

Breastfeeding advocates have been more reluctant to build on the fact that breastfeeding becomes deeply embedded in women's identity, knowing how varied and personal are women's relations to breastfeeding and to mothering. Breastfeeding does not fit well into identity construction, who we are or who we want to be. That turns the dance into a race, creating anxiety that is harmful to breastfeeding at the individual level. The Similac video, "Sisterhood of Motherhood" exploited these stereotypes of breastfeeding mothers to make their point. North American groups like La Leche League and other peer support groups have faced criticism when they make assumptions about the values of mothers who join their groups, accused of promoting limited approaches to breastfeeding or being intolerant of different nurturing styles (cf. Carter 1995; Blum 1999; Faircloth 2013). Yet La Leche League accepted a transmasculine parent as a potential group leader (Macdonald et al. 2016). For a group that emerged from the efforts of conservative suburban Catholic white women, it must have been a stretch to adjust gendered language and accommodate chestfeeding into their vocabulary, documents, and programs. But they did. Breastfeeding promotion campaigns still try to find the most suitable images to attract and appeal to the target population—the romantic idealist, the career woman, the earth-mother/hippie, the health consumer.

Much intellectual effort has been spent deconstructing advertising campaigns for infant formula or breastfeeding promotion (cf. Wolf 2010; Hausman 2011). But these cultural studies approaches focus on the most trivial aspects of advertising and fail to consider the broader political context and the importance of the social relationships created through infant feeding. Even within the discipline of anthropology, few acknowledge the foundational role breastfeeding and nurture plays in the development of human sociality. Instead we apologize for making women feel guilty for not breastfeeding. (Recall the disclaimer in the study of arsenic levels in infant formula.)

As a result of self-censorship, we are unable to fully explore breastfeeding in relation to specific problems such as allergies, childhood obesity, autism, and cancers, perhaps motivated by the uncertainty of how to raise the issue without offending or blaming mothers who did not breastfeed. For example, breastfeeding requires infants to develop the ability to read social cues, focus attention, and interact intensively with others. Could lack of breastfeeding reduce the need or the ability to read social cues? What would be the implications of this argument for autism research? While research explores possible links between autism and gut ecology, few studies mention mode of feeding, a factor that influences gut ecology.

Without an adequate vocabulary for talking about nurture, there will continue to be silences because we are unable or unwilling or uncertain how to incorporate breastfeeding into these current conversations without becoming entangled in discussions of guilt and the right to choose.

The World Is Still Not Doing Well

Framing breastfeeding in the broad ecological and historical context of nurture takes us back to the big questions affecting the human condition raised in Chapter 1, such as climate change and poverty. By changing the question from breast or bottle to how humans nurture others, we might be able to wriggle our way back to the big questions.

On the surface, decisions about how to feed a newborn appear to be small personal lifestyle choices made by mothers in private, unlike the larger more dramatic public decisions around carbon emissions or income distribution. Loss of nurturing practices also threatens the human condition. Naomi Klein (2014: 7) argues that climate change could become a catalyzing force for positive change in the world. The same could be said for breastfeeding. As with climate change, we have not done the things that we need to do to support breastfeeding because these things conflict with deregulated capitalism and complacent consumerism. She argues that addressing climate change threatens an elite minority that controls our economy, our politics, and our media (Klein 2014: 18). Supporting breastfeeding also challenges many entrenched practices and reveals the values that appear to be guiding policy priorities. Efforts to limit the promotion of artificial baby milks, much like climate change advocacy, have been attacked as plots to steal our freedoms and undermine the free enterprise system, with activists denounced as Nazis or Marxists (cf. Palmer 1988; Klein 2014: 32). Climate change deniers attacked the evidence, much like the current attacks on lactation science.

Banks are said to be "too big to fail," but what about human lactation? We bail out banks but not mothers. Why should nurturing practices that shape who we are as a species and as individuals be so under-resourced, underappreciated, and unsupported? When we support nurturing practices, tweak a few structures to make breastfeeding easier for women, we take a giant step toward solving other problems facing our species and our planet. As long as maternity entitlements are viewed as a luxury available only to privileged workers, we are unlikely to make the huge shift in priorities necessary to protect nurturing practices. Societies based on competition, growth, and consumption threaten the planet; but they also make it difficult to nurture the next generation, a necessity for the continuation of the species. Overworked people have less time to engage in low consumption activities like gardening and cooking (Klein 2014: 93). And breastfeeding. Cutting back on working hours would benefit the climate and nurture.

Solving the big problems requires examining the human record, using ethnographic, biomedical, evolutionary, and historical evidence. Where can we locate these broader ecological framings that stress relationships of reciprocity and interconnection with the natural world (Klein 2014: 182)? Although First Nations in Canada and indigenous groups throughout the world have been ravaged by extractive industries and the destruction of nurturing customs around infant care and child socialization, their underlying holistic ideologies of sustainability and nurture link the processes of regenerating the earth and reproducing people:

> That woman is the first environment is an original instruction. In pregnancies our bodies sustain life ... At the breast of women, the generations are nourished. From the bodies of women flows the relationship of those generations both to society and to the natural world. In this way is the earth our mother, the old people tell us. In this way, we as women are earth. (Katsi Cook, Mohawk midwife, cited in Klein 2014: 419)

The gender essentialism of mother earth makes anthropologists and others uncomfortable, but, as Klein argues,

> Protecting and valuing the earth's indigenous systems of reproducing life and the fertility of all its inhabitants, may lie at the center of the shift in worldview that must take place if we are to move beyond extractivism. A worldview based on regeneration and renewal rather than domination and depletion. (2014: 424)

Insufficient milk and chemical residues in human milk, along with infertility, may be warnings of broader ecological problems to come. We are living in a world where policy makers (who are usually adult males) look first at adult males instead of pregnant women and infants.

The Dance of Nurture represents an alternative worldview embedded in interdependence rather than hyper-individualism, reciprocity rather than dominance, and cooperation rather than hierarchy (cf. Klein 2014: 462). Can supporting breastfeeding help us find community on this troubled planet? Not likely; that would sentimentalize mothering and romanticize breastfeeding. But supporting nurturing customs wherever they occur might help.

One place to start would be to support family and education systems that produce people who nurture and care about others, and fully develop people's talents. Put more effort and resources into nurturing infants, children, and others, educate for empathy; breastfeeding is one small part of that education for empathy. Nurture the next generation as you were nurtured; pay it forward. Nurturing practices thrive in the customs surrounding birth and the postpartum. Their absence is also glaringly obvious in many parts of the world. Other researchers can document the possible effects of generations of failed nurture. We hope this book offers participants new "arenas in which to gather" (Latour 2004: 246) by providing a middle ground, a useful framework and some necessary vocabulary for exploring the subject of infant feeding in a way that acknowledges the key role it has and continues to play in the human story.

Notes

1. This argument was inspired by a presentation by Katazyna Cweiertka at a food conference at University of Lund, Sweden, in April 2014.
2. You can get this quote attributed to Ruth Benedict engraved on a mug from a website on quotable quotes, but not the citation.
3. South Asian women's groups and other NGOs objected to the very idea that breastfeeding empowers women, the theme of the 1995 WBW action folder.

References

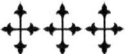

Almroth, Stina. 1978. "Water Requirements of Breast-Fed Infants in a Hot Climate." *American Journal of Clinical Nutrition* 31(7): 1154–57.
Altorki, Soraya. 1980. "Milk-Kinship in Arab Society: An Unexplored Problem in the Ethnography of Marriage." *Ethnology* 19(2): 233–44.
American Academy of Pediatrics. 2012. "Breastfeeding and the Use of Human Milk. Policy Statement." *Pediatrics* 129(3): 827–41.
Andaya, Barbara. 2006. *The Flaming Womb*. Honolulu: University of Hawaii Press.
Apple, Rima. 1980. "To Be Used Only under the Direction of a Physician: Commercial Infant Feeding and Medical Practice, 1870–1940." *Bulletin of the History of Medicine* 54: 402–17.
———. 1987. *Mothers and Medicine*. Madison: University of Wisconsin Press.
———. 2006. *Perfect Motherhood: Science and Childrearing in America*. New Brunswick, NJ: Rutgers University Press.
Arendt, Hannah. 1998. *The Human Condition*. Chicago: University of Chicago Press.
Baker, Phillip, Julie Smith, and Libby Salmon. 2016. "Global Trends in Commercial Milk-Based Formula Consumption: Is an Unprecedented Infant and Young Child Feeding Transition Underway?" *Public Health Nutrition* 19(14): 2540–50.
Ball, H. L. 2016. "Bed-sharing by Breastfeeding Mothers: Who Bed-shares and What Is the Relationship with Breastfeeding Duration?" *Acta Paediatrica* 105(6): 628–34.
Ball, H. L., E. Hooker, and P. J. Kelly. 1999. "Where Will the Baby Sleep: Attitudes and Practices of New and Experiences Parents Regarding Cosleeping with Their Newborn Infants." *American Anthropologist*. 101(1): 143–51.
Ball H. L., and L. E. Volpe. 2013. "SIDS Risk Reduction and Infant Sleep Location: Moving the Discussion Forward." *Social Science & Medicine:* 79: 84–91.
Bandy, Lauren. 2014. "Toddler Milk Formula: The Hello Kitty of Packaged Food." *Euromonitor International*. Retrieved 6 September 2015 from blog.euromonitor.com/2014/02/toddler-milk-formula-the-hello-kitty-of-packaged-food.
Barennes, Hubert, et al. 2008. "Misperceptions and Misuse of Bear Brand Coffee Creamer as Infant Food: National Cross-Sectional Survey of Consumers and Paediatricians in Laos." *British Medical Journal* 337: a1379. Retrieved 13 January 2016 from http://www.bmj.com/content/337/bmj.a1379.full.pdf.

Barston, Suzanne. 2012. *Bottled Up: How The Way We Feed Babies Has Come to Define Motherhood and Why It Shouldn't*. Berkeley: University of California Press.
Bartick, Melissa, and Arnold Reinhold. 2010. "The Burden of Suboptimal Breastfeeding in the United States: A Pediatric Cost Analysis." *Pediatrics* 125e: 1048–56.
Bartlett, Alison. 2000. "Thinking Through Breasts: Writing Maternity." *Feminist Theory* 1(2): 173–88.
———. 2002. "Breastfeeding as Headwork: Corporeal Feminism and Meanings for Breastfeeding." *Women's Studies International Forum* 25(3): 373–82.
———. 2005. "Scandalous Practices and Political Performances: Breastfeeding in the City." In *Motherhood, Power and Oppression*, edited by Andrea O'Reilly, Marie Porter, and Patricia Short, 57–73. Toronto: Women's Press.
Bartlett, Alison, and Rhonda Shaw. 2010. "Mapping the Ethics and Politics of Contemporary Breastmilk Exchange." In *Giving Breastmilk: Body Ethics and Contemporary Breastfeeding Practice*, edited by Rhonda Shaw and Alison Bartlett, 1–8. Toronto: Demeter Press.
Bateson, Gregory. 1972. *Steps to an Ecology of Mind*. New York: Ballantine Books.
Bateson, Gregory, and Margaret Mead. 1942. *Balinese Character*. New York: Academy of Sciences.
Bauman, Zygmunt. 1997. *Postmodernity and Its Discontents*. Cambridge: Polity Press.
Baumslag, Naomi. 1989. *Breastfeeding: The Passport to Life*. New York: NGO Committee on UNICEF.
Beasley, Annette. 1996. *Breastfeeding for the First Time*. Palmerston North, New Zealand: Department of Social Anthropology, Massey University.
Benedict, Ruth. 1934. *Patterns of Culture*. Boston: Houghton Mifflin.
Bentley, Amy. 2014. *Inventing Baby Food*. Oakland: University of California Press.
Berger, Peter. 1997. "The Four Faces of Global Culture." *The National Interest* 49: 23–29.
Bergmann, Karl E., et al. 2003. "Early Determinants of Childhood Overweight and Adiposity in a Birth Cohort Study: Role of Breast-Feeding." *International Journal of Obesity and Related Metabolic Disorders* 27: 162–72.
Bessire, Lucas, and David Bond. 2014. "Ontological Anthropology and the Deferral of Critique." *American Ethnologist* 41(3): 440–56.
Bethune, Brian. 2014. "The End of Neighbours." *Maclean's Magazine*, 8 August.
Bishop, Matthew, and Michael Green. 2009. *Philanthrocapitalism: How Giving Can Save the World*. New York: Bloomsbury.
Black, Robert E., et al. 2013. "Maternal and Child Nutrition: Building Momentum for Impact." *The Lancet* 382(9890): 372–75.
Blackmore, Willy. 2015. "Food Industry Money Talks, and It Says Coke and Kraft Singles Are Healthy." Retrieved 22 March 2015 from http://www.takepart.com/article/2015/03/17.
Bliss, Eula. 2014. *On Immunity: An Inoculation*. Minneapolis, MN: Graywolf Press.
Bloch, Maurice. 1999. "Commensality and Poisoning." *Social Research* 66(1): 133–49.
———. 2005. "Where Did Anthropology Go? Or the Need for Human Nature." In *Essays on Cultural Transmission*, edited by Maurice Bloch, 1–20. Oxford: Berg Publishers.
Blum, Linda. 1993. "Mothers, Babies and Breastfeeding in Late Capitalist America: The Shifting Contexts of Feminist Theory." *Feminist Studies* 19(2): 291–311.
———. 1999. *At the Breast: Ideologies of Breastfeeding and Motherhood in the Contemporary United States*. Boston: Beacon Press.
Bourdieu, Pierre. 1990. *The Logic of Practice*. Translated by Richard Nice. Stanford, CA: Stanford University Press.

Bramwell, Ros. 2011. "Blood and Milk: Constructions of Female Bodily Fluids in Western Society." *Women & Health* 34(4): 89–101.
Breakey, Gail F., and Emmanuel Voulgaropoulos. 1968. *Laos Health Survey: Mekong Valley.* Honolulu: University of Hawaii Press.
Brumberg, Joan. 1988. *Fasting Girls: The Emergence of Anorexia Nervosa as a Modern Disease.* Cambridge, MA: Harvard University Press.
Bruner, Jerome. 1986. *Actual Minds, Possible Worlds.* Cambridge, MA: Harvard University Press.
Burnier, Daniel, Lise Dubois, and Manon Girard. 2011. "Exclusive Breastfeeding Duration and Later Intake of Vegetables in Preschool Children." *European Journal of Clinical Nutrition* 65: 196–202.
Carignan, Courtney, et al. 2015. "Estimated Exposure to Arsenic in Breastfed and Formula-Fed Infants in a United States Cohort." *Environmental Health Perspective* 5(123): 500–6.
Carsten, Janet. 2004. *After Kinship.* Cambridge: Cambridge University Press.
———. 1995. "The Substance of Kinship and the Heat of the Hearth: Feeding, Personhood and Relatedness among Malays in Pulau Langawi." *American Ethnologist* 22(2): 223–241.
Carter, Pam. 1995. *Feminism, Breasts and Breastfeeding.* New York: St Martin's Press.
Castle, Mary Ann, et al. 1988. "Infant Feeding in Bogota, Colombia." In *Feeding Infants in Four Societies,* edited by Beverly Winicoff, Mary Ann Castle, and Virginia Hight Laukaran, 43–66. New York: Greenwood Press.
Chee, Bernadine. 2000. "Eating Snacks, Biting Pressure: Only Children in Beijing." In *Feeding China's Little Emperors,* edited by Jun Jing, 48–70. Stanford, CA: Stanford University Press.
Chodorow, Nancy. 1999. *The Reproduction of Mothering: Psychoanalysis and the Sociology of Gender.* Berkeley: University of California Press.
Claeyes, Priscilla, and Nadia Lambek. 2014. "Introduction: In Search of Better Options: Food Sovereignty, the Right to Food and Legal Tools for Transforming Food Systems." In *Rethinking Food Systems,* edited by Nadia Lambek et al., 1–25. Dordrecht: Springer.
Clancy, Kathryn, Katie Hinde, and Julienne Rutherford. 2013. *Building Babies: Primate Development in Proximate and Ultimate Perspective.* New York: Springer.
Clarke, Morgan. 2009. *Islam and New Kinship: Reproductive Technology and the Shariah in Lebanon.* New York: Berghahn Books.
Cochrane Summaries. 2009. *Probiotics in Infants for Prevention of Allergic Disease and Food Hypersensitivity.* Retrieved from http://summaries.cochrane.org/CD006475/probiotics-in-infants-for-prevention-of-allergic-disease-and-food-hypersensitivity.
Code, Lorraine. 2006. *Ecological Thinking. The Politics of Epistemic Location.* Oxford: University of Oxford Press.
Coloson, Suzanne, Judith H. Meek, and Jane M. Hawdon. 2008. "Optimal Positions for the Release of Primitive Neonatal Reflexes Stimulating Breastfeeding." *Early Human Development* 84: 441–49.
Connerton, Paul. 2009. *How Modernity Forgets.* New York: Cambridge University Press.
Corsini, Carlo A. 1991. "Breastfeeding, Fertility and Infant Mortality: Lessons from the Archives of the Florence Spedale degli Innocenti." In *Historical Perspectives on Breastfeeding,* by Sara F. Matthews Grieco and Carlo A. Corsini, 63–85. Florence, Italy: UNICEF, Instituto degli Innocenti.

Coveney, John. 2000. *Food, Morals and Meaning: The Pleasures and Anxiety of Eating*. London: Routledge.
Cowan, Cindy. 2011. "La Leche League International." In *The 21st Century Motherhood Movement*, edited by Andrea O'Reilly. Bradford, Canada: Demeter Press.
Cowley, Stephen, Sheshni Moodley, and Agnese Fiori-Cowley. 2004. "Grounding Signs of Culture: Primary Intersubjectivity in Social Semiosis." *Mind, Culture, and Activity* 11(2): 109–32.
Csordas, Thomas. 1994. *The Sacred Self*. Berkeley: University of California Press.
Damasio, Antonio R. 1994. *Descartes' Error: Emotion, Reason, and the Human Brain*. New York: Penguin Books.
Daniels, Cynthia. 2006. *Exposing Men*. New York: Oxford University Press.
David, Lawrence A., et al. 2014. "Diet Rapidly and Reproducibly Alters the Human Gut Microbiome." *Nature* 505 (7484): 559–63.
Davidson, Deborah, and Debra Langan. 2006. "The Breastfeeding Incident: Teaching and Learning Through Transgression." *Studies in Higher Education* 31(4): 439–52.
Davis-Floyd, Robbie, and Elizabeth Davis. 1996. "Intuition as Authoritative Knowledge in Midwifery and Home Birth." *Medical Anthropology Quarterly* 10(2): 237–69.
Debucquet, Gervaise, and Valerie Adt. 2015. "The Naturalist Discourse Surrounding Breastfeeding among French Mothers." In *Ethnographies of Breastfeeding*, edited by Tanya Cassidy and Abdullahi El Tom, 79–98. London: Bloomsbury.
DeLoache, Judy S., and Alma Gottlieb. 2000. *A World of Babies: Imagined Childcare Guides for Seven Societies*. Cambridge: Cambridge University Press.
Derrida, Jacques. 1981. *Plato's Pharmacy*. London: The Athlone Press.
de Schutter, Olivier. 2011. *Report Submitted by the Special Rapporteur on the Right to Food*. New York: United Nations General Assembly.
Descola, Philippe. 2013. *Beyond Nature and Culture*. Chicago: University of Chicago Press.
Dettwyler, Katherine A. 1988. "More than Nutrition: Breastfeeding in Urban Mali." *Medical Anthropology Quarterly* 2(2): 172–83.
———. 1994. *Dancing Skeletons: Life and Death in West Africa*. Prospect Heights, IL: Waveland Press.
———. 2004. "When to Wean: Biological versus Cultural Perspectives." *Clinical Obstetrics and Gynecology* 47: 712–23.
DeVault, M. 1991. *Feeding the Family*. Chicago: University of Chicago Press.
Diamond, Jared. 1997. *Guns, Germs and Steel: The Fates of Human Societies*. New York: Norton.
———. 2005. *Collapse: How Societies Choose to Fail or Succeed*. New York: Penguin Group.
———. 2012. *The World Until Yesterday*. New York: Viking.
Diener, Marissa. 2000. "Gifts from the Gods: A Balinese Guide to Early Child Rearing." In *A World of Babies: Imagined Childcare Guides for Seven Societies*, edited by Judy S. DeLoache and Alma Gottlieb, 91–116. Cambridge: Cambridge University Press.
Dietler, Michael. 2001. "Theorizing the Feast: Rituals of Consumption, Commensal Politics, and Power in African Contexts." In *Feasts: Archaeological and Ethnographic Perspectives of Food, Politics and Power*, edited by Michael Dietler and Brian Hayden, 65–114. Washington, DC: Smithsonian Institution Press.
Dimitrov, Radoslav. 2005. "Hostage to Norms: States, Institutions and Global Forest Politics." *Global Environmental Politics* 54: 1–24.

Doan, T., et al. 2007. "Breast-feeding Increases Sleep Duration of New Parents." *The Journal of Perinatal and Neonatal Nursing.* 21(3): 200–6.

———. 2014. "Nighttime Breastfeeding Behavior Is Associated with More Nocturnal Sleep Among First-time Mothers at One Month Postpartum." *Journal of Clinical Sleep Medicine* 10(3): 313–19.

Dougherty, Janet, and Charles Keller. 1982. "Taskonomy: A Practical Approach to Knowledge Structures." *American Ethnologist* 9(4): 763–74.

Douglas, Mary. 1973. *Natural Symbols: Explorations in Cosmology.* New York: Vintage Books.

Douglas, Mary, and Baron Isherwood. 1996. *The World of Goods: Towards an Anthropology of Consumption.* London: Routledge.

Dunkelman, Marc J. 2014. *The Vanishing Neighbor.* New York: Norton.

Dunsworth, Holly, and Leah Eccleson. 2015. "The Evolution of Difficult Childbirth and Helpless Hominin Infants." *Annual Review of Anthropology* 44: 55–69.

Eberhardt, Nancy. 2006. *Imagining the Course of Life: Self Transformation in a Shan Buddhist Community.* Honolulu: University of Hawaii Press.

The Economist. 2007. "Globalization: The Rise of Inequality." 20 January.

Elliott, Terry, and Penny Van Esterik. 1986. "Infant Feeding Style in Urban Kenya." *Ecology of Food and Nutrition* 18(3): 183–95.

Erikson, Erik. 1964. *Insight and Responsibility: Lectures on the Ethical Implications of Psychoanalytic Insight.* New York: Norton.

EU Project. 2004. *Promotion of Breastfeeding in Europe: A Blueprint for Action.* Report for the European Commission, Directorate Public Health and Risk Assessment.

Euromonitor International. 2001. *Euromonitor Passport Market Information Database for Baby Food.* Euromonitor International Ltd, London. Retreived from http://www.euromonitor.com/baby-food.

———. 2011. *Euromonitor Passport Market Information Database for Baby Food.* Euromonitor International Ltd, London. Retreived from http://www.euromonitor.com/baby-food.

European Society for Pediatric Gastroenterology, Hepatology and Nutrition. 2011. *Supplementation of Infant Formula with Probiotics and/or Prebiotics: A Systematic Review and Comment by the ESPGHAN Committee on Nutrition.* Retrieved from http://espghan.med.up.pt/position_papers/JPGN_CoN_Infant_formula_probotics_prebiotics.pdf.

Fadiman, Anne. 1997. *The Spirit Catches You and You Fall Down.* New York: Farrar, Straus and Giroux.

Fairbanks, Lynn, and Katie Hinde. 2013. "Behavioral Responses of Mothers and Infants to Variation in Maternal Condition: Adaptation, Compensation and Resilience." In *Building Babies: Primate Development in Proximate and Ultimate Perspective,* edited by Kathryn Clancy, Katie Hinde, and Julienne Rutherford, 281–302. New York: Springer.

Faircloth, Charlotte. 2013. *Militant Lactivism.* New York: Berghahn Books.

Faith, Myles S., and Julia Kerns. 2005. "Infant and Child Feeding Practices and Childhood Overweight: The Role of Restriction." *Maternal and Child Nutrition* 1(3): 164–68.

Faizal, Elly. 2013. "Government Urged to Stop Daffodil Study." *The Jakarta Post,* 19 January.

Fergusson, David, and L. Woodward. 1999. "Breastfeeding and Later Psychosocial Adjustment." *Paediatric and Perinatal Epidemiology* 13(2): 144–57.

Ferrieres, Madeleine. 2006. *Sacred Cow, Mad Cow: A History of Food Fears.* Translated by Jody Gladding. New York: Columbia University Press.

Fifield, Adam. 2015. *A Mighty Purpose: How Jim Grant Sold the World on Saving Children.* New York: Other Press.
Fildes, Valerie. 1986. *Breasts, Bottles and Babies: A History of Infant Feeding.* Edinburgh: Edinburgh University Press.
Fisher, Jennifer, et al. 2000. "Breast-Feeding through the First Year Predicts Maternal Control in Feeding and Subsequent Toddler Energy Intakes." *Journal of American Dietetic Association* 100(6): 641–46.
Foley, Kathy. 2015. "The Ronggeng, the Wayang, the Wali and Islam: Female or Transvestite Male Dancers-Singers-Performers and Evolving Islam in West Java." *Asian Theatre Journal* 32(2): 356–86.
Food and Agriculture Organization of the United Nations/World Health Organization. 2008. *Enterobacter sakazakii (Cronobacter spp.) in Powdered Follow-Up Formulae* (Microbiological Risk Assessment Series No. 15). Rome.
Fouts, Hillary, et al. 2012. "A Biocultural Approach to Breastfeeding Interactions in Central Africa." *American Anthropologist* 114(1): 123–36.
Fuentes, Agustin. 2013. "Blurring the Biological and Social in Human Becomings." In *Biosocial Becomings: Integrating Social and Biological Anthropology,* edited by T. Ingold and G. Paalson, 42–58. Cambridge: Cambridge University Press.
———. 2015. "Integrative Anthropology and the Human Niche: Toward a Contemporary Approach to Human Evolution." *American Anthropologist* 117(2): 302–15.
———. 2016. "The Extended Evolutionary Synthesis, Ethnography, and the Human Niche: Toward an Integrated Anthropology." *Current Anthropology* 57(S13): 13–26.
Gannon, Susanne, and Babette Mueller-Rockstroh. 2005. "Narrating Breasts: Constructions of Contemporary Motherhood(s) in Women's Breastfeeding Stories." In *Motherhood, Power and Oppression,* edited by Andrea O'Reilly, Marie Porter, and Patricia Short, 41–55. Toronto: Women's Press.
Geddes, Donna T., et al. 2008. "Tongue Movement and Intra-Oral Vacuum in Breastfeeding Infants." *Early Human Development* 84: 471–77.
Geertz, Clifford. 2000. *Available Light: Anthropological Reflections on Philosophical Topics.* Princeton, NJ: Princeton University Press.
Gettler, L. T., and J. J. McKenna. 2011. "Evolutionary Perspectives on Mother–Infant Sleep Proximity and Breastfeeding in a Laboratory Setting." *Am J Phys Anthropol.* 144(3): 454–62.
Giles, Fiona. 2012. "Re-instating Pleasure in Reality: Promoting Breastfeeding through Ars Erotica." In *Beyond Health: Beyond Choice: Breastfeeding Constraints and Realities,* edited by Paige Hall Smith, Bernice Hausman, and Miriam Labbok, 215–25. New Brunswick, NJ: Rutgers University Press.
Giles, Jim. 2011. "Social Science Lines Up Its Biggest Challenges." *Nature* 470, 18–19. Retrieved from http://www.nature.com/news/2011/110202/full/470018a.html.
Gleason, Tracy, and Darcia Narvaez. 2014. "Childhood Environments and Flourishing." In *Ancestral Landscapes in Human Evolution,* edited by Darcia Narvaez, Kristin Valentino, Agustin Fuentes, James McKenna and Peter Gray, 335–48. Oxford: Oxford University Press.
Golding, William. 1954. *Lord of the Flies.* London: Faber and Faber.
Goldman, Armond S. 2012. "Evolution of Immune Functions of the Mammary Gland and the Protection of the Infant." *Breastfeeding Medicine* 7(3): 132–42.
Goldschmidt, Walter. 1990. *The Human Career.* Cambridge: Blackwell.

———. 2006. *The Bridge to Humanity: How Affect Hunger Trumps the Selfish Gene*. New York: Oxford University Press.
Goodale, Mark, and Sally Merry, eds. 2007. *The Practice of Human Rights*. Cambridge: Cambridge University Press.
Goody, Jack. 1982. *Cooking, Cuisine and Class*. Cambridge: Cambridge University Press.
Gordon, Jane. 1989. "Choosing to Breastfeed: Some Feminist Questions." *Resources for Feminist Research* 18(2): 10–12.
Gordon, Mary. 2005. *Roots of Empathy*. Toronto: Thomas Allen.
Gottschang, Suzanne Zhang. 2007. "Maternal Bodies, Breast-Feeding, and Consumer Desire in Urban China." *Medical Anthropology Quarterly* 21(1): 64–80.
Graeber, David. 2011. *Debt: The First 5000 Years*. New York: Melville House Books.
Gribble, Karlen D. 2014. "'I'm Happy to Be Able to Help': Why Women Donate Milk to a Peer via Internet Based Milk Sharing Networks." *Breastfeeding Medicine* 9(5): 251–56.
Grieco, Sara F. Matthews. 1991. "Breastfeeding, Wet Nursing and Infant Mortality in Europe (1400–1800)." In *Historical Perspectives on Breastfeeding*, by Sara F. Matthews Grieco and Carlo A. Corsini, 15–60. Florence, Italy: UNICEF, Instituto degli Innocenti.
Grimmet, Richard, and Paul Kerr. 2012. "Conventional Arms Transfers to Developing Nations 2004–2011." *US Congressional Research Service Report to Congress*, August 24. Retrieved from fas.org/sgp/crs/weapons.
Groleau, Danielle, Margot Souliere, and Laurence Kirmayer. 2006. "Breastfeeding and the Cultural Configuration of Social Space among Vietnamese Immigrant Women." *Health and Place* 12(4): 516–26.
Gussler, Judy. 1980. "The Insufficient Milk Syndrome: A Biocultural Explanation." *Medical Anthropology* 4(2): 145–74.
Guttman, Nurit, and Deena Zimmerman. 2000. "Low-Income Mothers' Views on Breastfeeding." *Social Science and Medicine* 50(10): 457–74.
Hanks, Jane. 1964. "Reflections on the Ontology of Rice." In *Primitive Views of the World*, edited by Stanley Diamond, 151–53. New York: Columbia University Press.
Haraway, Donna. 1989. *Primate Visions: Gender, Race and Nature in the World of Modern Science*. New York: Routledge.
Harries-Jones, Peter. 1995. *A Recursive Vision: Ecological Understanding and Gregory Bateson*. Toronto: University of Toronto Press.
Harris, Gillian. 2000. "Developmental, Regulatory and Cognitive Aspects of Feeding Disorders." In *Feeding Problems in Children*, edited by Angela Southall and Anthony Schwartz, 77–88. Oxford: Radcliffe Medical Press.
Hartmann, Peter, et al. 1996. "Breast Development and Control of Milk Synthesis." *Food and Nutrition Bulletin* 17(4): 292–304.
Hauck, F., et al. 2011. "Breastfeeding and Reduced Risk of Sudden Infant Death Syndrome: A Meta-Analysis." *Pediatrics*. 128(1): 103–10.
Hausman, Bernice. 2003. *Mother's Milk: Breastfeeding Controversies in American Culture*. New York: Routledge.
———. 2007. "Things (Not) to Do with Breasts in Public: Maternal Embodiment and the Biocultural Politics of Infant Feeding." *New Literary History* 38(3): 479–504.
———. 2011. *Viral Mothers: Breastfeeding in the Age of HIV/AIDS*. Ann Arbor: University of Michigan Press.

Hausner, Helene, et al. 2008. "Differential Transfer of Dietary Flavour Compounds into Human Breast Milk." *Physiology and Behaviour* 95(1–2): 118–24.

Haw, Jennie. 2014. "From the Incinerator to the Bank: A Feminist Qualitative Study of Private Cord Blood Banking in Canada." PhD diss., York University.

Hefner, Robert. 1990. *The Political Economy of Mountain Java*. Berkeley: University of California Press.

Heiberg Endresen, Eli, and Elisabet Helsing. 1995. "Changes in Breastfeeding Practices in Norwegian Maternity Wards: National Surveys 1973, 1982 and 1991." *Acta Paediatrica* 84(7): 719–24.

Helsing, Elisabet. 1990. "Supporting Breastfeeding: What Governments and Health Workers Can Do—European Experiences." *International Journal of Gynecology and Obstetrics* 31: 69–76.

Hendricks, Glenn, Bruce Downing, and Amos Deinard, eds. 1986. *The Hmong in Transition*. New York: Centre for Migration Studies of New York.

Henrich, Joseph, Steven J. Heine, and Ara Norenzayan. 2010. "Most people are not WEIRD." *Nature* 466(7302): 29.

Hesselmar, Bill, et al. 2013. "Pacifier Cleaning Practices and Risk of Allergy Development." *Pediatrics* 131(6): 1–9. Retrieved 29 January 2016 from www.pediatrics.org/cgi/doi/10.1542/peds.2012-3345.

Hinde, Katie. 2013. "Lactational Programming of Infant Behavioral Phenotype." In *Building Babies: Primate Development in Proximate and Ultimate Perspective,* edited by Kathryn Clancy, Katie Hinde, and Julienne Rutherford, 187–207. New York: Springer.

Hinde, Katie, and Bruce German. 2012. "Food in an Evolutionary Context." *Journal of the Science of Food and Agriculture* 92: 2219–23.

Hinde, Katie, and John Capitanio. 2010. "Lactational Programming? Mother's Milk Energy Predicts Infant Behaviors and Temperament in Rhesus Macaques." *American Journal of Primatology* 72(6): 522–29.

Hinde, Katie, and Lauren Milligan. 2011. "Primate Milk Synthesis: Proximate Mechanisms and Ultimate Perspectives." *Evolutionary Anthropology* 20: 9–23.

Hinde, Katie, and Zachery T. Lewis. 2015. "Mother's Littlest Helpers." *Science* 348(6242): 1427–28.

Hofmeyer, Amanda. 1995. *Breastfeeding and Human Rights*. Penang, Malaysia: World Alliance for Breastfeeding Action.

Holland, Nina, Claire Robinson, and Rod Harbinson. 2012. *Conflicts on the Menu: A Decade of Industry Influence at the European Food Safety Authority (EFSA)*. Brussels: Corporate Europe Observatory.

Holman, Darryl J., and Michael A. Grimes. 2003. "Patterns for the Initiation of Breastfeeding in Humans." *American Journal of Human Biology* 15: 765–80.

Homer-Dixon, Thomas. 2006. *The Upside of Down: Catastrophe, Creativity and the Renewal of Civilization*. Toronto: Alfred A Knopf.

Horne, R., et al. 2004. "Comparison of Evoked Arousability in Breast and Formula Fed Infants." *Arch Dis Child*. 89(1): 22–25.

Hörnell, Aarts, et al. 1999. "Breastfeeding Patterns in Exclusively Breastfed Infants: A Longitudinal Prospective Study in Uppsala, Sweden." *Acta Paediatrica* 88: 203–11.

Horton, Susan, et al. 2010. *Scaling Up Nutrition, What Would It Cost?* Washington, DC: World Bank.
———. 1996. "Breastfeeding Promotion and Priority Setting in Health." *Health Policy and Planning* 11(2): 156–68.
Howell, Nancy. 2010. *Life Histories of the Dobe !Kung.* Berkeley: University of California Press.
Hrdy, Sarah Blaffer. 1999. *Mother Nature: A History of Mothers, Infants and Natural Selection.* New York: Pantheon Books.
———. 2009. *Mothers and Others.* Cambridge, MA: Harvard University Press.
Huang, Y., et al. 2013. "Influence of Bedsharing Activity on Breastfeeding Duration Among US Mothers." *JAMA Pediatrics* 167(11): 1038–44.
Huber, Joan. 2007. *On the Origins of Gender Inequality.* Boulder, CO: Paradigm Publishers.
Ingold, Tim. 2000. *The Perception of the Environment: Essays in Livelihood, Dwelling and Skill.* London: Routledge.
———. 2007. *Lines: A Brief History.* New York: Routledge.
———. 2011. *Being Alive.* New York: Routledge.
Ingold, Tim, and Gisli Palsson. 2013. *Biosocial Becomings.* Cambridge: Cambridge University Press.
International Baby Food Action Network. 2012. "The Scaling up Nutrition (SUN) Initiative: IBFAN's Concern about the Role of Businesses" (Discussion paper). Retrieved from http://www.ibfan.org.
———. 2013a. Legal Update, January 2013. Penang, Malaysia.
———. 2013b. Legal Update, July 2013. Penang, Malaysia.
———. 2015. *Formula for Disaster: Weighing the Impact of Formula Feeding vs Breastfeeding on Environment.* Retrieved from http://ibfan.org/docs/climate-change-2015-English.pdf.
International Baby Food Action Network-ASIA. 2013. "The Need to Invest in Babies." IBFAN-ASIA/BPNI, Delhi. Retrieved from www.ibfanasia.org.
Ireson-Doolittle, Carol, and Geraldine Moreno-Black. 2004. *The Lao: Gender, Power and Livelihood.* Boulder, CO: Westview Press.
Jablonka, Eva, and Marion J. Lamb. 2005. *Evolution in Four Dimensions: Genetic, Epigenetic, Behavioral, and Symbolic Variation in the History of Life.* Cambridge, MA: MIT Press.
Janowski, Monica. 2007. "Introduction: Feeding the Right Food: The Flow of Life and the Construction of Kinship in Southeast Asia." In *Kinship and Food in South East Asia,* edited by Monica Janowski and Fiona Kerlogue, 1–23. Copenhagen: NIAS Press.
Janowski, Monica, and Fiona Kerlogue, eds. 2007. *Kinship and Food in South East Asia.* Copenhagen: NIAS Press.
Jelliffe, Derrick. 1972. "Commerciogenic Malnutrition?" *Nutrition Reviews* 30(9): 199–205.
Jennings, Betty, and Margaret Edmundson. 1980. "The Postpartum Period: After Confinement, the Fourth Trimester." *Clinical Obstetrics and Gynecology* 23(4): 1093–1104.
Johnson, Sally, et al. 2009. "Expressing Yourself: A Feminist Analysis of Talk Around Expressing Breastmilk." *Social Science and Medicine* 69(6): 900–7.
Jones, Gareth, et al. 2003. "How Many Child Deaths Can We Prevent This Year?" *Lancet* 362: 65–71.
Jones, Martin. 2007. *The Feast: Why Humans Share Food.* Oxford: Oxford University Press.

Jung, Courtney. 2015. *Lactivism: How Feminists and Fundamentalists, Hippies and Yuppies, and Physicians and Politicians Made Breastfeeding Big Business and Bad Policy*. New York: Basic Books.

Kaartinen, Timo. 2007. "Nurturing Memories: The Cycle of Mortuary Rituals in an East Indonesian Village." In *Kinship and Food in South East Asia*, edited by Monica Janowski and Fiona Kerlogue, 149–69. Copenhagen: NIAS Press.

Kahn, Miriam. 1986. *Always Hungry, Never Greedy: Food and the Expression of Gender in a Melanesian Society*. Cambridge: Cambridge University Press.

Kaufman, Sharon, and Lynn Morgan. 2005. "The Anthropology of the Beginnings and Ends of Life." *Annual Review of Anthropology* 34: 315–41.

Keck, Margaret, and Kathryn Sikkink. 1998. *Activists Beyond Borders*. Ithaca, NY: Cornell University Press.

Keim, Sarah A., et al. 2013. "Microbial Contamination of Human Milk Purchased via the Internet." *Pediatrics* 132: e1227-e35.

Kerlogue, Fiona. 2007. "Food and the Family: Assimilation in a Malay Village." In *Kinship and Food in South East Asia*, edited by Monica Janowski and Fiona Kerlogue, 54–70. Copenhagen: NIAS Press.

Kerner, Susanne, Cynthia Chow, and Morten Warmind, eds. 2015. *Commensality: From Everyday Food to Feast*. London: Bloomsbury.

Kertzer, David. 2008. *Amalia's Tale: A Poor Peasant, an Ambitious Attorney, and a Fight for Justice*. Boston: Houghton Mifflin Harcourt.

Khatibh-Chhidi, Jane. 1992. "Milk Kinship in Shi'ite Islamic Iran." In *The Anthropology of Breast-Feeding*, edited by Vanessa Maher, 109–32. Oxford: Berg Publishers.

Kimura, Aya Hirata. 2013. *Hidden Hunger*. Ithaca, NY: Cornell University Press.

King, Barbara, and Stuart Shanker. 2003. "How Can We Know the Dancer from the Dance? The Dynamic Nature of African Ape Communication." *Anthropological Theory* 3(1): 5–26.

Kinnally, Erin. 2013. "Genome-Environment Coordination in Neurobehavioral Development." In *Building Babies: Primate Development in Proximate and Ultimate Perspective*, edited by Kathryn Clancy, Katie Hinde, and Julienne Rutherford, 155–68. New York: Springer.

Kirsch, Thomas. 1973. *Feasting and Social Oscillation: A Working Paper on Religion and Society in Upland Southeast Asia*. Ithaca, NY: Southeast Asia Program Publication, Cornell University.

Kitzinger, Sheila. 1995. *Ourselves as Mothers*. Reading, MA: Addison-Wesley.

Kjernes, Unni, Mark Harvey, and Alan Warde. 2007. *Trust in Food: A Comparative and Institutional Analysis*. New York: Palgrave Macmillan.

Klausner, William. 2000. *Thai Culture in Transition*. Bangkok: Siam Society.

Klein, Naomi. 2007. *The Shock Doctrine: The Rise of Disaster Capitalism*. New York: Metropolitan Books.

———. 2012. "Occupy Movement Now Most Important Thing in the World." *CCPA Monitor* 18(7): 10–11.

———. 2014. *This Changes Everything*. Toronto: Random House.

Klima, Alan. 2002. *The Funeral Casino*. Princeton, NJ: Princeton University Press.

Koerber, Amy. 2006. "From Folklore to Fact: The Rhetorical History of Breastfeeding and Immunity, 1950–1997." *Journal of Medical Humanities* 27(3): 151–66.

Kramer, Michael. 1981. "Do Breastfeeding and Delayed Introduction of Solid Foods Protect Against Subsequent Obesity?" *Journal of Pediatrics* 98(6): 883–87.

Kushwaha, Komal, et al. 2014. "Effect of Peer Counselling by Mother Support Groups on Infant and Young Child Feeding Practices: The Lalitpur Experience." *PLoS ONE* 9(11): e109181.

Kuzawa, Christopher, and Elizabeth Quinn. 2009. "Developmental Origins of Adult Function and Health: Evolutionary Hypotheses." *Annual Review of Anthropology* 38: 131–47.

Kwiatkowski, Lynn. 1998. *Struggling with Development: The Politics of Hunger and Gender in the Philippines*. Boulder, CO: Westview Press.

Labbok, Miriam. 2012. "Breastfeeding in Public Health." In *Beyond Health, Beyond Choice: Breastfeeding Constraints and Realities*, edited by Paige Hall Smith, Bernice Hausman, and Miriam Labbok, 36–50. New Brunswick, NJ: Rutgers University Press.

Labbok, Miriam, David Clark, and Armond Goldman. 2004. "Breastfeeding: Maintaining an Irreplaceable Immunological Resource." *Nature Reviews* 4(7): 565–72.

Laderman, Carol. 1983. *Wives and Midwives: Childbirth and Nutrition in Rural Malaysia*. Berkeley: University of California Press.

Lambek, Nadia. 2014. "Respecting and Protecting the Right to Food: When States Must Get Out of the Kitchen." In *Rethinking Food Systems*, edited by Nadia Lambek et al., 101–22. Dordrecht: Springer.

Lansing, Stephen. 1995. *The Balinese*. Fort Worth, TX: Harcourt Brace.

———. 2007. *Priests and Programmers: Technologies of Power in the Engineered Landscape of Bali*. Princeton, NJ: Princeton University Press.

Latham, Michael. 2008. "The First Food Crisis: How to Reduce the Unacceptable Levels of Malnutrition through Improved Breastfeeding." Lecture, World Alliance for Breastfeeding Action, Penang, Malaysia.

Latham, Michael, K. Okoth Agunda, and Terry Elliot. 1988. "Infant Feeding in Nairobi, Kenya." In *Feeding Infants in Four Societies*, edited by Beverly Winikoff, Mary Ann Castle, and Virginia Hight Laukaran. 67–93. New York: Greenwood Press.

Latham, Michael, et al. 1986. "Infant Feeding in Urban Kenya: A Pattern of Early Triple Nipple Feeding." *Journal of Tropical Pediatrics* 32: 276–80.

Latour, Bruno. 1993. *We Have Never Been Modern*. Cambridge, MA: Harvard University Press.

———. 2004. "Why Has Critique Run out of Steam? From Matters of Fact to Matters of Concern." *Critical Inquiry* 30: 225–48.

Laughlin, Charles. 1991. "Pre- and Perinatal Brain Development and Enculturation." *Human Nature* 2(3): 171–213.

Law, Jules. 2000. "The Politics of Breastfeeding." *Signs* 25(2): 407–50.

Lears, Jackson. 1981. *No Place of Grace: Antimodernism and the Transformation of American Culture 1880–1920*. New York: Pantheon Books.

Lee, Dorothy. 1986. *Valuing the Self: What We Can Learn from Other Cultures*. Prospect Heights, IL: Waveland Press.

Lévi-Strauss, Claude. 1966. *The Savage Mind*. Chicago: University of Chicago Press.

Lewis, Stephen. 2005. *Race Against Time*. Toronto: Anansi Press.

Leys, Ruth. 2011. "The Turn to Affect: A Critique." *Critical Inquiry* 37(3): 434–72.

Lhotska, Lida, Anne Bellows, and Veronika Scherbaum. 2012. "Conflicts of Interest and Human Rights-Based Policy Making: The Case of Maternal, Infant and Young Children's Health and Nutrition." *Right to Food and Nutrition Watch* 6: 31–36.

Lieberman, Leslie Sue. 2008. "Diabesity and Darwinian Medicine: The Evolution of an Epidemic." In *Evolutionary Medicine and Health*, edited by Wenda Trevathan, E. O. Smith and James McKenna. 72–95. New York: Oxford University Press.
Lock, Margaret. 2001. "The Tempering of Medical Anthropology: Troubling Natural Categories." *Medical Anthropology Quarterly* 15(4): 478–92.
Lomax, Alan. 1978. *Cantometrics: An Approach to the Anthropology of Music*. University of California Extension Media Center.
MacDonald, Trevor, et al. 2016. "Transmasculine Individuals' Experiences with Lactation, Chestfeeding and Gender Identity: A Qualitative Study." *BMC Pregnancy and Childbirth* 16: 106.
Machado, Christopher. 2013. "Maternal Influences on Social and Neural Development in Macaque Monkeys." In *Building Babies: Primate Development in Proximate and Ultimate Perspective*, edited by Kathryn Clancy, Katie Hinde, and Julienne Rutherford, 259–80. New York: Springer.
Maher, Vanessa. 1992. *The Anthropology of Breastfeeding*. Oxford: Berg Publishers.
Mahon-Daly, Patricia, and Gavin Andrews. 2002. "Liminality and Breastfeeding: Women Negotiating Space and Two Bodies." *Health and Place* 8: 61–76.
Marchione, Thomas, and Elisabet Helsing. 1984. "Rethinking Infant Nutrition Policies under Changing Socio-Economic Conditions." *Acta Paediatrica Scandinavica*, Supplement 314.
Marchione, Thomas, and Ellen Messer. 2010. "Food Aid and the World Hunger Solution: Why the US Should Use a Human Rights Approach." *Food and Foodways* 18(1–2): 10–27.
Markens, Susan, C. H. Browner, and Nancy Press. 1997. "Feeding the Fetus: On Interrogating the Notion of the Maternal-Fetal Conflict." *Feminist Studies* 23(2): 351–72.
Marmot, Michael. 2004. *The Status Syndrome: How Social Standing Affects Our Health and Longevity*. New York: Henry Holt.
Martin, Aryn, and Michael Lynch. 2009. "Counting Things and People: The Practices and Politics of Counting." *Social Problems* 56(2): 243–66.
Martin, Emily. 2001. *The Woman in the Body: A Cultural Analysis of Reproduction*. Boston: Beacon Press.
———. 2013. "The Potentiality of Ethnography and the Limits of Affect Theory." *Current Anthropology* 54(s7): s149–58.
Martin, Melanie, and David Sela. 2013. "Infant Gut Microbiota: Developmental Influences and Health Outcomes." In *Building Babies: Primate Development in Proximate and Ultimate Perspective*, edited by Kathryn Clancy, Katie Hinde, and Julienne Rutherford, 233–57. New York: Springer.
Martucci, Jessica. 2015. *Back to the Breast: Natural Motherhood and Breastfeeding in America*. Chicago: University of Chicago Press.
Mathews, Anne. 2015. "'Impersonal Perspectives' on Public Health Guidelines on Infant Feeding and HIV in Malawi." In *Ethnographies of Breastfeeding*, edited by Tanya Cassidy and Abdullahi El Tom, 145–55. London: Bloomsbury.
Maxted, Anna. 2011. "Protect Us from the Breastapo." *The Telegraph*, 11 May.
McGoey, Linsey. 2015. *No Such Thing as a Free Gift: The Gates Foundation and the Price of Philanthropy*. London: Verso Books.
McKenna, James. 2000. "Cultural Influences on Infant and Childhood Sleep Biology and the Science That Studies It: Toward a More Inclusive Paradigm." In *Sleep and Breathing*

in Children: A Developmental Approach, edited by Gerald Loughlin, John Carroll, and Carole Marcus, 90–130. New York: Marcel-Dekker.
McKenna, James, and Lee Gettler. 2007. "Mother-Infant Co-Sleeping with Breastfeeding in the Western Industrial Context." *Textbook of Human Lactation,* edited by Thomas Hale and Peter Hartmann, 271–302. Amarillo: Hale Publishing.
McKenna, James J., Helen L. Ball, and Lee T. Gettler. 2007. "Mother–infant Cosleeping, Breastfeeding and Sudden Infant Death Syndrome: What Biological Anthropology Has Discovered about Normal Infant Sleep and Pediatric Sleep Medicine." *American Journal of Physical Anthropology.* 134 (S45): 133–61.
———. 2016. "There Is No Such Thing as Infant Sleep, There Is No Such Thing as Breastfeeding, There Is Only Breastsleeping." *Acta Paediatrica* 105: 17–21.
McMahon, Martha. 1995. *Engendering Motherhood.* New York: Guilford Press.
McTeer, Heather. 2012. "Fat, Young and Poor: Why Breastfeeding is a Critical Weapon in the Fight Against Childhood Obesity." *Breastfeeding Medicine* 7(3): 325–26.
Mead, Margaret. 1949. *Coming of Age in Samoa.* New York: Mentor Books.
Mennella, Julie. 2001. "Alcohol's Effect on Lactation." *Alcohol Research and Health* 25(3): 230–34.
Mennella, Julie, et al. 2009. "Early Milk Feeding Influences Taste Acceptance and Liking During Infancy." *American Journal of Clinical Nutrition* 90: 780S–788S.
Mennella, Julie, Coren Jagnow, and Gary Beauchamp. 2001. "Prenatal and Postnatal Flavor Learning by Human Infants." *Pediatrics* 107(6): 1–6.
Mennella, Julie, and G. Beauchamp. 1991. "The Transfer of Alcohol to Human Milk." *New England Journal of Medicine* 325: 981–85.
Merchant, Carolyn. 1980. *The Death of Nature: Women, Ecology and the Scientific Revolution.* San Francisco: Harper and Row.
Merry, Sally. 2001. "Changing Rights, Changing Culture." In *Culture and Rights,* edited by Jane Cowan, Marie-Bénédicte Dembour, and Richard Wilson, 31–55. Cambridge: Cambridge University Press.
———. 2006. *Human Rights and Gender Violence: Translating International Law into Local Justice.* Chicago: University of Chicago Press.
———. 2011. "Measuring the World: Indicators, Human Rights, and Global Governance." *Current Anthropology* 52: S83-S95.
Miles, Margaret. 1991. *Carnal Knowing.* New York: Vintage Books.
Milligan, Lauren. 2013. "Do Bigger Brains Mean Better Milk?" In *Building Babies: Primate Development in Proximate and Ultimate Perspective,* edited by Kathryn Clancy, Katie Hinde, and Julienne Rutherford, 209–32. New York: Springer.
Minchin, Maureen. 2015. *Milk Matters: Infant Feeding and Immune Disorder.* Geelong, Australia: Milk Matters.
Montague, Ashley. 1971. *Touching: The Human Significance of the Skin.* New York: Columbia University Press.
Montgomery-Downs H. E., H. M. Clawges, and E. E. Santy. 2010. "Infant Feeding Methods and Maternal Sleep and Daytime Functioning." *Pediatrics* 126(6): e1562–68.
Moran, Victoria, and Fiona Dykes. 2009. "Complex Challenges to Implementing the Global Strategy for Infant and Young Child Feeding." In *Infant and Young Child Feeding,* edited by Fiona Dykes and Victoria Moran, 197–201. Oxford: Blackwell Publishing.

Morris, David. 1998. *Illness and Culture in the Postmodern Age*. Berkeley: University of California Press.
Morris, Ian. 2013. *The Measure of Civilization*. Princeton, NJ: University of Princeton Press.
Morris, Jenny. 2001. "Impairment and Disability: Constructing an Ethics of Care Which Promotes Human Rights." *Hypatia* 16(4): 1–16.
Mosby, Ian. 2013. "Administering Colonial Science: Nutrition Research and Human Biomedical Experimentation in Aboriginal Communities and Residential Schools, 1942–1952." *Social History* 46(91): 145–72.
Moss, Michael. 2013. *Salt, Sugar and Fat: How the Food Giants Hooked Us*. Toronto: McClelland and Stewart.
Murphy, Elizabeth. 2004. "Anticipatory Accounts." *Symbolic Interaction* 27(2): 129–54.
Murphy, Elizabeth, Susan Parker, and Christine Phipps. 1998. "Food Choices for Babies." In *The Nation's Diet*, edited by Anne Murcott, 250–66. London: Longman.
Musher-Eizenman, Dara, et al. 2009. "Child and Parent Characteristics Related to Parental Feeding Practices. A Cross-cultural Examination in the US and France." *Appetite*. 52 (1): 89–95.
Narvaez, Darda, Kristin Valentino, Agustin Fuentes, James McKenna and Peter Gray, editors. 2014. *Ancestral Landscapes in Human Evolution*. Oxford: Oxford University Press.
Nathoo, Tasnim, and Aleck Ostry. 2009. *The One Best Way? Breastfeeding History, Politics, and Policy in Canada*. Waterloo, Canada: Wilfred Laurier Press.
Nestle, Marion. 2003. *Safe Food: Bacteria, Biotechnology and Bioterrorism*. Berkeley: University of California Press.
Neville, Margaret, et al. 2012. "Lactation and Neonatal Nutrition: Defining and Refining the Critical Questions." *Journal of Mammary Gland Biology Neoplasia* 17(2): 167–88.
Newson, Lesley. 2013. "Cultural Evolution and Human Reproductive Behavior." In *Building Babies: Primate Development in Proximate and Ultimate Perspective*, edited by Kathryn Clancy, Katie Hinde, and Julienne Rutherford, 481–503. New York: Springer.
Nichter, Mark. 2008. *Global Health: Why Cultural Perceptions, Social Representations and Biopolitics Matter*. Tucson: University of Arizona Press.
Nicklaus, Sophie. 2009. "Development of Food Variety in Children." *Appetite* 52(1): 253–55.
Nicklaus, Sophie, et al. 2004. "A Prospective Study of Food Preferences in Childhood." *Food Quality and Preference* 16(7–8): 805–18.
Niedenthal, Paula, et al. 2012. "Negative Relations between Pacifier Use and Emotional Competence." *Basic and Applied Social Psychology* 34(5): 387–94.
Nunez-de la Mora, Alejandra, and Gillian Bentley. 2008. "Early Life Effects on Reproductive Function." In *Evolutionary Medicine and Health*, edited by Wenda Trevathan, E. O. Smith, and James McKenna, 149–68. New York: Oxford University Press.
Oberg, Charles, et al. 1986. *A Cross-Cultural Assessment of Maternal-Child Interaction*. New York: Center for Migration Studies of New York.
O'Connor, Richard A. 1995. "Agricultural Change and Ethnic Succession in Southeast Asian States: A Case for Regional Anthropology." *Journal of Asian Studies* 54(4): 968–96.
———. 2009. "Place, Power and People: Southeast Asia's Temple Tradition." *Arts Asiatiques* 64: 2–9.
———. 2011. "Discussant's Remarks: Reviving Ethnology to Understand the Rice Neolithic." *Rice* 4(3–4): 187–89.
O'Connor, Richard A., and Penny Van Esterik. 2012. "Breastfeeding as Custom Not Culture: Cutting Meaning Down to Size." *Anthropology Today* 28(5): 13–16.

———. 2015. *From Virtue to Vice: Negotiating Anorexia*. New York: Berghahn Books.
Onstad, Katrina. 2006. "Breastfeeding Sucks." *Chatelaine,* November, 59–60.
Ortner, Sherry. 1998. "Generation X: Anthropology in a Media-Saturated World." *Cultural Anthropology* 13(3): 414–40.
Palmer, Brian. *The Importance of Breastfeeding as It Relates to Total Health*. Retrieved 21 March 2012 from http://www.brianpalmerdds.com/bfing_import.htm.
Palmer, Gabrielle. 1988. *The Politics of Breastfeeding*. London: Pandora.
Palmquist, Aunchalee. 2015. "Demedicalizing Breastmilk: The Discourses, Practices and Identities of Informal Milk Sharing." In *Ethnographies of Breastfeeding,* edited by Tanya Cassidy and Abdullahi El Tom, 23–44. London: Bloomsbury.
Palou, Andreu, and Catalina Picó. 2009. "Leptin Intake during Lactation Prevents Obesity and Affects Food Intake and Food Preferences in Later Life." *Appetite* 52(1): 249–52.
Parkes, Peter. 2001. "Alternative Social Structure and Foster Relations in the Hindu Kush: Milk Kinship Allegiance in Former Mountain Kingdoms of Northern Pakistan." *Comparative Studies in Society and History* 43(1): 4–36.
———. 2004. "Milk Kinship in Southeast Europe." *Social Anthropology* 12(3): 341–58.
Parkin, David. 2007. "The Visceral in the Social: The Crowd as Paradigmatic Type." *Holistic Anthropology,* edited by David Parkin and Stanley Ulijaszek, 234–54. New York: Berghahn Books.
Pataki, Amy. 2006. "Loving Lessons." *Toronto Star,* 9 June.
Patel, Raj. 2012. *Stuffed and Starved: The Hidden Battle for the World Food System*. Brooklyn, NY: Melville House Books.
Peake, Linda, and Martina Rieker. 2013. *Rethinking Feminist Interventions into the Urban*. New York: Routledge.
Peletz, Michael. 1988. *A Share of the Harvest*. Berkeley: University of California Press.
Pelto, Gretel, Yuanyuan Zhang, and Jean-Pierre Habicht. 2010. "Premastication: The Second Arm of Infant and Young Child Feeding for Health and Survival?" *Maternal and Child Nutrition* 6(1): 4–18.
Pentland, Alex. 2014. *Social Physics: How Good Ideas Spread—The Lessons from a New Science*. New York: Penguin Press.
Perez-Escamilla, Rafael, et al. 2012. "Scaling up of Breastfeeding Support Programs in Low and Middle Income Countries: The Breastfeeding Gear Model." *Advances in Nutrition* 3: 790–800.
Petchesky, Rosalind. 2005. "Rights of the Body and Perversions of War: Sexual Rights and Wrongs Ten Years Past Beijing." *International Social Science Journal* 184: 301–18.
Phuttakeo, Pornpai, et al. 2009. "Factors Influencing Breastfeeding in Children Less Than 2 Years of Age in Lao PDR." *Journal of Pediatrics and Child Health* 45: 487–92.
Pile, Steve. 2010. "Emotion and Affect in Recent Human Geography." *Transactions of the Institute of British Geographers*. 35(1): 5–20.
Pinker, Steven. 2011. *The Better Angels of Our Nature*. New York: Viking.
Pollan, Michael. 2006. *The Omnivore's Dilemma*. New York: Penguin Press.
Porter, Catherine. 2012. *Stella*. Toronto: Star Dispatches.
Post, James. 1985. "Assessing the Nestlé Boycott: Corporate Accountability and Human Rights." *California Management Review* 27(2): 113–31.
Powe, C. E., C. D. Knott, and N. Conklin-Brittain. 2010. "Infant Sex Predicts Breast Milk Energy Content." *American Journal of Human Biology* 22(1): 50–54.

Praet, Istvan. 2013. "Humanity and Life as the Perpetual Maintenance of Specific Efforts: A Reapraisal of Animism." *Biosocial Becomings*, edited by Tim Ingold and Gisli Palsson, 191–210. Cambridge: Cambridge University Press.

Prentice, Ann. 1996. "Constituents of Human Milk." *Food and Nutrition Bulletin* 17(4): 305–15.

Probyn, Elspeth. 2000. *Carnal Appetites: Foodsexidentities*. New York: Routledge.

Proctor, Robert. 2008. "Agnotology: A Missing Term to Describe the Cultural Production of Ignorance." In *Agnotology*, edited by Robert Proctor and Londa Schiebinger, 1–33. Stanford, CA: Stanford University Press.

Proctor, Robert, and Londa Schiebinger, eds. 2008. *Agnotology*. Stanford: Stanford University Press.

Quaritch Wales, Horace Geoffrey. 1931. *Siamese State Ceremonies*. London: Bernard Quaritch.

Quinn, Elizabeth. 2014. "Too Much of a Good Thing: Evolutionary Perspectives on Infant Formula Fortification in the United States and Its Effects on Infant Health." *American Journal of Human Biology* 26(1): 10–17.

———. 2015. *Milk Remembers: Immune Factors in Milk "Remember" Childhood Environments*. Retrieved 1 April 2015 from http://biomarkersandmilk.blogspot.ca/2015/01/milk-remembers-immune-factors-in-milk.html.

———. 2016. "Infancy by Design: Maternal Metabolism, Hormonal Signals, and the Active Management of Infant Growth by Human Milk." In *Costly and Cute*, edited by Wenda Trevathan and Karen Rosenberg, 87–107. Albuquerque: University of New Mexico Press.

Raphael, Dana. 1976. *The Tender Gift*. New York: Schoken Books.

Raum, Otto. 1940. *Chaga Childhood*. Oxford: Oxford University Press.

Ravelli, Anita, et al. 1999. "Obesity at the Age of 50 Years in Men and Women Exposed to Famine Prenatally." *American Journal of Clinical Nutrition* 70: 811–16.

Raynor, Steve. 2006. "Jack Beale Memorial Lecture on Global Environment. Wicked Problems: Clumsy Solutions—Diagnoses and Prescriptions for Environmental Ills." Institute for Science, Innovation, and Society, ANSW Sydney Australia. Retrieved 16 July 2014 from http://eureka.bodleian.ox.ac.uk/93/.

Research and Markets. 2011. *Baby Food and Paediatric Nutrition Market: Global Analysis and Forecast from 2007–2017*. Retrieved from http://www.researchandmarkets.com/reports/1991904/baby_food_and_pediatric_nutrition_market_global.

Reynolds, Frank, and Mani Reynolds. 1982. *Three Worlds According to King Ruang: Thai Buddhist Cosmology*. Berkeley, CA: Asian Humanities Press.

Richter, Judith. 2005. *Conflict of Interest and Policy Implementation: Reflections from the Fields of Health and Infant Feeding*. Geneva: International Baby Food Action Network-Geneva Infant Feeding Association.

———. 2012. "WHO Reform and Public Interest Safeguards: An Historical Perspective." *Social Medicine* 6(3): 141–50.

Riles, Annelise. 2001. *The Network Inside Out*. Ann Arbor: University of Michigan Press.

Riordan, Jan, and Kathleen Auerbach. 1993. *Breastfeeding and Human Lactation*. Boston: Jones and Bartlett. Robertson Smith, William. 1889. *The Religion of the Semites*. London: Adair and Charles Black.

Rodin, Judith. 2014. *The Resilience Dividend*. New York: Public Affairs/Perseus.

Rollins, Nigel C., et al. 2016. "Why Invest, and What It Will Take to Improve Breastfeeding Practices." *The Lancet* 387: 491–504.

Romero-Gwynn, Eunice. 1989. "Breastfeeding Patterns Among Indochinese Immigrants in Northern California." *Journal of Diseases of Childhood* 143: 804–8.

Rossano, Matt J. 2009. "Ritual Behaviour and the Origins of Modern Cognition." *Cambridge Archaeological Journal* 19(2): 243–56.

Rouch, Mira, and Grant O'Neil. 2000. "Sustaining Identities? Prolegomena for Inquiry into Contemporary Foodways." *Social Science Information* 39(1): 181–92.

Saleh, El-Sayed, et al. 2013. "Predictors of Postpartum Depression in a Sample of Egyptian Women." *Neuropsychiatric Disease and Treatment* 13(9): 15–24.

Sandberg, Sheryl. 2013. *Lean In: Women, Work, and the Will to Lead*. New York: Random House.

Sandlos, Lisa. 2014. "Shimmy, Shake, or Shudder?: Behind-the-Scenes Performances of Competitive Dance Moms." In *Performing Motherhood: Artistic, Activist, and Everyday Enactments,* edited by Amber Kinser, Kryn Freehling-Burton, and Terri Hawkes, 99–120. Bradford, Canada: Demeter Press.

Schechner, Richard. 1985. *Between Theatre and Anthropology*. Philadelphia: University of Pennsylvania Press.

Schegloff, Emanuel A. 2006. "Interaction: The Infrastructure for Social Institutions, the Natural Ecological Niche for Language, and the Arena in Which Culture Is Enacted." In *Roots of Human Sociality: Culture, Cognition and Interaction,* edited by Nicholas J. Enfield and Stephen C. Levinson, 70–96. New York: Berg Publishers.

Scheper-Hughes, Nancy. 1995. "The Primacy of the Ethical: Propositions for a Militant Anthropology." *Current Anthropology* 36(3): 409–20.

Schmied, Virgina, and Deborah Lupton. 2001. "Blurring the Boundaries: Breastfeeding and Maternal Subjectivity." *Sociology of Health and Illness* 23(2): 234–50.

Schmitt, Raymond. 1986. "Embodied Identities: Breasts as Emotional Reminders." *Studies in Symbolic Interaction* 7(A): 229–89.

Schorske, Carl E. 1998. *Thinking with History: Explorations in the Passage to Modernism*. Princeton, NJ: Princeton University Press.

Schrauwers, Albert. 1999. "Negotiating Parentage: The Political Economy of 'Kinship' in Central Sulawesi, Indonesia." *American Ethnologist* 26(2): 310–23.

Schweder, Richard, Lene Arnett Jensen, and William M. Goldstein. 1995. "Who Sleeps by Whom Revisited: A Method for Extracting the Moral Goods Implicit in Practice." In *Cultural Practices as Contexts for Development,* edited by Jacqueline Goodnow, Peggy J. Miller, and Frank Kessel, 21–40. San Francisco: Jossey-Bass.

Scott, James. 2009. *The Art of Not Being Governed: An Anarchist History of Upland Southeast Asia*. New Haven, CT: Yale University Press.

Scott, Jennifer. 2009. "The Next Breast Thing." *Canadian Living,* February, 14.

Seaman, Andrew. 2015. "Breastfeeding May Protect Babies from Arsenic Exposure." *Reuters,* 23 February. Retrieved from http://www.reuters.com/article/us-breastfeeding-arsenic-idUSKBN0LR0CW20150223.

Seligman, Adam, et al. 2008. *Ritual and Its Consequences: An Essay on the Limits of Sincerity*. New York: Oxford University Press.

Sellen, Daniel. 2001. "Comparison of Infant Feeding Patterns Reported for Nonindustrial Populations with Current Recommendations." *Journal of Nutrition* 131(10): 2707–15.

———. 2002a "Anthropological Approaches to Understanding the Causes of Variation in Breastfeeding and Promotion of Baby-Friendly Communities." *Nutritional Anthropology* 25(1): 19–29.

Sellen, Daniel. 2002b "Sub-Optimal Breast Feeding Practices: Ethnographic Approaches to Building 'Baby Friendly' Communities." In *Integrating Population Outcomes, Biological Mechanisms and Research Methods in the Study of Human Milk and Lactation,* edited by Margarett Davis et al., 223–32. New York: Kluwer Academic/Plenum Publishers.

———. 2006. "Lactation, Complementary Feeding, and Human Life History." In *The Evolution of Human Life History,* edited by Kristen Hawkes and Richard Paine, 155–96. Santa Fe, NM: School of American Research Press.

———. 2007. "Evolution of Infant and Young Child Feeding: Implications for Contemporary Public Health." *Annual Review of Nutrition* 27: 123–47.

Sengupta, Amit, ed. 2011. *Global Health Watch 3.* London: Zed Books.

Shaikh, Ulfat, and Omar Ahmed. 2006. "Islam and Infant Feeding." *Breastfeed Medicine* 1(3): 164–67.

Shaw, Rhonda. 2003. "Theorizing Breastfeeding: Body Ethics, Maternal Generosity and the Gift Relation." *Body and Society* 9(2): 55–73.

Shepherd, Gordon. 2012. *Neurogastronomy.* New York: Columbia University Press.

Shim, Jae Eun, et al. 2011. "Associations of Infant Feeding Practices and Picky Eating Behaviors of Preschool Children." *Journal of the American Dietetic Association* 111(9): 1363–68.

Silk, Joan. 2002. "The Form and Function of Reconciliation in Primates." *Annual Review of Anthropology* 31: 21–44.

Smale, Mary. 2000. "Beginning with Breastfeeding: Breast-Fed Infants and Their Mothers." In *Feeding Problems in Children,* edited by Angela Southall and Anthony Schwartz, 123–40. Oxford: Radcliffe Medical Press.

Smith, Dorothy. 1999. *Writing the Social.* Toronto: University of Toronto Press.

———. 2005. *Institutional Ethnography: A Sociology for People.* Walnut Creek, CA: AltaMira Press.

Smith, Julie. 2007. "The Contribution of Infant Food Marketing to the Obesogenic Environment in Australia." *Breastfeeding Review* 15(1): 23–35.

———. 2013. "Lost Milk?: Counting the Economic Value of Breast Milk in Gross Domestic Product." *Journal of Human Lactation* 29(4): 537–46.

Smithson, Michael. 2008. "Social Theories of Ignorance." In *Agnotology,* edited by Robert Proctor and Londa Schiebinger, 209–229. Stanford, CA: Stanford University Press.

Solemn Papal Audience. 1996. "Discourse by Pope John Paul II." *Food and Nutrition Bulletin* 17(4): 289–91.

Southall, Angela, and Anthony Schwartz, eds. 2000. *Feeding Problems in Children.* Oxford: Radcliffe Medical Press.

Spitz, Alison, Nancy Lee, and Herbert Peterson. 1998. "Treatment for Lactation Suppression: Little Progress in One Hundred Years." *American Journal of Obstetrics and Gynecology* 179(6): 1485–90.

Spock, Benjamin. 1968. *The Common Sense Book of Baby and Child Care.* 3rd ed. New York: Hawthorne Books.

Stahlie, Teunis Dirk. 1962. *Thai Children under Four.* Bangkok, Thailand.

Stearns, Peter N. 1999. *Battleground of Desire: The Struggle for Self-Control in Modern America.* New York: New York University Press.

Stocking, George. 1992. *The Ethnographer's Magic and Other Essays in the History of Anthropology.* Madison: University of Wisconsin Press.

Stockwell, A. J. 1998. "Conceptions of Community in Colonial Southeast Asia." *Transactions of the Royal Historical Society* 8(1998): 337–55.
Strathearn, Lane, et al. 2009. "Does Breastfeeding Protect against Substantiated Child Abuse and Neglect?" *Pediatrics* 123(2): 483–93.
Strathern, Marilyn. 2000. *Audit Cultures: Anthropological Studies in Accountability, Ethics and the Academy*. London: Routledge.
Stuart-Macadam, Patricia, and Katherine Dettwyler, eds. 1995. *Breastfeeding: Biocultural Perspectives*. New York: Aldine de Gruyter.
Stuebe, Alison. 2009. "The Risks of Not Breastfeeding for Mothers and Infants." *Reviews in Obstetrics & Gynecology* 2(4): 222–31.
Sutlive, Vinson. 1978. *The Iban of Sarawak*. Arlington Heights, IL: AHM Publishing.
Symonds, Patricia. 2004. *Calling the Soul in a Hmong Village*. Seattle: University of Washington Press.
Taggart, James. 2012. "Interpreting the Nahuat Dialogue on the Envious Dead with Jerome Bruner's Theory of Narrative." *Ethos* 40(4): 411–30.
Tan, Jingzhi, and Brian Hare. 2013. "Bonobos Share with Strangers." *PLoS One* 8(2013): e51922.
Tapias, Maria. 2006. "'Always Ready and Always Clean?' Competing Discourses of Breast-Feeding, Infant Illness and the Politics of Mother-Blame in Bolivia." *Body & Society* 12(2): 83–108.
Tarulevicz, Nicole. 2013. *Eating Her Curries and Kway: A Cultural History of Food in Singapore*. Urbana: University of Illinois Press.
Taylor, Shelley. 2002. *The Tending Instinct*. New York: Henry Holt.
Telle, Kari. 2007. "Nurturance and the Spectre of Neglect: Sasak Ways of Dealing with the Dead." In *Kinship and Food in South East Asia,* edited by Monica Janowski and Fiona Kerlogue, 121–48. Copenhagen: NIAS Press.
Thaler, Richard, and Cass Sunstein. 2008. *Nudge: Improving Decisions about Health, Wealth, and Happiness*. New York: Penguin Book.
Thompson, Charis. 2005. *Making Parents: The Ontological Choreography of Reproductive Technologies*. Cambridge, MA: MIT Press.
Thompson, Clair, et al. 2016. "Contrasting Approaches to Doing Family Meals: A Qualitative Study of How Parents Frame Children's Food Preferences." *Critical Public Health* 26(3): 322–32.
Thorley, Virginia. 2011. "Middleclass Mothers as Activists for Change." In *The 21st Century Motherhood Movement,* edited by Andrea O'Reilly, 219–32. Bradford, Canada: Demeter Press.
Tomori, Cecilia. 2014. *Nighttime Breastfeeding: An American Cultural Dilemma*. New York: Berghahn Books.
Trevarthen, Colwyn. 1979. "Communication and Cooperation in Early Infancy: A Description of Primary Intersubjectivity." In *Before Speech: The Beginning of Interpersonal Communication,* edited by Margaret Bullowa, 530–71. Cambridge: Cambridge University Press.
Trevathan, Wenda, E. O. Smith, and James McKenna, eds. 2008. *Evolutionary Medicine and Health*. New York: Oxford University Press.
Trevathan, Wenda, and Karen Rosenberg, eds. 2016. *Costly and Cute: Helpless Infants and Human Evolution*. Albuquerque: University of New Mexico Press.
Tuttle, Cynthia, and Kathryn Dewey. 1994. "Determinants of Infant Feeding Choices among Southeast Asian Immigrants in Northern California." *Journal of the American Dietetic Association* 94: 282–84.

UNICEF. 2006. *1990–2005. Celebrating the Innocenti Declaration on the Protection, Promotion and Support of Breastfeeding: Past Achievements, Present Challenges and Priority Actions for Infant and Young Child Feeding.* Florence, Italy: Innocenti Research Centre.

UNIFEM. 1995. *Putting Gender on the Agenda: A Guide to Participating in UN World Conferences.* New York.

US Senate Hearing. 1978. *Hearing before the Subcommittee on Health and Scientific Research of the Committee on Human Resources,* 95th Congress (28 May 1978).

Uvnes-Moberg, Kerstin. 2005. *The Oxytocin Factor: Tapping the Hormone of Calm, Love and Healing.* Boston: Da Capo Press.

Van Esterik, Penny. 1973. "Thai Tonsure Ceremonies: A Reinterpretation of Brahmanic Ritual in Thailand." *Journal of the Steward Anthropological Society* 4(2): 79–121.

———. 1982. "Interpreting a Cosmology: Guardian Spirits in Thai Buddhism." *Anthropos* 77: 1–15.

———. 1986. "Feeding Their Faith: Recipe Knowledge among Thai Buddhist Women." *Food and Foodways* 1(1): 198–215.

———. 1988. "To Strengthen and Refresh: Herbal Therapy in Southeast Asia." *Social Science and Medicine* 27(8): 751–61.

———. 1989. *Beyond the Breast-Bottle Controversy.* New Brunswick, NJ: Rutgers University Press.

———. 1999. "Right to Food; Right to Feed: Right to Be Fed: The Intersection of Women's Rights and the Right to Food." *Agriculture and Human Values* 16: 225–32.

———. 2000. *Materializing Thailand.* Oxford: Berg Publishers.

———. 2002. *Risks, Rights and Regulation: Communicating About Risks and Infant Feeding.* Penang, Malaysia: World Alliance for Breastfeeding Action.

———. 2011. "Genealogies of Nurture: Of Pots and Professors." *The Journal of the Burma Research Society* 15(1): 21–42.

———. 2012a. "Breastfeeding and HIV/AIDS: Critical Gaps and Dangerous Intersections." In *Giving Breast Milk,* edited by Rhonda Shaw and Alison Bartlett, 151–62. Toronto: Demeter Press.

———. 2012b. "Breastfeeding Across Cultures: Dealing with Difference." In *Beyond Health, Beyond Choice,* edited by Paige Hall Smith, Bernice Hausman, and Miriam Labbok, 53–63. New Brunswick, NJ: Rutgers University Press.

———. 2015. "Commensal Circles and the Common Pot." In *Commensality: From Everyday Food to Feast,* edited by Susanne Kerner, Cynthia Chou, and Morten Warmind, 31–42. London: Berg Publishers.

Van Esterik, Penny, and Laksmi Menon. 1996. *Being Mother-Friendly: A Practical Guide for Working Women and Breastfeeding.* Penang, Malaysia: World Alliance for Breastfeeding Action.

Van Oosterhout, Dianne. 2007. "Constructing Bodies, Constructing Identities: Nurture and Kinship Ties in a Papuan Society." In *Kinship and Food in South East Asia,* edited by Monica Janowski and Fiona Kerlogue, 170–95. Copenhagen: NIAS Press.

Victora, Cesar, et al. 2016. "Breastfeeding in the 21st Century: Epidemiology, Mechanisms, and Lifelong Effect." *Lancet* 387(10017): 475–90.

Volkman, Toby. 1985. *Feasts of Honor.* Urbana: University of Illinois Press.

von Kries, Rüdiger, et al. 1999. "Breast Feeding and Obesity: Cross Sectional Study." *British Medical Journal* 319(7203): 147–50.

WABA-UNICEF. 2002. *HIV and Infant Feeding: a Report of a WABA-UNICEF Colloquium*. Arusha, Tanzania.
Walker, Marsha. 1993. "A Fresh Look at the Risks of Artificial Infant Feeding." *Journal of Human Lactation* 9(2): 97–107.
Wall, Glenda. 2001. "Moral Constructions of Motherhood in Breastfeeding Discourse." *Gender and Society* 15(4): 592–610.
Walters, Dylan, et al. 2016. "The Cost of Not Breastfeeding in Southeast Asia." *Health Policy and Planning* 31(8): 1107–16.
Ward, Carol. 2003. "The Evolution of Human Origins." *American Anthropologist* 105(1): 77–88.
Ward, Jude DeJager. 2000. *La Leche League: At the Crossroads of Medicine, Feminism and Religion*. Chapel Hill: University of North Carolina Press.
Washburn, Sherwood. 1960. "Tools and Human Evolution." *Scientific American* 203: 62–75.
Weber, Max. 1963. *The Sociology of Religion*. Boston: Beacon Press.
Weiner, Annette. 1976. *Women of Value, Men of Renown: New Perspectives in Trobriand Exchange*. Austin: University of Texas Press.
Weiss, Allen, ed. 1997. *Taste, Nostalgia*. New York: Lusitania Press.
Wessing, Robert. 1978. *Cosmology and Social Behaviour in a West Javanese Settlement*. Athens: Ohio University Center for International Studies, Southeast Asia Programs.
Whitaker, Elizabeth. 2000. *Measuring Mama's Milk: Fascism and the Medicalization of Maternity in Italy*. Ann Arbor: University of Michigan Press.
Whitehouse, Harvey. 2007. "Towards an Integration of Ethnography, History, and the Cognitive Science of Religion." In *Religion, Anthropology, and Cognitive Science*, edited by H. Whitehouse and J. Laidlaw. Durham, NC: Carolina Academic Press.
Whittaker, A. 1999. "Birth and the Postpartum in Northeast Thailand: Contesting Modernity and Tradition." *Medical Anthropology* 18(3): 215–42.
Whittemore, Robert D., and Elizabeth A. Beverly. 1996. "Mandinka Mothers and Nurslings: Power and Reproduction." *Medical Anthropology Quarterly* 10(1): 45–62.
WHO/UNICEF. 1990. *Innocenti Declaration on the Protection, Promotion and Support of Breastfeeding*. Florence, Italy.
Widstrom, A. M., et al. 1987. "Gastric Suction in Healthy Newborn Infants: Effects on Circulation and Developing Feeding Behavior." *Acta Paediatrica Scandinavica* 76(4): 566–72.
Wikan, Unni. 2000. "With Life in One's Lap: The Story of an Eye/I (or Two)." In *Narrative and the Cultural Construction of Illness and Healing*, edited by Cheryl Mattingly and Linda Garro, 212–36. Berkeley: University of California Press.
Williams, Cicily. 1939. "Milk and Murder." Address to the Singapore Rotary Club. International Organization of Consumers Unions, Penang.
Williams, Raymond. 1985. *Keywords: A Vocabulary of Culture and Society*. Rev. ed. New York: Oxford University Press.
Wilson, Bee. 2012. *Consider the Fork: A History of How We Cook and Eat*. New York: Basic Books.
Wittgenstein, Ludwig. 1984. *Culture and Value*. Chicago: University of Chicago Press.
Wolf, Jacqueline. 2001. *Don't Kill Your Baby: Public Health and the Decline in Breastfeeding in the Nineteenth and Twentieth Centuries*. Columbus: Ohio State University Press.
———. 2003. "Low Breastfeeding Rates and Public Health in the United States." *The American Journal of Public Health* 93(12): 2000–11.

Wolf, Joan. 2010. *Is Breast Best? Taking on the Breastfeeding Experts and the New High Stakes of Motherhood.* New York: NYU Press.

Wolf, Naomi. 1993. *Fire with Fire: The New Female Power and How to Use It.* Toronto: Vintage.

Wood, Karen, and Penny Van Esterik. 2010. "Infant Feeding Experiences of Women Who Were Sexually Abused in Childhood." *Canadian Family Physician* 55: 136–41.

Woolridge, Michael. 1996. "Problems of Establishing Lactation." *Food and Nutrition Bulletin* 17(4): 316–23.

World Health Organization. 1979. *Joint WHO/UNICEF Meeting on Infant and Young Child Feeding: Statement and Recommendations.* Geneva: Author.

———. 2000. "Effects of Breastfeeding on Infant and Child Mortality Due to Infectious Diseases in Less Developed Countries: A Pooled Analysis." *Lancet* 355: 451–55.

———. 2003. *Global Strategy for Infant and Young Child Feeding.* Geneva: Author.

World Health Organization, UNICEF, and International Baby Food Action Network. 2016. *Marketing of Breast-Milk Substitutes: National Implementation of the International Code. Status Report.* Geneva: World Health Organization.

Worthman, Carol. 1993. "Biocultural Interactions in Human Development." In *Juvenile Primates: Life History, Development, and Behavior,* edited by Michael Perira and Lynn Fairbanks, 339–58. New York: Oxford University Press.

Wrangham, Richard. 2009. *Catching Fire: How Cooking Made Us Human.* New York: Basic Books.

Young, Iris. 2005. *On Female Bodily Experience: Throwing Like a Girl and Other Essays.* New York: Oxford University Press.

Yovsi, Relindis D., and Heidi Keller. 2003. "Breastfeeding: An Adaptive Process." *Ethos* 31(2): 147–71.

Zhen, Li, et al. 2016. "Prevalence and Charaterization of Chronobacter sakazakii in Retail Milk-Based Infant and Baby Foods in Shaanxi, China." *Foodborne Pathogens and Disease.* 13(4): 221–27.

Zihlman, Adrienne, and Debra Bolter. 2004. "Mammalian and Primate Roots of Human Sociality." In *The Origins and Nature of Sociality,* edited by Robert W. Sussman and Audrey R. Chapman, 23–52. New York: Aldine de Gruyter.

Index

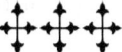

activism, 2, 18, 169, 183, 187, 189, 201, 217
   activist NGOs. *See* IBFAN; WABA
   lactivism, 200
activity, 17, 20–21, 33, 36–37, 39, 42n4, 71, 73, 81, 94–5, 105, 110, 122, 146–47, 193, 218
advocacy, 170, 199–203
AFASS (affordable, feasible, acceptable, sustainable, safe), 170, 188–89. *See also* AIDS
affect, 67
   affect hunger, 47, 60
   affect theory, 216
agnotology, 11
AIDS, 84, 169–71, 174
alcohol, 78, 80, 104
allergies, 52, 63, 148, 215, 219
   food allergies, 70
American Academy of Pediatrics, 82,
anthropology, 2, 13–20, 32–35, 145, 153, 215
   applied, 217
   early years, 8
   integrated, 47
   postmodern, 9
   subfields, 47, 196, 216
   visual, 121
   See also New Ethnology
attachment, 57, 67, 154, 200, 218
audit culture, 178

Bali, 41, 111, 116, 119, 121, 134
biocultural hybrid, 4, 30, 36–37, 45–47, 56, 60, 109, 196–97
bioculturalism, 30, 46
   weak vs. strong, 47–49
birth, 14, 36, 55–56, 61–63, 67, 80, 112, 115–16, 124, 130, 144, 160, 209
   cesarean, 62–63, 80, 130
   primate, 58
bottle feeding, 19, 49, 61, 66, 68–69, 75, 78, 84, 87, 88, 98–99, 101, 103, 139, 205
breastfeeding
   and appetite control, 64, 94, 103
   complex, 49–52
   exclusive, 3, 76, 84, 91, 101, 129, 160, 170, 173, 190, 218
   and food security, 117
   and human evolution, 53–56
   as human heritage, 212–14
   as modern dance, 154–55
   obstacles to, 172, 176, 213
   in popular media, 153
   as ritual dance, 70–71
   studied realistically, 29–31
   studied reductively, 25–29
   style, 21, 39, 135n2
   and world religions, 112–13, 127
breastmilk, 16, 20, 27, 39, 52, 70, 74, 80–85, 90, 92, 115, 117, 125, 130, 134, 147–48, 150, 153, 155, 171, 174, 181, 204, 213
   composition, 50–51, 63–65, 82, 146

volume, 147
water in, 52
breastmilk substitutes, 13, 19, 23, 50, 62, 75, 84, 88, 129, 152, 176, 186. *See also* bottle feeding; formula
breastsleeping, 52, 67, 89. *See also* cosleeping
Burma, 113, 118

Cambodia, 118
Cartesian dualism, 11, 18, 196
   Descartes, 25
   See also breastfeeding: studied reductively
Chicago, 137–39
Chronobacter sakazakii, 182. *See also* Enterobacter sakazakii
class, 28, 85, 100, 138, 149, 159
Code of Marketing of Breast Milk Substitutes, 173, 176, 185, 188, 199, 211
colonialism, 13, 132
colostrum, 52, 63–64, 80–81, 101, 115–16, 129, 134
commensality, 15, 73–75, 79, 97, 99–102, 114, 117, 121, 152–53
   commensal circles, 73, 76, 88, 91, 106
   embodied commensality, 76–77, 96, 98
   encultured commensality, 77, 88
   political commensality, 126
   religious commensality, 127
complementary foods, 59, 64, 88–91
   commercial baby foods, 92–94
constitution, 28, 30–31, 45, 49, 77, 86, 216
   definition of, 30
   infant constitution, 75, 81–83, 95, 110, 122, 148
   maternal constitution, 29, 36, 80
coregulation, 21, 51, 61, 64, 77, 79–80, 83, 88–89, 105, 145, 151, 154. *See also* person-making
cosleeping, 52, 67–68, 154. *See also* breastsleeping
crisis, 9, 52, 140–41, 160, 179
culture, 2, 26–28, 32–33, 35–40, 42n3, 45, 47, 57–59, 77, 105, 121, 142, 162–63, 173, 185, 213
custom, 23, 35–36, 39, 41, 52, 58, 65, 72, 77, 79, 86, 105, 114–16, 144, 149, 152, 198, 216

dance, 3–4, 7, 16, 18, 20–22, 46, 51, 67, 70–73, 96, 98, 105–6, 134, 154–55, 191, 195, 197, 216, 219
death, 52, 58–59, 65, 102, 105, 115–16, 119, 122–23, 126, 130, 134, 145, 163, 167, 171
dental and oral development, 61–62
DES (diethylstilbestrol), 80

eating disorders, 2–3, 101–2
ecology, 30, 39, 66, 95, 193, 217
   gut ecology, 62–63, 220
emergent system, 25, 30–31, 33, 41, 48
Enterobacter sakazakii, 63, 182. *See also* Chronobacter sakazakii
epigenetics, 15, 45, 55, 216
evolution, 11–13, 34, 38–39, 45–47, 49, 51, 53–56, 65, 69

fathers, 19, 131, 214
feminism, 169, 175, 206–9
fetus, 63, 74, 78, 80, 124
First Nations, 13, 17, 66, 72n1, 86, 207, 221
food sharing, 10, 73–75, 77, 97, 100, 105, 109, 130, 149, 190. *See also* commensality
formula, 41, 49–50, 52, 70, 75, 80, 84, 87–89, 92
   composition, 26, 50, 63, 87, 155, 203
   promotion and marketing, 129, 132, 164, 178, 186
   risk of, 68, 98, 103, 181–83, 185, 211
   soy, 87
   See also bottle feeding

GAIN (Global Alliance for Improved Nutrition), 179–84
Gates foundation, 184
GRAS (generally recognized as safe), 87

health professionals, 18, 202
   and global health, 207
   modernity and, 141, 161
   promotion of formula through, 187
Hinde, Katie, 51, 54, 57–58, 62
HIV. *See* AIDS
Hmong, 111, 116, 130–31, 134, 136n5

Hrdy, Sarah, 11, 45, 53, 57, 168, 198, 214, 218
human niche, 47, 57, 59
human rights, 210–11
humoral system, 79

IBFAN (International Baby Food Action Network), 20, 187, 199–200, 204
ILCA (International Lactation Consultant Association), 175
ILSI, (International Life Sciences Institute), 181
immune system, 48, 52, 58, 61–64, 70, 85, 153–54, 184
infant feeding complex, 73
Ingold, Tim, 17, 45, 47, 65, 71, 149, 204, 216
Innocenti Declaration, 171–74, 177, 190
Innocenti +15, 172–77, 188
instinct, 39
insufficient milk, 58, 182, 192, 221
intangible cultural heritage, 212–14

Java, 83, 116, 125, 127, 135

KAP (knowledge, attitude, practice), 161, 218

La Leche League, 1, 66, 148, 175, 219
Lao PDR, 86, 88, 118, 120, 126, 129–31, 143
leptin, 64, 83
life cycle, 7, 11, 16, 18, 24, 28, 39–41, 46, 73, 77, 100, 105, 113, 121–22, 143, 153–54, 197, 203, 215–16
  definition, 30

machine metaphor, 24, 29, 41
maternity entitlements, 13, 19, 145–46, 199, 207–8, 220
MCH (Maternal and Child Health), 167–68
McKenna, James, 52, 56, 67–68, 154
meal format, 82, 90, 97, 113, 126
medical anthropology, 216
microbiome, 62–63, 75, 153
milk, human. *See* breastmilk

milk sharing, 85, 151, 153
milk sibling, 84
modernity, 142–45
modernization, 14, 135, 140, 146, 171
mommy blogs, 3, 18
mommy wars, 19, 194–95
mother–infant dyad, 28, 50, 52, 61, 67, 69, 95–96, 116, 132, 169, 191, 201

neoliberalism, 178, 198, 217
neoteny, 53, 69
Nestlé boycott, 199
New Ethnology, 4, 31, 33, 38, 41, 111, 165–66, 215–17
nurturing practices, 4, 10–12, 14, 16, 21, 39, 45–46, 57, 64–66, 72, 86, 104, 107, 110–15, 119, 121, 128, 135, 147, 160, 180, 190, 194–99, 213, 220
obesity, 49, 64, 102–4, 219. *See also* appetite control
obstetrical dilemma, 55
oxytocin, 30, 48, 64, 71

pacifiers, 62, 67, 148
person-making, 59, 73, 105, 114, 117, 219
Philanthrocapitalists, 184
Philippines, 120, 130–31, 187
placenta, 36, 64, 77, 80–81, 116, 119, 124, 137
plasticity, 45, 53–55, 58, 61, 64, 67, 70, 111
policy, ii, 4, 16, 18, 20, 75–76, 82, 89, 103, 110–11, 149, 155, 159, 160–66, 168–69, 171–77, 183, 187–91, 200, 207–9, 215–17, 220–21
POPS (persistent organic pollutants), 181, 204–5
PPP (public-private partnerships), 176–79, 184, 199. *See also* GAIN
pregnancy, 28, 36, 58, 65, 76–80, 82, 95, 116–17, 127, 135, 144–45, 148, 168, 170, 197
premastication, 76, 85–86, 147
primates, 16–17, 38, 53–54, 57–61, 94, 139, 149, 194, 202, 218
prolactin, 64, 80
pumps, 145, 149–51, 195, 209

Quinn, E. A., 46, 48–52, 64–65, 197, 203

race, 13, 28
rice, 21, 41, 89–90, 97, 109, 112–18, 120–29, 132–35, 151–52, 155
risk, 181–82
 chemical contamination, 99
 HIV transmission, 170
 poisoning, 126
 See also formula, risk of
ritual, 38, 59–61, 70–71, 76–77, 114, 116–17, 120, 127, 130, 145
root crops, 112, 133

scheduled feeding, 75, 138, 140
scientific motherhood, 138
Sellen, Daniel, 46, 58–59, 94–95, 110, 160–62
serotonin, 53, 71
Shan, 120–21
SIDS (sudden infant death syndrome), 52, 68
sleeping, 52, 67–68, 95. *See also* cosleeping; breastsleeping
sociality, 53–57, 73, 197, 219
social universal, 4, 34, 196
social womb, 36, 57–58, 60, 68, 72, 83, 109, 115–17, 126, 132, 145, 160, 165, 167, 191, 196–97, 216
 definition, 30
Southeast Asia, 3, 21, 81, 86, 100, 109

SRH (Sexual and Reproductive Health), 169
stem cells, 63, 66, 73
SUN (Scaling Up Nutrition), 180–81

taste, 64, 67, 76, 78, 82, 91, 93, 95, 98–104, 129, 132, 149, 152, 197
Thailand, 3, 86, 102, 113, 116, 118, 120, 122, 129, 134, 143

UNESCO, 213–14
UNICEF, 20, 87, 129, 160–61, 172, 175, 179, 184, 188, 192n2, 195, 199
UNIFEM, 175

Van Esterik, Penny, stories, 1, 69, 81, 146, 162, 173, 201, 204, 206, 211
Vietnam, 131

WABA (World Alliance for Breastfeeding Action) 20, 184, 189, 199–200, 207, 211. *See also* advocacy
WIC (Women, Infants and Children), 131
women's movement, 206–10
World Breastfeeding Week, 189
weaning, 20, 59, 82, 87, 93–96, 105, 123, 151, 205
WEIRD (Western, educated, industrial, rich, democratic), 19, 149–50, 216
wet nursing, 76, 84, 112, 125, 153, 168
WHO (World Health Organization), 20, 160–61, 164, 172, 175, 184, 188, 199

www.ingramcontent.com/pod-product-compliance
Lightning Source LLC
Chambersburg PA
CBHW070917030426
42336CB00014BA/2456